NATIVE AMERICAN HERBALIST'S BIBLE

13 BOOKS IN 1

Naturally Improve Your Wellness with 500+ Herbal Remedies and Medicinal Herbs. Create Your Own Herbal Dispensatory and Apothecary Table.

By

Aiyana Tessay

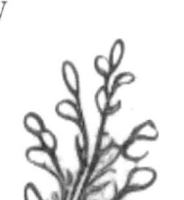
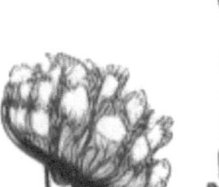

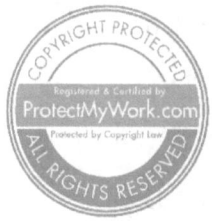

13 BOOKS IN 1

BOOK 1: HISTORY AND INTRODUCTION TO HERBALISM

BOOK 2: NATIVEAMERICAN HERBAL DISPENSATORY

BOOK 3: NATIVE AMERICAN HERBAL ENCYCLOPEDIA

BOOK 4: NATIVE AMERICAN HERBAL APOTHECARY

BOOK 5: ESSENTIAL OILS

BOOK 6: MEDICINAL HERBS

BOOK 7: MEDICINAL PLANTS

BOOK 8: NATIVE AMERICAN HERBAL RECIPES VOL. I

BOOK 9: NATIVE AMERICAN HERBAL RECIPES VOL.II

BOOK 10: NATIVE AMERICAN HERBAL REMEDIES VOL. I1

BOOK 11: NATIVE AMERICAN HERBAL REMEDIES VOL. II1

BOOK 12: NATIVE AMERICAN HERBAL REMEDIES
FOR YOUR CHILD'S HEALTH

BOOK 13: NATIVE AMERICAN CRYSTALS
AND STONES FOR HEALING.

TABLE OF CONTENTS

Thank You for Your Purchase!
From Aiyana Tessay to You

Dear Herbal Enthusiasts,

I am Aiyana Tessay, and I would like to extend my deepest gratitude for selecting **"Native American Herbalists Bible: 13 Books in 1."**

This work is a manifestation of my profound respect for the ancestral wisdom of Native American herbalism and is dedicated to you and all who are drawn to the ancient practices of natural healing.

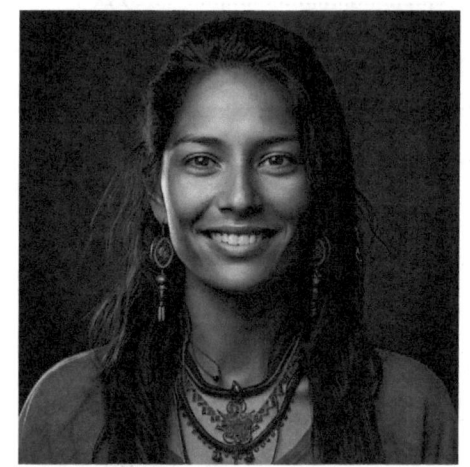

Your choice to explore this extensive compilation reflects a dedication to understanding and adopting natural, holistic health practices that have been nurtured by generations of Native American herbalists. Within these pages, I have woven together traditional knowledge with extensive research and a passionate commitment to the preservation and application of indigenous herbal medicine.

Whether you are an adept herbalist or a newcomer eager to uncover the richness of Native American natural remedies, this book aims to equip you with the insights and skills needed to tap into the ancient wisdom of the Earth for healing and wellness.

Before you dive deep into the world of Native American herbal remedies, I wish to share a review that has greatly moved me:

"This book is an incredible guide that immerses us in the wealth of herbal wisdom from Native American cultures. Which can help us to naturally improve wellness through herbal remedies and medicinal herbs.

It also contains a world of knowledge about the healing properties of plants. The way it presents the recipes and remedies clarifies their practical application and helps you understand all their benefits.

With an immense variety of information on medicinal herbs, their uses and how to prepare effective remedies. Each section is supported by practical examples and tips that allow you to explore the power of herbalism." – ***Julian***

Unfortunately, the significance of reader feedback and its power to amplify our voices and share our knowledge more broadly is often overlooked. Now, as you embark on this enlightening journey, should you find inspiration in these teachings, I kindly ask you to consider leaving your honest feedback on Amazon.

Your support in spreading the word about this book is incredibly precious. Remember, every review counts and plays a crucial role in guiding and inspiring fellow readers.

Leaving feedback is simple, and I treasure each piece of insight. Just go to the ORDERS section of your Amazon account and click on the "Write a product review" button, or scan this QR Code:

Should you feel any aspect of the book might be enhanced, your constructive feedback is warmly welcomed at **info@herbulharmony.com**.

Diving into the **"Native American Herbalists Bible: 13 Books in 1"** opens the door to more than knowledge; it invites you to a life enriched by the powerful synergy of holistic well-being and ancestral wisdom. As you turn each page, I encourage you to engage, discover, and immerse yourself in the transformative essence of Native American herbalism.

For ongoing updates, additional resources, and to join a community of like-minded individuals, please visit **www.herbfulharmony.com**.

Stay healthy and inspired,
Let's walk this path together,
Aiyana Tessay

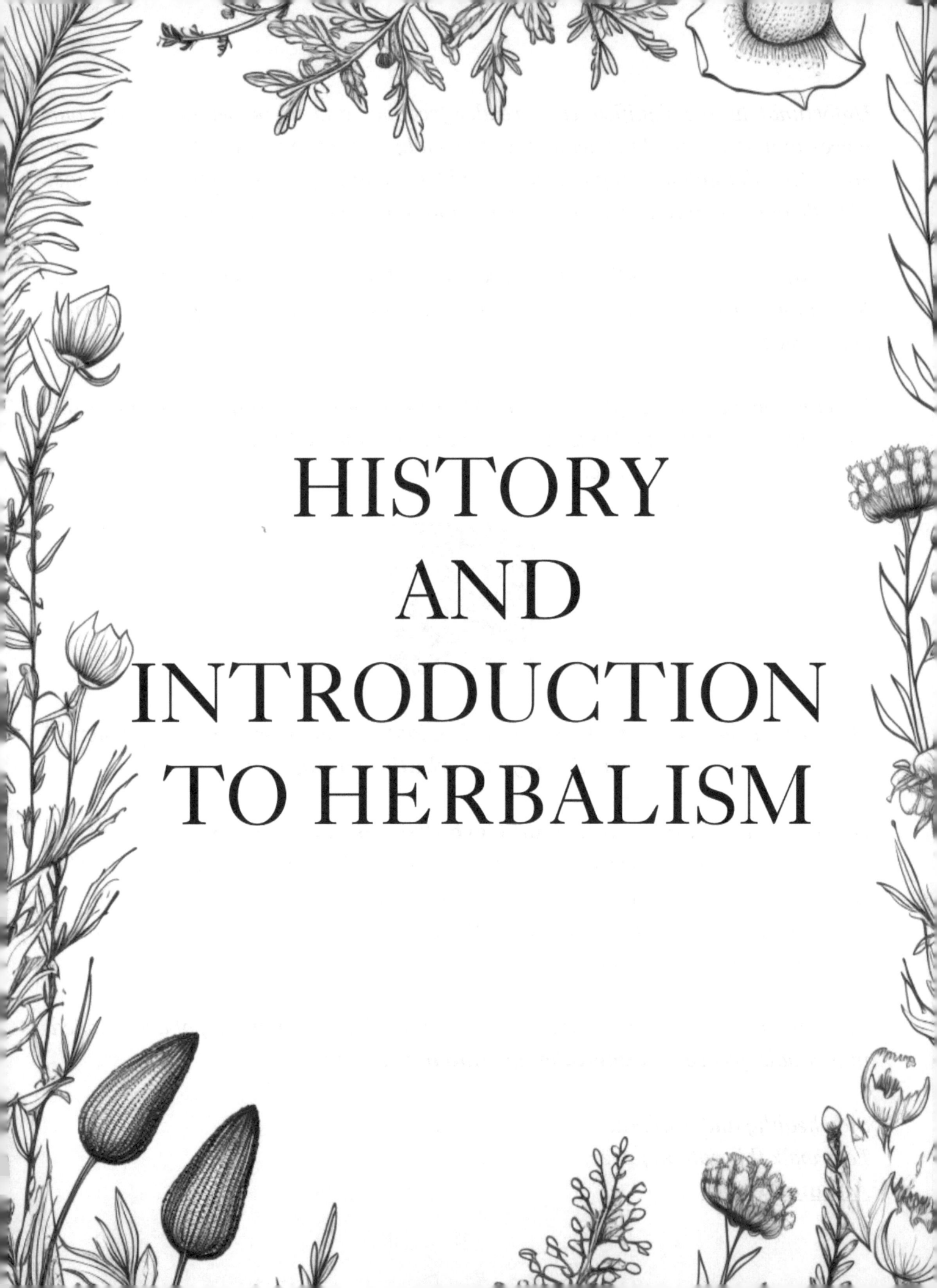

HISTORY AND INTRODUCTION TO HERBALISM

INTRODUCTION

Herbal medicine has been used since ancient times and predates written history, oral traditions, and even the presence of humans. Herbalism, in its broadest sense, involves using herbs to rebalance the body. Herbalism can also be defined as incorporating herbs such as vegetables and fruits into one's diet. Herbal medicine is the earliest recognized form of medicine and serves as the foundation for all other medical practices. It encompasses the scientific study of plants, including their energetic aspects, flavors, activities, patterns, and affinities.

The practice of herbalism involves intertwining various pearls of wisdom with the intention and awareness of promoting healing, balance, and harmonizing disharmonious tendencies with the assistance of plants and practical magic. Herbalism is utilized to treat common ailments and enhance overall health and well-being. It is one of the oldest and most potent forms of medicinal practices and is experiencing increasing popularity due to the growing interest in natural healing and health.

Many of us may have learned gardening and gathering wild and medicinal foods from our parents or grandparents. However, the "back to the land" movement is rapidly spreading in Connecticut, and many residents are enthusiastic about participating. For beginners, the best place to start is in their homes, communities, and gardens.

According to the World Health Organization, medicinal plant preparations continue to be the primary source of healthcare for 80 percent of the world's population. Humans have been using plants for medicine and nutrition since the beginning of our existence, and we have coexisted with them for centuries. Surprisingly, this close relationship has led to a co-evolution where people naturally prefer to use plant remedies and consume wild foods.

An example of an herbal remedy used today is chamomile, which is often used to promote sleep. It is also common to incorporate a bit of extra garlic into daily meals to help combat the common cold that circulates in the office. Even when we apply the juice of an aloe plant to treat a kitchen burn, we are practicing herbalism.

Ancient herbals

The Sumerians of ancient Mesopotamia preserved the oldest written evidence of medicinal plants on clay tablets nearly 5,000 years ago. These tablets contained a dozen herbal formulas comprising over 250 different plants. The Ebers Papyrus, written around 1500 BCE and containing over 850 herbal remedies, was not the earliest Egyptian herbal publication, but it is one of the oldest surviving written herbals.

Ayurveda, a 5,000-year-old ancient healing system that originated in India and its surroundings, has valuable documented medical literature dating back to around 400 BCE. One of the ancient texts, the Charaka Samhita, lists over 300 herbs, many of which are still used in Ayurvedic and Western medicine today.

Chi'en Nung, an almost legendary Chinese monarch, is credited with compiling the Pen Ts'ao Ching, a fundamental materia medica for traditional Chinese medicine. It covers nearly 350 plants and is believed to describe ancient procedures dating back to 2700 BCE, over 5,000 years ago. Several plants described in the Pen Ts'ao Ching are still used in Traditional Chinese Medicine today, and many more can be found in the materia medicas of modern herbalists.

Around 450 BCE, a Greek philosopher named Empedocles wrote "Nature & its Purifications," which established his "Four Roots Theory." This theory studied Earth, water, air, and fire and served as a foundation for Western medical expertise in energetics. Around 400 BCE, Plato, a classical Greek philosopher, expanded on these principles in his work "The Four Elements." Hippocrates, a Greek physician, further refined them into "The Four Humors," which included the human foundation. Hippocrates is also known for separating medicine from religion or spirituality, and his principles, known as The Hippocratic Oath, have had a long-lasting influence on Western medicine.

Herbalism in the Stone Age

Herbalism has a long history with humans and humanoid species. Herbaceous plants have existed for 125 million years, while the first humanoid beings appeared only about 5 million years ago. Until about 12,000 years ago, all peoples were hunter-gatherers, marking the longest period of human civilization. It was a lengthy and fruitful clinical trial aimed at determining the therapeutic properties of plants.

During this period, plants that provided the best food, medicines, colors, poisons, weapons, fuels, textiles, and hallucinogenic and spiritual experiences emerged, influencing minds, bodies, and society.

The introduction of agriculture approximately 10,000 years ago and the establishment of more stable communities in later human history paved the way for a much more scientific approach to herbal medicines. Herbal medicine has been practiced for over 5,000 years, with only a few fragments of information on preliterate herbal medicine available.

According to archaeological evidence, the use of medicinal plants dates back to the Paleolithic period, approximately 60,000 years ago. Studies of Neanderthal tooth plates revealed that Neanderthals consumed poplar, yarrow, and chamomile plants. The discovery of Ötzi, a 5,300-year-old ice man from the Final Neolithic-First Period, provides evidence of ancient knowledge of herbs. He was found frozen and almost hairless, with a backpack containing food, tools, and medicinal plants.

In his possession, he had:

- Dried blackthorn berries, which appear to have metabolic stimulant, immunological boosting, carminative, antimicrobial, and anti-inflammatory properties, in addition to being high in vitamin C.

- A birch polypore, a fungus known for its antiviral, vermifuge, and antibacterial properties.

Th fact that the blackthorn berries had been dried since the previous autumn indicates that they had been specifically used for a purpose, thus validating Ötzi's empirical knowledge of plants and their medicinal benefits.

Native American Medicine's History

Native American healing practices have a long history, with indigenous tribes throughout North America discovering the therapeutic properties of herbs, roots, and other natural plants for treating various medical conditions. However, Native American healing methods encompassed more than just remedies.

With over 2,000 indigenous tribes in North America, healing traditions varied significantly, incorporating diverse rituals, rites, and healing knowledge. While specific healing criteria were not universal, most tribes believed that health manifested as a result of spiritual, mental, and physical strength, representing an ongoing process.

By maintaining harmony with themselves, others, their natural surroundings, and their Creator, they believed they could ward off diseases and ailments. Thoughts and behaviors were believed to have consequences, such as illness, disability, misfortune, or trauma, and individuals were responsible for their own well-being. Only by restoring balance could one regain their health.

Herbal remedies played a prominent role in these healing practices, extending beyond concepts of harmony and spirituality. Indigenous tribes often sourced herbs and other natural substances from their immediate environment, resulting in a wide array of medicinal treatments. In some cases, scarce items were obtained through long-distance trade. The value placed on herbs and medicinal plants was significant.

Many medicinal remedies were passed down orally from generation to generation, never documented in writing, resulting in many being lost to history. Only a small percentage of healers, such as the Cherokee, recorded their formulas and methods.

When the first Europeans arrived in the United States over 500 years ago, they were astonished to witness Native Americans recover from injuries and illnesses that they deemed fatal. Traditional Native American herbal remedies often outperformed those used by the European immigrants. However, Native Americans were not prepared for the "illnesses of civilization" brought by the Europeans, such as smallpox and measles, which decimated their populations over the subsequent centuries.

As a result, not only did the Native Americans suffer, but the wealth of knowledge held by their healers was lost to the grave. Despite this loss, a significant portion of this knowledge has been preserved and continues to be used by both Native Americans and non-native individuals.

Many modern medicines are derived from plants and herbs that have been used by Native Americans for centuries. More than 200 botanicals, many of which were originally discovered and utilized by Native Americans, have found their way into pharmaceutical applications.

Prohibition of Religious Rights

In 1882, the federal government implemented a ban on Native American religious freedoms, which had a significant impact on traditional medical practices. Secretary of the Interior Henry M. Teller deemed them an "enormous impediment to civilization" and prohibited "pagan dances and rituals" on reservations. The following year, Hiram Price, Commissioner of Indian Affairs, stated, "There is no good reason why any

Indian should be allowed to engage in practices which are equally repugnant to common human decency and morality; moreover, the maintenance of good order on the reservations requires that active measures be taken to discourage and, if possible, eliminate the demoralizing impact of pagan rites."

The government intervened to prevent the holding of the "Ghost Dance," a widespread movement that envisioned a peaceful resolution to white American expansion and advocated for clean livelihoods, honest existence, and cross-cultural cooperation among Native Americans. This intervention culminated in the Wounded Knee Massacre on Dec. 29, 1890. When the U.S. Seventh Cavalry was dispatched to the Lakota Sioux reservations of Pine Ridge and Rosebud to suppress the dance and apprehend the participants, approximately 150 Native American women, men, and children were killed.

Despite accusations against the Seventh Cavalry soldiers for the killing of innocent people, they were all pardoned. Only two years later, Thomas J. Morgan, Commissioner of Indian Affairs, authorized fines and up to six months of imprisonment for those who frequently engaged in religious dances and worked as medicine men, further repressing Native beliefs. However, due to the challenges of enforcing these new regulations, Native Americans continued practicing their traditions.

Prior to 1900, Native Americans relied on their medicine men for all ailments and diseases. This began to change in the early 20th century when the Indian Health Service established hospitals and clinics. While spiritual harmony remained an important aspect of their culture, many Native Americans started using modern medicine, especially for "white man's" diseases that traditional healers couldn't cure.

Surprisingly, the ban on Native American spiritual rituals remained in effect until 1978 when the American Indian Religious Freedom Act was passed. Unfortunately, as a result of this decades-long ban, many Native American healing techniques were forced underground or abandoned altogether. Presently, many tribes fiercely protect the knowledge of their healers and refuse to share it with non-Indigenous individuals, believing that sharing such knowledge diminishes the spiritual power of medicine.

Healing Rituals and Ceremonies

Through symbolic healing ceremonies and rituals, participants were often brought into harmony with themselves, their tribes, and the environment. Ceremonies were utilized to facilitate the reunification of groups of people rather than for individual healing. Certain tribes, such as the Sioux and the Navajo, employed a medicine wheel, the sacred hoop, as well as singing and dancing in multi-day rituals.

Individual healing rituals could involve dancing, painting, modifying feathers, drumming, and using rattles. In some cases, sacred stones were rubbed on specific body parts.

Sweat lodges and sweat baths were commonly utilized by Native Americans for cleansing and purification. These practices aimed to restore balance and promote healing by eliminating negative influences and refreshing the body.

Baths could range from simple practices of reclining beneath a blanket in the hot sun to more elaborate structures, such as small conical constructions covered in branches, blankets, or hides. Hot stones were placed in water inside the lodge to create a steam bath, where the healer would pray, sing, and drum together with others to cleanse the spirits.

Sweat lodges served various purposes, including healing, gathering large crowds before spiritual events, and bringing clarity to a situation. Sage, the most potent purifying herb, was burned in different cultures until it smoldered and released clouds of smoke. It was applied to the skin and believed to cleanse both the soul and body. This practice was referred to as "sweeping the smoke."

Spirituality and Connection

The incorporation of spirituality into the healing process is a key distinction between Native American healing and conventional medicine, both in the past and present. Native Americans believe in the interconnectedness of all things on Earth, where spirits can either contribute to or cause illness. Therefore, it is crucial to restore an individual's physical and emotional wholeness, as well as their connection to their communities and surroundings. Alongside herbal remedies, rituals, dances, prayers, and chanting were commonly utilized by the community to assist those who were unwell.

Modern medicine solely relies on science and a mechanistic understanding of the body, but many Native Americans believe that the spirit is an essential component of healing.

Healers within Native American tribes were known by various names, such as healers, medicine men/women, but the term "shamans" was not used by Native Americans. These healers aimed to seek assistance from the spiritual realm, particularly from the "Creator" or "Great Spirit," for the betterment of individuals or communities.

In addition to being a doctor, the healer also held a role similar to that of a priest. They believed that diseases could be caused by supernatural, human, or natural factors, and the healer was prepared to address illnesses resulting from any of these causes. Healers employed peculiar and sometimes terrifying masks to frighten away the spirits believed to be causing the disease or suffering.

Exorcism rituals involving drumming, rattles, and swaying around the patient were also used to banish demons. These exorcism rights were combined with practical techniques that involved the use of plant and animal ingredients. Suction tube cups were commonly used by healers alongside herbal remedies for purging and cleansing.

Many medicine people were born into families with a lineage of healers, while others may have been inspired to pursue a medical career through dreams. Aspiring healers would undergo an extensive apprenticeship alongside an experienced practitioner before becoming qualified to work independently.

Being a respected member of the community and a medical practitioner was a full-time commitment, ensuring the well-being and balance of both individuals and the tribe. Healers received everything they needed for their services, including food, lodging, and any other assistance required. Gifts were given to healers in exchange for services such as herbal medicine, midwifery, bone setting, and counseling.

Healers utilized natural tools such as fur, bone, skins, shells, crystals, feathers, and roots. These tools were used to invoke the spirit of the tree or animal from which they were derived. Feathers, associated with wind and air, were commonly used for communication with the Great Spirit. In certain cases, the healer would enter a trance state and seek guidance from "spirit guides."

Inherited diseases, such as congenital disabilities and retardation, were seldom addressed. Other conditions were typically not treated if a healer believed they resulted from the patient's behavior and were meant to serve as life lessons.

Healers kept their tools and remedies in a medicine bundle made of cloth or tightly knotted skin. There were three types of bundles: personal bundles for individual healers, tribe bundles, and special-purpose bundles for festivals and rituals.

The contents of each medicine bundle were considered sacred, and it was traditionally taboo to inquire about the ingredients of a personal bundle. Tribe bundles were often referred to as "grandmothers" due to their ability to nourish and nurture the tribe. Medicine pipes, symbolizing the ebb and flow of life, were a common tool found in medicine bundles. It is believed that the smoke released from the pipes carries petitions to the Great Spirit.

Individual healing was regarded as a private matter between the patient and the healer. Moreover, the patient's preferences were always respected within the context of their cultural customs.

Native American Medicine Today

Today, medical thinking is shifting towards a paradigm that acknowledges and respects all aspects of an individual, including their spiritual and emotional states. As a result, both Native and non-Native individuals are showing a growing interest in Native American medicinal practices.

Many people are turning to natural medicinal herbs due to concerns about the toxicity, addictive properties, and side effects of pharmaceutical drugs. Native American products of superior quality have been used for centuries to treat various diseases. While this may not always be the case, herbal remedies often have lower toxicity levels and therefore tend to produce fewer unpleasant side effects compared to many pharmaceutical drugs.

When selecting herbal remedies, it is important to choose products that have undergone meticulous creation and testing, contain the highest quality organic ingredients, and adhere to rigorous pharmaceutical manufacturing standards.

Just like any other medication, herbal medicines should be taken precisely as directed.

The Native American Connection to Nature

Nature's importance in Native American culture has been well-documented throughout history and continues to be recognized today. Religion, daily rituals, mythology, literature, cuisine, medicine, art, and many other aspects of American Indian culture are all influenced by the natural environment. Their way of life is intimately connected to the land and the environment.

It is easy to comprehend the significance of nature in all forms of Native American culture once you grasp the critical role it plays in their society. I have shared a concise yet comprehensive explanation of how nature shapes and defines the worlds of indigenous peoples. This material provides an informative and engaging way to immerse yourself in the unique and captivating world of Native American art and gain a true appreciation for it.

Spirituality and religion

Native Americans had learned to coexist with nature rather than fight against it, and this harmonious relationship was deeply ingrained in their culture. Native American religions emphasized their spiritual connection to the natural Creator(s).

As demonstrated by the wisdom of the Iroquois Confederacy, Native Americans understood the long-term consequences of their actions on the Earth and the impact they would have on future generations. Their ancestors relied solely on the resources of the land, and it is our duty to honor and respect that profound relationship.

Just like their ancestors, contemporary Native Americans strive to ensure a secure and prosperous future for their children.

Nature's elements hold profound significance.

In the American Indian worldview, nature features are both symbolic and multifunctional, permeating every aspect of their lives and creations.

Totems serve as sources of power and strength for Native Americans, while symbols in their writings and artwork facilitate understanding and connection with the larger world. If symbols represent their language, then nature serves as their lexicon.

Trees, for instance, embody more than just life and healing; they also embody permanence and longevity. Different tree types play distinct roles. The Cherry tree signifies rebirth and compassion, aiding digestion, while the Elm tree is associated with the development of wisdom and willpower. It can also be used for treating wounds.

The presence of Animal Spirits exemplifies the inseparable link between nature and Native American customs and traditions. Individuals often connect with a spirit animal, a guide that significantly influences their identity and way of life. In addition to personal spirit animals, tribes often select Spirit Creatures as Tribe Totems, representing the most influential and prevalent animals in their respective territories. These

Spirit Creatures provide vital resources and spiritual revelations to help people navigate through life.

For example, the Bat symbolizes the protector of the night, representing death and rebirth, while the Turtle symbolizes the guardian of Mother Earth and embodies perseverance. The Wolf, known as the Pathfinder, leads with wisdom and a spirit of leadership.

In Native American culture, nature serves as the underlying foundation upon which all spiritual and earthly existence is built. The artistic expression of this worldview by Native American artists sets them apart from their contemporaries and allows their work to reach a broader audience. Understanding the significance of nature in their culture enables viewers to appreciate and comprehend the profound and unique creations crafted by American Indian artists.

Despite residing in different regions of what is now the United States, many Native American tribes shared a collective wisdom rooted in the recognition and understanding of the interdependence of all ecological components. Humans, rocks, plants, and even animals relied on one another for survival and the well-being of their environmental niche.

Every action we take as human beings has an impact on our surroundings. This fundamental concept equated Native Americans with the animals they hunted for sustenance and the berries they gathered from the bushes.

They were mindful of the consequences of their actions, approaching nature with a level of respect and reverence that often goes unnoticed in modern societies.

Native Americans made modest alterations to their ecological niches, clearing land for settlements and fields. However, these minimal changes did not result in permanent damage to the environment. Archaeological excavations have uncovered remnants of their settlements, demonstrating their ability to coexist harmoniously with nature.

This approach to interacting with nature led to numerous conflicts when European settlers arrived in America with divergent land management philosophies. The Pilgrims and other early immigrants viewed America as a land to conquer, expressing fear in their writings and letters regarding this unfamiliar new world and its inhabitants.

Presently, Native Americans, along with individuals from diverse cultural backgrounds, strive to restore traditional land management practices. By recognizing ourselves as integral parts of the system, we become responsible stewards of the environment. Engaging in a blame game by pointing fingers at politicians, nations, or our neighbors down the street will not lead us far.

To overcome this challenge, we must collectively work towards finding ways to coexist with nature, fostering a harmonious relationship that benefits both humanity and the natural world.

Native Americans hold a deep reverence for the natural world.

In American Indian culture, nature is revered above all else. This concept is intricately intertwined with their spiritual beliefs, which are fundamental aspects that shape their perspective and way of life.

Native Americans believe that every object and element of the Earth, whether living or non-living, possesses a distinct spirit that is part of the greater soul of the universe. This belief is rooted in Animism, a religion characterized by its belief in and reverence for the underlying spirituality present in all things.

Animism encompasses all living beings, natural phenomena, and non-living entities. This includes humans, plants, animals, as well as natural elements and geographic features like rivers, mountains, and thunderstorms.

Native American culture places great value on the essence of the land and acknowledges its vital contributions.

Cultural evolution does not involve science.

While there exist numerous contradictory legends and discussions about the origins of the Earth, science typically serves as the discipline employed to explain the workings of the universe and specific phenomena. Although the process of photosynthesis is now a well-established and widely accepted theory for plant growth, Native Americans perceived a blooming flower as a gift from a land imbued with its own spirit.

Throughout history, many Native American individuals, both in the past and present, turned to nature to interpret phenomena that eluded full comprehension. They held the belief that spirits governed the Earth and its natural elements. Consequently, they developed reverence for the wind, animals, plants, and water, among other things.

All Native American cultures share the conviction that life is sacred and originates from the land, thereby elevating Mother Earth to a divine status. This concept permeates every piece of art they create.

Climate change

Climate change is a significant problem that affects the entire planet, and many American communities are recognizing the value of Native American knowledge in addressing these challenges.

The Houma Nation, who have inhabited the marshes and coastal areas of the Louisiana Gulf Coast for centuries, have witnessed the devastating impact of climate change. Their way of life, centered around fishing, shrimping, and other subsistence activities, has been severely impacted.

Due to climate change and industrialization, the Louisiana coast has experienced extensive erosion, leading to rapid landscape changes and the depletion of fish and shellfish populations. Consequently, the Houma people are concerned about their ability to pass on their traditional way of life to future generations.

Indigenous coastal communities have long recognized the importance of preserving coastal marshes, as these habitats serve as breeding grounds for numerous fish and crustacean species, which are vital for their livelihoods. These communities have actively engaged in planting marsh grasses and trees to maintain these habitats.

However, the efforts to preserve these habitats have been hindered by the construction of canals by oil companies and commercial fisheries. These canals have disrupted the natural cycle of the waterways, leading to a significant decline in fish reproduction and negatively impacting the delicate ecosystem.

Foraging

Plant gathering in the wild is a wonderful way to reconnect with nature while supplementing our food supply. When we forage for wild foods, we can appreciate everything nature has to offer and the effort that goes into providing food for all members of the group.

Indigenous peoples teach us that foraging does not deplete the crop. They practiced sustainable harvesting by only gathering about one-third of the crop, allowing the remaining plants to grow and reproduce. This ensured an abundant supply for future generations and subsequent foraging expeditions.

Foraging held great value as a skill among Native Americans and early American colonists. It provided not only food and flavoring ingredients but also medicinal resources. According to Iroquois archives, they obtained over eighty varieties of wild edibles.

Self-Restraint

Many Native American tribes embrace a unique concept of self-control. This notion of self-control originates from communal living and harmonizing with the natural world, which often presents unforeseen changes. In a collaborative culture where collective strength equates to survival, self-control proves advantageous.

Native peoples safeguarded the lives of future generations by practicing restraint in their utilization of natural resources. They bequeathed a legacy for future descendants to uphold, refraining from plundering the planet for personal gain.

The Seventh Generation ideology of the Iroquois Confederacy exemplifies this approach. It mandates that tribal decision-makers assess the consequences of their actions and choices for progeny up to seven generations into the future.

The Haudenosaunee Confederacy's governance traces its roots back to 1142 AD and earned admiration from Benjamin Franklin, who incorporated elements of its principles into the Constitution. This network emphasizes the interconnections between animals, humans, and the environment, which shape our lives and the lives of future generations.

Agriculture

Native Americans are not primarily thought of as farmers. The common stereotype depicts them as brave warriors riding horses and living in teepees on the Great Plains.

However, many Native American societies had highly developed sustainable agricultural systems capable of producing crops for large populations. Prior to European contact, the Cherokee had developed and cultivated at least 15 different types of corn.

Spirituality also played a significant role in food production. For the Iroquois, the Three Sisters crops were corn, squash, and beans. These three crops were traditionally grown together in gardens, forming a complementary and mutually beneficial group.

The Three Sisters represented the spirits of young women known collectively as Our Life. Offerings and prayers of thanksgiving were made to these Three Sisters to express gratitude and appreciation for the bountiful crops.

This sense of gratitude is crucial for long-term sustainability, something that is often lacking in modern civilizations. The Wampanoag, a tribe known for their assistance to the Pilgrims in their first year, taught them various organic farming techniques and relied on nature for support.

Just like animals, plants require nourishment, and the Wampanoag supplemented their diet with wood ash and fish scraps. These organic farming methods not only sustained their land but also enriched it, setting a sustainable precedent.

Regenerative agriculture and permaculture

Regenerative agriculture and permaculture are agricultural techniques that emphasize natural and holistic practices. It is worth noting that Native Americans and tribal nations own half of Arizona's farmland.

The Hopi people are renowned for their dryland farming, and the arid environment of the Southwest is well-suited for this ancient farming method. Presently, Hopi farmers sow their crops deeper than previously recommended and rely on minimal irrigation.

Ramona Farms, one of Arizona's largest Native-owned farms, is owned by the Button family of the Akimel O'odham (River People, Pima) tribe from the Gila River Indian Community. In addition to cultivating commercial crops such as alfalfa and cotton, they have taken steps to revive several ancient plants historically grown by tribes in the Southwest.

They are now successfully cultivating bafv, a type of tepary bean that thrives in drought conditions. This is yet another example of their harmonious collaboration with the environment, land, and cultural heritage.

The Healing Spirit

All Native American tribes possess extensive oral mythologies of creation that connect them to the divine, particularly to living spirits. Deities collectively created the indigenous peoples in the region, including the Quechan, Navajo, and Apache. The great spirits of wisdom, understanding, and healing that dwell in nature and have always influenced the history and culture of these three prominent tribes are revered by all three communities.

Native Americans believe that their healing practices and customs are grounded in four principles:

• Spirituality (Great Father, Mother Earth, Creator)

• Environment (balance, nature, daily life)

• Community (clan, family, tribe/nation)

• Self (inner peace and passions, thoughts and values).

There are two methods of receiving spiritual healing. One involves consuming a beverage made from parts of the gemsbok, which grants power upon ingestion. As the dance commences, one starts to quiver and vibrate naturally.

During the dance, the spirit begins to move towards the base of the spine, causing the stomach to tremble and the body to shake and vibrate due to the perceived heat. The movement of the feet initiates this process, igniting an internal fire that induces trembling. Sometimes, the vibration occurs spontaneously when one relaxes while lying down, signifying the arrival of the spirit. Otherwise, it is necessary to dance to summon the spirit. When the light is witnessed in such a dance, it is believed that one has transcended into the spiritual realm.

At times, the light can transport individuals to the realms of their ancestors and the Great God. If this occurs, others may think one has collapsed or fainted and attempt to awaken them.

The Great God does not possess a fixed color; it changes with each instance. The Great God is not excessively old, but simply aged. The Great God can assume any form. The light that manifests during the dance resembles a flickering light. The body is struck by a beam of light, eliciting shivers and trembling.

When someone is unwell, the healer begins to tremble. The healer then endeavors to alleviate the suffering of the sick person. Their anguish manifests as small bullets, which the healer extracts and discards. The anguish sometimes enters the hands, travels to the stomach, and eventually exits through the mouth. In other instances, it simply falls into the palm of the hand and is discarded. The healer must scream to alleviate their suffering.

Patients may be horrified as they have never encountered anything like this before. When the spirit first touches them, fear arises. Due to their trepidation, they anticipate a dreadful experience that will ultimately transform their lives.

Occasionally, the spirit materializes abruptly. At that point, one must cease their activities and request that the women chant. The spirit will briefly shake them, facilitating healing. This can transpire at any time.

Every Bushman healer undergoes the same sensations from the spirit. In other words, all Bushman medicines follow similar procedures after the initial stage, which may differ. Gender does not affect the spirit; the same applies to everyone.

Native Americans do not rely on medicine to help them perceive the spirit or witness the light; they receive all the strength they need from the spirit. When they become filled with the spirit, they experience immense joy as they may be able to communicate with the deceased.

Some young individuals make an effort to educate themselves about drugs. However, when possessed by the spirit, they become fearful and cease attending dances. Nonetheless, some continue their learning.

Shamanism

The shaman, a person thought to acquire various talents through ecstatic religious experiences, is the focal point of the religion known as shamanism. The skills of shamans differ from culture to culture, but they are typically believed to have the ability to heal the sick, communicate with the afterlife, and, in some cases, guide the souls of the departed to the afterlife. The word "shamanism" is derived from the Manchu-Tungus term "saman," and it can be interpreted as "one who knows" since it originates from the verb "to know." Historical ethnographies have described shamans as men, women, and transgender individuals of all ages, even from infancy.

Shamanistic practices are prevalent in indigenous societies where the roles of healer, religious authority figure, counselor, and advisor are combined. Examples of such groups include American Indians, Arctic Peoples, Australian Aborigines, and African tribes like the San, who have maintained their ancient civilizations well into the twentieth century. Shamanism often coexists with animism, a religion that believes in the presence of numerous spirit creatures on Earth who can aid or hinder human endeavors.

Shamanism holds a prominent place in the religious life of the Inuit and Yupik (Eskimo) people. In these communities, the primary responsibilities of shamans are healing and undertaking trance-based underwater journeys to the Mother of Animals in order to procure an abundance of game and assist childless women in conceiving. Any breach of taboo or the enslavement of a soul by a spirit results in sickness. In the former case, the shaman expels all impurities through group confessions, while in the latter, the shaman descends to heaven or the depths of the sea to retrieve the sick person's soul and reunite it with their body.

Shamanism plays a fundamental role in the religious life of many American Indian tribes. A shaman is defined by supernatural abilities acquired through direct personal experience. Whether these powers are obtained naturally or through a deliberate vision quest, aspiring shamans must overcome specific initiatory challenges. Shamans in these communities wield their influence in a way that impacts the entire society. Healing is the primary responsibility of a shaman, but they may also be involved in other magical-religious events such as community hunts, secret societies, or mystical movements like the Ghost Dance.

Scholars generally agree that one becomes a shaman through inheritance, training, or an inward calling or vocation, although each term has its own qualifications. In this context, "inheritance" refers to the passing of a deceased shaman's soul and the so-called shaman's illness. Since shamans are believed to be taught by spirits, the term "instruction" does not usually imply the study of specific facts and unambiguous doctrines. The inner "calling" is, in fact, the summons of a spirit who has chosen and compelled the individual to pursue this vocation. The classification of the spirit that selects the shaman describes the qualitative categories by which shamans are distinguished: small, medium, and great. On the other hand, the shaman's professional competence is clearly based on personal attributes such as mental prowess, dramatic flair, and the ability to effectively manifest their will. All these factors contribute to the excellence of the shaman's performance and the art they practice.

Shamans are said to be born into their roles, evident through distinct defining features that set them apart from ordinary individuals. For instance, a shaman may possess more bones, such as extra teeth or fingers, than regular people. However, simply desiring to become a shaman is not enough, as it is supernatural beings who choose the individual rather than the other way around. Adolescence is typically when spirits become increasingly visible in ashaman's life, although there can be exceptions. The spirits can cause the chosen person to weep, faint repeatedly, and experience visions that can persist for weeks.

The beings or entities that have chosen the shaman eventually reveal themselves in a vision or dream, disclosing their intentions. The shaman must undergo this initiation to acquire their abilities. The spirits make various promises to the hesitant aspiring shaman before tormenting them if they refuse. These torments, known as "shaman illness," can persist for months or even years until the person accepts their calling as a shaman.

When the applicant finally surrenders, they usually enter a three-day and three-night sleep. During this "long slumber," the spirits divide the applicant into pieces and count their bones to see if they possess an "extra bone" (according to mythology). If they do, they are now considered a shaman. Certain groups, such as the Manchu-Tungus and Mongols, formally and publicly initiate shamans. They introduce the shaman to supernatural beings, and the shaman ascends the "tree-up-to-the-heavens," a pole symbolizing this ascent.

The shaman must be well-versed in all things humans require in their everyday lives but cannot learn on their own. A shaman foresees distant events in time and space, locates lost animals, forecasts fishing and hunting opportunities, and assists in increasing the gain. They are healers and psychopomps, individuals who travel to the afterlife with the departed. They fulfill all these obligations by speaking directly with the spirits whenever they desire.

The shaman can carry out their responsibilities by communicating with spirits at any time and entering a trance. Trances of possession, in which the spirit seizes the shaman's body, and wandering trances, in which the shaman's soul enters the world of spirits, are two varieties of wandering trances. In the first, the possessed person goes into a trance-like state, demonstrating superhuman power and wisdom: they quiver, struggle, rage, and eventually pass out. After absorbing the spirit, the shaman regains consciousness and becomes its mouthpiece— "they turn into the spirit that entered them."

A shaman's regalia frequently comprises animal-like parts, most commonly deer, bears, or birds. Examples include an antler headdress and a ring with bird feathers pierced into it. Symbolic footwear includes iron deer hooves, bear paws, and bird claws. Tofalar, Soyet, and Darhat shamans wear clothes decorated with human bones—arms, ribs, and finger bones. When performing the rite, the Goldi-Ude tribe's shamans wear a single shirt and a front and back apron portraying snakes, frogs, lizards, and other creatures.

The shaman's primary tool is the drum, which often has only one membrane. It is usually oval, but it can also be circular. Certain peoples paint decorations on the exterior and interior of the membrane; for example, the Tatars of Abakan decorate the membrane with images of the Upper and Lower Worlds. The handle is usually shaped like a cross. The pounding surface is fur-coated, while the drumstick is made of wood or horn. The drumstick is occasionally painted with human and animal patterns, and rattling rings are frequently strung.

During the trance created by the drum's sound, the spirits move to the shaman or into the drum, or the shaman's soul travels to the world of the spirits. In the latter case, the shaman rides the drum like an animal, with the drumstick serving as their lash. The shaman occasionally travels by river, utilizing the drum as a canoe and the drumstick as an oar. All of this is revealed in the shaman's song. Along with the drums, Buryat shamans sometimes travel with sticks shaped like a horse's head.

The following are some characteristics of shamanism:

- A community accepts the existence of specialists who can engage directly with the transcendence realm and, as a result, can heal and divine; these individuals, known as shamans, are considered immensely helpful to society in communicating with the spirit world.

- A shaman's mental characteristics, such as intuition, sensitivity, mercuriality, or eccentricity, are usually accompanied by a physical impairment, such as lameness, an extra finger or toe, or more teeth than the typical number.

- Shamans are claimed to be assisted by a playful spirit being or group of spirits, as well as a dormant guardian spirit in the form of a person, animal, or another sex.

- The unusual talents and societal role of the shaman are considered to be the result of a decision made by one or more supernatural entities. The chosen one, usually an adolescent, may reject the call for years. The resistance of the shaman candidate is crushed by spirit torture, which manifests as physical or mental illness, and they are forced to accept the vocation.

- Depending on the belief system, the shaman may be introduced simultaneously on a transcendent or realistic level. The applicant's corpse is hacked into pieces by spirits from a Yonder World or undergoes a similar experience while lying in a trance state, appearing as if dead. The spirits are trying to determine whether the shaman's body contains more bones than the typical human. After waking, a symbolic initiation process, including climbing a World Tree, is occasionally performed.

- The shaman is known to be capable of communicating directly with spirits by entering a trance state at will. This is accomplished in two ways: allowing the soul to leave the body and enter the spirit realm or acting as a megaphone for the spirit-being, similar to a medium.

- One distinctive feature of shamanism is the conflict of two shamans in the shape of animals, usually reindeer or horned cattle. Combat rarely has a clear goal, yet it is a task that the shaman must fulfill. The victor will live happily ever after, while the loser will perish.

- To enter a trance and perform magical battles and healing processes, the shaman uses artifacts such as a drum, headgear, robe, metal rattler, mirror, drumstick, and staff. The materials and designs of these tools are critical for distinguishing and categorizing the various types and species of shamanism.

- Different folklore (oral and written) and shaman songs have arisen as a result of improvisations on traditional formulae used to lure or imitate animals.

The shaman's extraordinary occupation inevitably distinguishes them socially. They have power because they believe they can communicate with the spirits. Furthermore, they are terrified since they believe their actions may benefit or harm others. Even a good shaman can inadvertently cause harm, and a cruel shaman in communication with spirits of the Lower World is extremely dangerous.

Due to their occupation, the shaman cannot go hunting or fishing or engage in gainful jobs. Some shamans make money by exploiting their unique status. Poor households traditionally paid the shaman one animal for their services, including some reindeer-raising, whereas affluent families paid two, three, or even four animals. Shamanic meaning is conveyed through dramatic dramatization and dance.

The shaman, clad in regalia, sings to the spirits with their voice. Although this song is improvised, it contains required imagery, similes, dialogue, and refrains. The performance always takes place at night. The stage is the area around the fire where the spirits are summoned; the theater is a cylindrical tent or yurt. The audience consists of clan members who have been invited and are waiting for the spirits to appear in awe.

The shaman's assistant, a stage lighter and designer, keeps the fire going to produce stunning shadows on the wall. All of these effects assist those in attendance in seeing everything that the shaman's repeated deed refers to. The shaman is an actor, dancer, singer, and conductor all at the same time. This figure is a wonderful sight, with their cloak flowing in the light of the fire where anything is possible. Ribbons fly around their regalia; their spherical mirror reflects flames and their adornments tinkle.

The sound of the drum captivates both the shaman and their audience. The fact that the audience members are not only objective observers but also devoted followers enables the shaman to achieve results, such as treating physical or mental ailments, which is a crucial component of this performance. Certain people, such as the Altai Kizhi, place a long tree into the smoke once it has opened at the tent's peak to symbolize the Tree of the World.

The shaman climbs the tree to the highest point of the Upper World, which they communicate to their listeners through the lyrics of their song.

A shaman commands immense respect and power as a healer, a mediator between humans and gods and spirits, and, in some locations, as the guide of the deceased to their new home. They also ensure that rituals are carried out appropriately, defend the tribe from evil spirits and magic, point out suitable hunting and fishing locations, increase fauna, and facilitate births. South American shamans might also assume the role of a sorcerer, transforming into animals and consuming their enemies' blood, for example.

The Native Healer

Native American healing perspectives, including the term "medicine," reflect a way of life that differs greatly from the Western medical paradigm. While healing and curing are often seen as interchangeable in Western medicine, they hold distinct meanings in Native American culture. In Native American culture, healing is more about reclaiming one's wholeness and restoring natural harmony rather than simply treating an illness.

A Native Healer is an indigenous individual who possesses extensive knowledge of the magical and chemical properties of various materials, referred to as medicines, as well as the ceremonies used to administer them. While the term is commonly associated with American Indian tribes, it can be used across various civilizations.

Traditionally, healers have taken on the responsibility of healing both the physical and mental ailments of individuals, as well as addressing the social ruptures that occur within a community due to tragedies like murders. Some healers undergo challenging initiation procedures to acquire supernatural abilities, while others learn through apprenticeships, and many pursue both paths.

Healers typically carry a kit containing various healing artifacts, such as specific bird feathers, shaped and marked stones, hallucinogens, pollen, therapeutic herbs, and other items. In some cases, these items are believed to have been extracted from the healer's own body during their initiation into the healing practice.

As a result, techniques like sucking, tugging, or other methods of removing harmful substances from the patient's body are commonly employed in the healing process. In situations where the offending material is metaphysical, the focus of the healing process is on restoring spiritual and mental well-being. In such cases, sleight of hand can be used to symbolically "remove" an object from the sufferer. The term "witch doctor" was coined by 18th-century Western observers to refer to individuals who diagnose and treat conditions attributed to the actions of witches or sorcerers, as these conditions often align with traditional belief systems that attribute illness and trouble to such influences.

The Red Path places emphasis on the spiritual aspects present in all things. It is characterized by values such as fostering a sense of belonging and mastery, promoting kindness, respecting individuality, and practicing selflessness. Healers on the Red Path receive teachings in healing rituals and ceremonies from knowledgeable and experienced mentors. The Medicine Wheel represents the Red Road as a path that extends from north to south, while the Black Road in the Medicine Wheel represents a path of conflict and destruction, running from west to east. According to Black Elk, humans walk both paths.

At the Seven Circles Heritage Center, artist Charlie Armstrong created a mural depicting existence from a Native American perspective, showcasing a life lived in harmony with nature, the disruptions and genocide that occurred with the arrival of Europeans, and a revival and return to traditional Native American ways that foster a renewed sense of spiritual connection and hope. The Medicine Wheel concept symbolizes the Red Path and encompasses the associated ideas.

The Medicine Wheel is used as a means to orient oneself in relation to the cardinal points and other aspects of life associated with them. The circle represents the whole, while the four spokes of the wheel point in different directions. The specific meanings associated with each direction may vary depending on the tribe.

In one traditional medicine wheel interpretation, the East is associated with the rising sun, spirituality, and the color red. The South is linked to the full sun, nature, and the color yellow. The West, where the sun sets, represents the physical elements of existence and the color black. The bitter winter winds blow from the North, bringing snow, and are connected to the color white and the cognitive aspects of life. The Medicine Wheel serves as a reminder that all aspects of life must be balanced, and neglecting vital areas can result in an imbalanced and more challenging life.

When considering wellness from a Native American perspective, individuals seeking a balance of the mental, physical, and spiritual components of life also take the community context into account. Native American medicine differs from Western medicine in its compassionate, intentional, and relationship-oriented approach, as evidenced by indigenous healing traditions. This viewpoint emphasizes the different types of energy present in interpersonal interactions, spiritual connections, and the relationship with the land and earth.

Herbs

Native Americans used to study the indigenous plants in their surroundings to identify which components of specific plants contributed to their healing. Unlike Western medicine's perspective, many people believe that the beneficial effects of herbal remedies are also influenced by the healer's spiritual connection to the plants. Therefore, synthetic drugs created in laboratories would not have the same properties. Healers regarded herbs as a way to restore balance in an individual's physical, emotional, spiritual, and intellectual aspects.

Healing Tools

Native American healers utilize various items in their practices:

• Pipes are ceremonially smoked to invoke the four elements and make a sacrifice to the Great Spirit.

• Birds and animals serve as totem messengers, appearing in real life or dreams to provide spiritual guidance.

• Dream catchers, also known as sacred hoops, were initially created as therapeutic amulets for children to prevent nightmares.

• Prayer flags or prayer ties made of cloth and tobacco are offered to The Great Spirit in exchange for blessings.

• Native and Hispanic healing approaches are blended and evolved, incorporating the use of herbs, sweat, food, and magick.

• Feathers, seashells, bones, animal skins, and other sacred artifacts are utilized to facilitate spiritual connection, prayer, healing, and protection. Feather Fetishes refer to a collection of feather amulets.

• Amulets and talismans associated with Native American rituals include shells, crystals, jewels, rattles, animal skins, feathers, Zuni fetishes, and bones.

Note: The text provided doesn't contain any grammatical, punctuation, or syntax errors.

Story Telling

Native American tribes have a rich tradition of relying on oral storytelling to pass down knowledge from one generation to the next. Through storytelling, tribal histories, origins, ceremonies, and healing practices have been preserved and shared. The power of storytelling extends beyond mere transmission of information; it plays a vital role in shaping one's identity, understanding of the world, and path to healing. These stories offer hope and instill trust in the healing journey for those who are suffering, and they themselves can serve as a form of medicine and aid in the recovery process. Indigenous healing stories hold equal validity to modern Western medical science, providing a unique way to comprehend the intricacies of the healing process.

Dance

The Sundance requires immense dedication from individuals who willingly endure hardships and suffering for the betterment of their community and to strengthen their resolve to persevere. This ceremony symbolizes the sacrifice of personal comfort for the collective good. Sun dancers adorn themselves with leather thongs attached to buffalo skulls, which are worn across their chests, shoulders, and backs. They dance until their bodies are liberated, representing liberation from the limitations of ignorance in the earthly realm. Other sacred dances include gourd dances and spirit dances. Engaging in these dances has been shown to decrease drug and alcohol consumption and misuse.

Native American Healing Methods

Native American healing practices exemplify significant cultural beliefs and influence the development of Native Americans' identities. These healing methods are rooted in traditions and concepts that often diverge from mainstream Western psychological principles, yet they can profoundly impact Native Americans' well-being. Native Americans engage in rituals that imbue symbolic meaning into their life experiences. To effectively work with Native Americans and foster intercultural adaptability in counseling practices, counselors must familiarize themselves with these diverse perspectives and understanding Native American viewpoints.

Many contemporary healing techniques and spiritual ceremonies employed by healers and metaphysical organizations draw from Native American traditions. Historical records indicate that each tribe had one or more elders trained in the healing arts, encompassing healers, herbalists, and spirit communicators. The specific tasks and forms of healing practices and spiritual rituals varied naturally among different tribes. Native American healing arts and practices reverently honor and acknowledge the Father Sky, Grandfather Sun, Mother Earth, and Grandmother Moon.

Various tribes and individuals who adopt a pan-Indian mindset observe several common Native American healing treatments.

Powwow

A powwow is a Native American gathering that serves social and religious purposes. It features a circular arena where Native Americans engage in drumming, singing, and dancing. Many attendees don traditional Native American attire, often designing and sewing the garments themselves. Wearing regalia and dancing in the arena circle is a symbolic expression of Native American unity, embodying the essence of the phrase "mitakuye oyasin," which translates to "we are all related."

The drum holds a special and spiritual significance for many Native Americans due to its round shape, symbolizing the entire world, and its rhythmic beat, which represents the heartbeat of the planet.

Pipe Ceremony

According to Lakota legend, White Buffalo Cow Woman bestowed the sacred pipe and other sacraments upon the Lakota people.

The pipe typically consists of a hardwood stem and a red catlinite bowl. When not used in a ritual, the pipe and stem are kept separate; their combination signifies the beginning of the ceremony, which must be carried through to completion. Instead of tobacco, various herbs like sage and red willow are used. Tobacco, rather than being smoked for pleasure, is intended to convey prayers to the Creator and the Great Mystery. Pipe rituals are often incorporated into various rites, including inipi. In a circle, participants engage in smoking and prayer, passing the pipe from one person to the next. The pipe ritual brings solace and comfort to those seeking healing.

Inipi/ Sweat Lodge

The sweat lodge, also known as the Inipi ceremony, is a purification rite. The Inipi can be conducted as an independent ceremony or as a prelude to other ceremonies like vision quests, weddings, or sundances. The lodge structure consists of a wooden A-frame, with tied willow branches forming a dome spacious enough for a few individuals. Around a small pit, adults gather where hot stones are placed. Tarps and blankets are then used to enclose the frame, leaving a small access and exit point, which may be secured.

During the Inipi ceremony, the door is closed. Many participants observe a fast prior to entering. Two crucial ceremonial roles are the sweat lodge leader, who oversees the entire process, and the fire keeper, who heats the stones before bringing them into the sweat lodge during the ceremony. Typically, a total of 28 stones are heated. The ceremony consists of four "doorways," with each doorway introducing seven stones. Once the doors are closed, songs and prayers are sung while water and herbs like sage, sweetgrass, and cedar are sprinkled onto the hot rocks, producing a dense and fragrant steam that fills the lodge.

Smudging

Smudging is a cleansing technique in which healers and individuals undergoing treatment waft the smoke from burning cedar, sweetgrass, or sage over themselves and their surroundings. Cedar and sage are known to dispel various forms of negative energy, while sweetgrass attracts positive energies. Smudging aids in the healing process by purging harmful negative energies and inviting beneficial ones. It is often integrated with other sacred rituals, such as inipi, to help individuals and spaces prepare for more profound spiritual experiences.

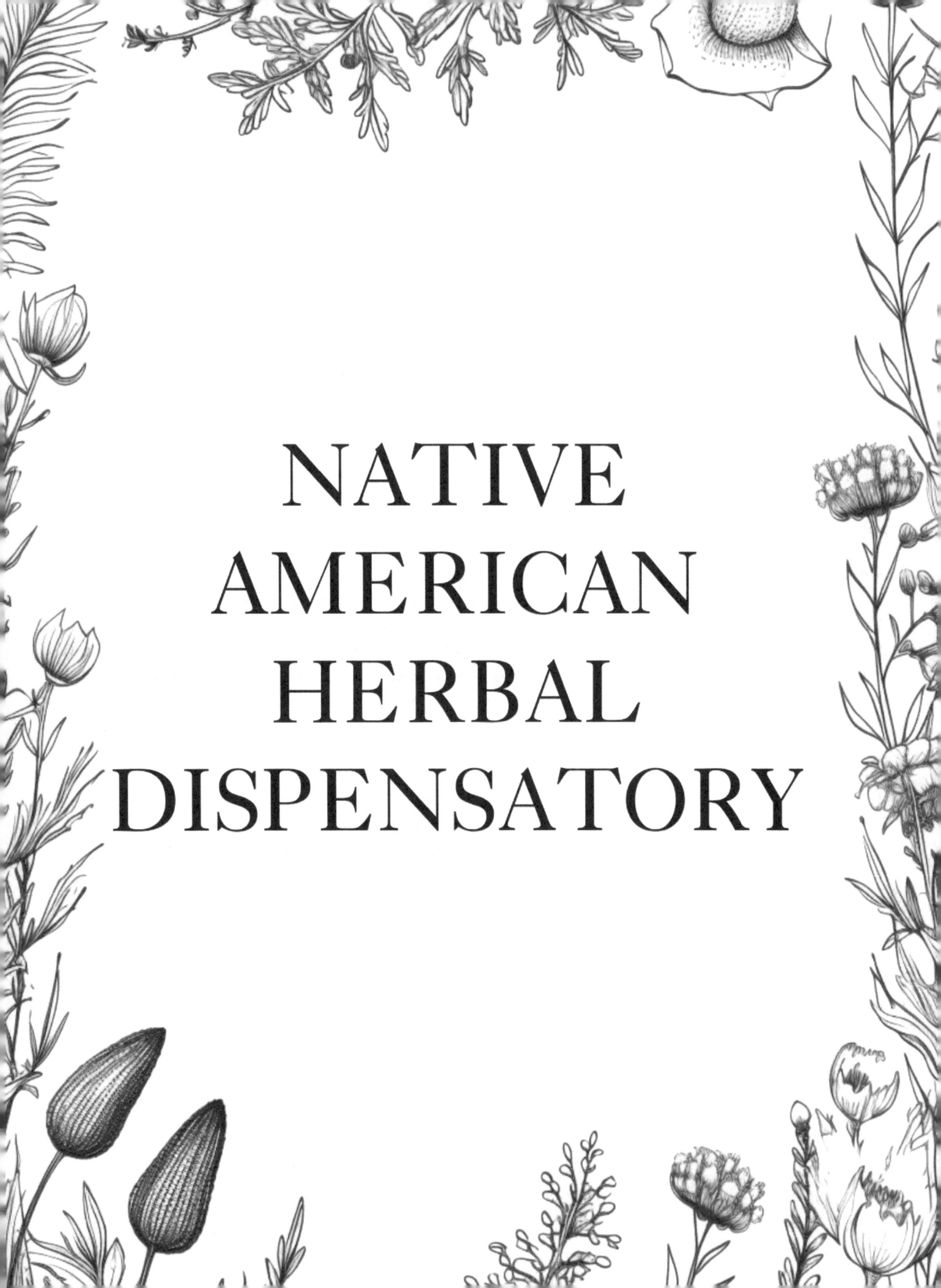

NATIVE AMERICAN HERBAL DISPENSATORY

INTRODUCTION

Native American healing traditions have a long and rich history predating recorded history. There is a growing interest in medicinal botanicals as part of alternative medicine in the United States. Native American societies, in particular, are becoming more aware of the usage of herbals by both practitioners and consumers. Many botanicals offered as nutritional supplements in the western world today were utilized for similar purposes by Native Americans. However, these supplements are among the 2,500 different vascular taxonomic plant species and 2,800 species of all taxa known to have been prized for their therapeutic capabilities by the continent's native populations. Since ancient times, cultures worldwide have relied on traditional natural medicine to meet their health needs. The global market for herbal treatments is expanding due to technological and medical breakthroughs in the current era. This industry is estimated to generate around $60 billion each year.

Native American healing activities demonstrate important cultural viewpoints and impact the formation of Native American culture. Such therapeutic procedures are founded on ideas and traditions that are generally beyond the norm of Western psychological ideals yet can significantly impact Native American well-being. The ceremonial celebration of Native Americans, according to Hammerschlag, attempts to invest symbolic importance in one's life events.

Native Americans are renowned for their medicinal plant knowledge. It is thought that plants and herbs were originally used for healing after observing animals devour such plants when they were ill. To safeguard these plants from overharvesting, the medicine men used to select every third plant they found. Native Americans had a spiritual perspective on life. To be healthy, a person should have a sense of purpose and follow a fair, harmonious, and balanced path. They believed that certain diseases were life lessons that the individual needed to learn and should not be intervened in. Many current medications and treatments are based on Native American interpretations of the numerous plants and herbs they have used for thousands of years.

It is an important aspect of alternative medicine and is useful in treating and preventing various common disorders. Nature's pharmacy is vast and full of herbs with powerful medical powers. With the right information and supervision, everyone can use herbs to relieve pain and promote recovery. Growing up in the hills of Montana, I heard stories about Native Americans curing various maladies using medicines created from wild plants that grew exclusively beyond our family's boundaries. Today, I enjoy growing aromatic herbs in my backyard and the hardwood woods behind my house. When I'm not feeling well, I'm often able to take care of myself with plants that I've chosen and prepared. Some herbal therapies involve using plant components in their natural state. By doing some study, ensuring that a certain plant is safe and appropriate for me, and sticking to any necessary precautions,

A huge supplement stack demonstrates that whoever consumes the most vegetables obtains a good diet. One reason herbalism has been so successful as a preventative and curative medicine is that the herbs we use today are often plants called "vegetables" throughout human history. So many of the illnesses we see today are caused by a lack of critical nutrients. On the most basic level, herbs can assist us in filling such gaps and keeping our bodies going strong.

Most likely, herbs are already a part of your self-care or beauty routine—you don't realize it. Examine the ingredient list on various facial creams and cleansers, shampoos and sprays, and even cough drops. Herbal extracts of many of the components discussed in this book are likely to be found. Acne, dry skin, and brittle hair, as well as fatigue, mild depression, and anxiety, are all common problems that can be avoided, reduced, or treated by using herb-infused creams, shampoos, teas, and other products. You may have realized that natural medicine is ineffective. It is not based on mathematics or historical notions that are no longer valid in today's

environment. The truth is that herbs (and meals) have been used for centuries to heal, restore, and protect people from injuries and illness for a reason. Begin to comprehend it by examining commonly used words, such as organic salad greens: Essential oils are volatile oils extracted from plant parts such as stalks, leaves, blossoms, and fruits that emit a specific healing odor. Antioxidants are molecules present in herbs, plants, and food that help combat the harmful oxidizing agents that kill cells.

NATIVE AMERICAN MEDICINE
Native American Healthcare

Native American healthcare is critical to the survival of Native Americans, as there are more than five million uninsured people in this community. People in the United States who are members of a Native tribe are more than twice as likely to be poor. Due to migration and external pressures, these tribes have gradually become smaller over time. Moreover, treaties were established between tribes that forced them to relocate without providing any provisions for others. Consequently, these Native tribes lacked doctors, clinics, hospitals, medical equipment, and resources. They could only carry with them what they could during their journeys.

The "Indian Health Service" (IHS), established during the administration of Franklin D. Roosevelt, was one of the initial measures taken to assist these tribes. The IHS aimed to provide medical treatment to off-reservation patients and educate them on becoming more "civilized." However, it encountered numerous challenges. Doctors did not take it seriously, and it failed to deliver quality healthcare to Native Americans in need. Additionally, it suffered from insufficient funding. Consequently, Native Americans were dying at an alarming rate due to contagious diseases such as smallpox and TB.

In order to address this issue, the government established the Indian Health Board (IHB) to collaborate with agencies like the IHS before they were disbanded. The GI Bill of 1944 also played a significant role in improving Native American healthcare by providing post-secondary education to Native American doctors, enabling them to practice within their tribes.

In 1955, the Indian Health Service (IHS) was established. However, it continues to face the same challenges it did in the past, including underfunding. One of the primary sources of underfunding is the lack of funding from Medicare or Medicaid, despite the critical role these programs play in supporting Native Americans.

Native American Beliefs on Religion and Healing

Religious Beliefs

Religion has always been an important part of the lives of all Aboriginal groups in North America. Religious ideas originated with their forefathers and continue to hold significant value. Each tribe has its own culture, including unique religious beliefs.

The beliefs of these Native American groups can be categorized into three groups: shamanism, spirituality, and animism.

Shamanism is a traditional Native American practice that incorporates local folk traditions. It derives from the Tungusic language of northeastern Asia, meaning the name of a priest who acts as an intermediary between his tribe's members and their gods/spirits.

Native Americans, also known as shamans, have existed in North America for hundreds, if not thousands, of years. During times of illness, Native American medicine men would perform rites and ceremonies. The shaman would also be present at significant life cycle events such as birth and puberty. A Native shaman may also be referred to as a medicine man, mystic, faith healer, or diviner. From the Native American perspective, shamanism is the belief that the Creator has bestowed healing powers upon their tribe or that the spirits possess special spiritual abilities.

Spirituality is the second belief system. It is often considered a form of religion, but it is more focused on an individual's relationship with God rather than a communal one. It emphasizes personal connections and one-on-one relationships rather than group dynamics. Spirituality has played an essential role in Native American society since ancient times. Most Native American tribes believe in a higher power.

Animism is the third belief system. It is a term used to describe the spiritual relationship between all things on the planet, including objects, plants, and animals. This belief encompasses the Native American idea that spirits exist within all things, creating a connection between the animate and inanimate universe. Natural objects, such as plants, rivers, or mountains, are believed to possess a spiritual essence that can freely move between the earthly realm and the spiritual realm.

One of the most significant aspects of Native American culture is their religion, which serves as a vital connection to a higher power and is an integral part of their daily lives.

Native American religion revolves around appreciating and respecting the natural forces that govern the planet. Each indigenous group had its own set of spiritual beliefs, which included specific ceremonies, rituals, festivals, and other events to honor and celebrate nature.

Native Americans held four fundamental beliefs: Creator, Creation, Divinity, and Sacredness. These concepts are reflected in various ways across different cultural traditions throughout North America, where indigenous civilizations have flourished for thousands of years.

Creation was seen as a complex process influenced by multiple spiritual forces, and Native Americans believed that these supernatural energies governed all aspects of nature.

In traditional Native American rituals, individuals sought guidance from spirits or requested assistance for illnesses or calamities that could harm their family, village, or tribe. Throughout history, the principles of Creator, Creation, Divinity, and Sacredness have been central to indigenous religions across North America.

• Creator: Everything in existence is created by a being whose intent, energy, and intelligence are perfectly aligned with everything else.

• Creation: The creation of the universe was a multi-step process that took a considerable amount of time. Indigenous people believed that their universe was created by many gods or spirits rather than a single entity.

• Divinity: Spiritual elements are inherently intertwined with humans, and maintaining harmony with these elements is of utmost importance. For instance, it was considered improper to kill an animal and leave its carcass for scavengers because the deceased animal possessed special spiritual qualities. Honoring the animal's power involved expressing gratitude and seeking permission from its spirit before taking its life for sustenance.

• Sacredness: Everything in nature, including plants, animals, rivers, and mountains, carries a sacred essence that must be

acknowledged and respected. This reverence for the sacred is one reason why many Native Americans practice vegetarianism.

In the past, Native Americans would worship by visiting sacred locations such as mountains or forests. They would construct altars or shrines in natural settings and depict images of the gods or spirits they wished to honor. Rituals, including music, singing, dancing, chanting, and praying, were performed. The primary purpose of these ceremonies was to enhance the spiritual strength of participants and foster a closer connection with their gods or spirits.

The majority of Native American rituals were conducted outdoors, as they believed the spiritual world encompassed all aspects of nature, including plants, mountains, and forests.

If you ask any Native American why they worship a higher force or divinity, they will tell you that their Creator, Wakan Tanka (meaning "Great Mystery"), guided them to believe in this spiritual path. Wakan Tanka is a widely used term among Native Americans to refer to the creator god or spirit of their tribe.

Like many indigenous groups throughout the Americas, North American Indians believe that every plant and animal possesses a spirit with its own distinct traits. Native Americans sought the company of these spirits or gods to gain knowledge and develop a closer relationship with their Creator.

In ancient traditions, it was considered taboo to create an image representing one of their gods or spirits. This prohibition existed because humans were believed to have excessive influence over them. It was also believed that creating such an image would make the deity or spirit envious, resulting in negative consequences rather than the desired assistance.

In addition to worshiping animal spirit guides and gods found throughout North America, many Native Americans maintained a connection with Earth Mother and her son Sky Father. Earth Mother, known as Spider-Woman among the Hopi, Zuni, and other tribes, played a significant role. The Pueblo people of New Mexico and Arizona refer to her as Kachina. Sky Father, known as Kujikai or Sky Horse, descended from Heaven to teach humanity how to coexist with one another and the Earth.

These two spiritual parents hold importance for all Native Americans, as their power and wisdom brought life into this world. They also nurtured Native Americans during infancy, often symbolized through rituals conducted in stone rooms called kivas.

Intersection of Traditional and Western Healing

Despite their names' resemblance, there is one significant distinction between them. Traditional healing is based on a wide range of ancient traditions that exist in various cultures and vary by place. This encompasses techniques such as shamanic healing, healing touch, and treatments like reflexology and reiki. However, Western healing is scientific and involves more standard Western medical procedures such as surgery and pharmaceutical drugs.

The origins of both treatment methods are unknown, and we cannot determine which is better at healing (although there are some speculations). However, it could be argued that traditional healing carries a lower risk of problems such as drug addiction or surgical complications compared to Western medicine.

Traditional vs. Modern Healing

Modern healthcare treatment is primarily scientific in nature, focusing less on the spiritual aspect of the human being. On the other hand, traditional medicine recognizes the independent nature of an individual's spirit from their physical manifestation. In this modern world, we have been raised to believe that everything in nature has a physical cause and physical effects, but this does not apply to the body, mind, and soul. The mental and spiritual aspects of individuals are just as vital as their physical well-being. Therefore, it makes sense to address all areas of existence when dealing with health issues.

You may have come across various treatments available for individuals with emotional disorders. This is because spiritual healing has proven to be quite effective in many diseases within the Western medical realm. For instance, individuals who have received spiritual healing from a traditional practitioner often gain access to hidden knowledge about their illness, which they can then share with their doctors. They can also discuss their family history and any other circumstances that may have contributed to the development of their ailment.

Furthermore, spiritual healing is far less invasive than Western procedures. For example, you would never have to undergo unnecessary surgery to cure your ailment. Unnecessary procedures are considered wasteful and a poor investment for patients. It's also worth noting that spiritual healing tends to be more cost-effective than Western procedures, and it does not come with negative side effects.

Traditional medicine has the ability to heal both the mind and body simultaneously without jeopardizing people's health or finances.

Healing Plants

Here are several healing plants and their potential uses.

Burdock: Burdock is a perennial herb found all over the world. Burdock root has several medicinal properties and can be consumed raw or cooked (often in conjunction with other herbs), brewed into tea, infused into bath water, or used externally. In China, it has been used for many years to treat high blood pressure.

Pennyroyal: Pennyroyal is a mint-scented, invasive weed that, if taken in excessive quantities, can be poisonous and even fatal. Herbal medicine has used it to treat various diseases, including pain, reduce fever, and alleviate allergy symptoms. It also has insecticidal effects and can be an excellent treatment for scabies or lice when combined with other herbs such as lemon balm or lavender oil.

Rosemary: Rosemary is a perennial herb with several medicinal uses, including topical application for joint pain relief and internal consumption for digestive issues. It belongs to the mint family and is often used in conjunction with other medicinal herbs such as mint, eucalyptus, basil, and oregano.

Cayenne pepper: Cayenne pepper is a perennial herb that thrives in warm areas worldwide. It has numerous medical applications and can be used both internally and externally. Cayenne pepper, when ingested raw or added to certain meals like eggs or salad dressing, can alleviate joint pain, indigestion, stomach ulcers, and high cholesterol. It can also be taken in pill or powder form. Topically, cayenne pepper can be applied to reduce pain, swelling, and promote healing. Some individuals use it directly on their skin (in the form of a lotion or ointment), while others boil it in water and use a towel to soak up the tea and apply it to the affected area.

Sacred Basil: Holy basil is a perennial herb that grows worldwide. It has long been used for therapeutic purposes in India, including improving digestion, easing diarrhea, and treating eye problems when prepared as herbal tea.

Comfrey: Comfrey is a perennial herb found all over the world. It can be consumed in various ways, both cooked and raw, and has several medicinal properties, including wound healing and relief from arthritis pain due to its anti-inflammatory properties.

Plantain: Plantain is a perennial herb that grows worldwide. It has been used as a medicinal herb for decades and has various applications, including relieving aches and pains when brewed as tea.

Agrimony: Agrimony is a perennial herb found throughout Europe and most of Asia. It has been used for generations as a remedy for palpitations and skin pallor, particularly in individuals with leprosy or those who have undergone removal of infected tissue due to the disease.

Yarrow: Yarrow is a perennial herb that thrives in Europe and the United States. Due to its antibacterial properties, it has been used to heal wounds. Traditionally, the fresh plant is applied directly to a wound to seal it shut or wrapped in fabric soaked in yarrow tea. Yarrow tea is made by steeping fresh yarrow leaves in hot water for a few minutes.

NATIVE AMERICAN MEDICINE IN OUR LIVES

Native Americans have existed since the beginning of time and continue to exist today. Native Americans identify with a specific tribe and must be born into the tribe to become a member. This form of society differs from others in that it was created by the people themselves rather than imposed by external forces. They were guided by spiritual leaders such as shamans, who treated diseases and disorders using herbs and other natural materials. Due to their deep connection with the land and natural resources, they had the ability to cure and treat diseases and illnesses. They could communicate with these natural objects, which they utilized for therapeutic purposes.

Native Americans believe that the earth is a sacred area dedicated to their creator, and it is where they live, hunt, and protect. They consider it their responsibility to care for the environment because it was created by the creator for people to use as they see fit. The Native American way of life was rooted in the relationship with the land; everything that occurred in nature had an impact on their lives. They used medicine to establish a connection with the land and its creatures.

Medicine is the term used to describe the remedies used by Native Americans. Plants, roots, shrubs, and other natural materials such as tree bark are commonly employed in their medicinal practices. They offer prayers to their creator before starting the production of their medicine. Native Americans believe that the plants were provided by the creator for therapeutic purposes, and they believe in the healing properties of these plants. Therefore, they utilize them to treat illnesses and diseases. They gather various herbs to create their medicine, and before using the remedies, they carefully gather all the necessary ingredients. This meticulous organization ensures that when the time comes to utilize these natural materials for making medicine, everything is in order and at least one ingredient is readily available. While plants are typically the primary components of their medicine, if certain ingredients are not available, Native Americans also utilize animal components to create remedies. Therefore, animal-derived medicines can be employed to treat ailments and diseases in a similar manner as plant-based medicines.

The medicines used by Native Americans for medical purposes were developed by the indigenous people themselves. The medicine usually consists of a combination of two different plants: one to cure an ailment and the other to prevent it. The choice of which combination to use depends on the specific condition or illness being treated or prevented. Typically, the treatment involves consuming a beverage containing the medicinal components. In some cases, the therapy is intended to be inhaled. Common ailments treated with this medicine include colds, sore throats, fevers, and headaches. Native Americans would consume the medicine to cure their ailments. It was believed that if the medicine was not used promptly upon falling ill, the outcome would be worse than the original ailment.

Traditional Remedies that are Healing Us Today

You may not realize it, but Indian wisdom has been passed down through generations and is well-known for its therapeutic abilities. Herbal medicine is the primary approach used by over 80% of the population to treat diseases and minor injuries. And it's not without good reason: traditional treatments have been proven in Western countries to effectively combat chronic ailments like asthma and arthritis.

Peppermint, turmeric, licorice root, and ginger were used by our ancestors in India and continue to be utilized today. These herbs can be purchased in tea form at your local grocery shop or health food store, or you can prepare them into a tea by boiling water and adding honey for flavor, just as your grandmother used to make.

New World Science

Medicine has been used since 2000 BCE in Ancient Egypt and China. Medicines are classified into three types: over-the-counter, prescription, and complementary.

The earliest records of herbal medicine, however, can be traced back to ancient China, India, and Persia. References to the use of herbs can be found in documents such as the "Yellow Emperor's Inner Canon," which dates between 600 BCE and 200 CE in China. Ayurvedic medicine, derived from natural herbs, has been practiced in India for thousands of years. There are also mentions in the Bible regarding the use of spices and herbs for healing.

Among today's most vital medicines are antibiotics, which were introduced in 1930 when Alexander Fleming discovered penicillin while working with bacterial cultures at St Mary's Hospital in London during World War II. Penicillin was named after the bacterium Penicillium, not because Fleming used it on himself! The generic name of penicillin refers not only to the fungus that produces it but also to the shape of its mushroom.

HERBAL MEDICINE

Herbal medicines, also known as phytomedicines, are components derived from plants or botanicals used to treat illnesses or maintain health. A herb is a plant or any component of a plant used for its scent, flavor, or therapeutic properties. Herbal medicine is a type of dietary supplement. In general, people utilize herbal remedies to try to preserve or improve their health. A herbal supplement is a plant-based substance meant for internal use.

Herbal medications contain active ingredients, many of which are still unknown. Even a single active component derived from plants is employed in various pharmaceutical treatments and pharmaceuticals. Herbalists believe that separating an active component from the rest of the plant reduces its effectiveness and makes it less toxic and unsafe.

Many prescription and over-the-counter drugs are also made from plant materials, including only purified compounds, and are regulated by the FDA. Herbal supplements can contain complete plants or plant parts. Herbal remedies are available in various forms, including dried, powdered, chopped, liquid, and capsules. They can be used in various ways, including:

- Consumed in the form of powders, pills, and tinctures.

- Applied to the skin as gels, creams, and lotions, or dissolved in bathwater.

For thousands of years, people have used herbal medicine and supplements. People in the United States are increasingly using herbal supplements, which are suitable for some individuals. Herbal medicines are frequently controversial since they are not thoroughly inspected by the FDA or other regulatory organizations. It is best to consult your doctor about any symptoms or illnesses you are experiencing and the use of herbal remedies.

Precautions to Take When Using Herbal Medicines:

Many believe that "natural" products are always safe, healthy, and useful, which is only sometimes true. In fact, herbal therapies are not subjected to the same rigorous testing as pharmaceuticals. Some plants, such as comfrey and ephedra, are poisonous, and some plants may interact with prescription and over-the-counter medications.

- Herbal medicines can be combined with prescription treatments or be effective on their own. Do not attempt to diagnose yourself. Consult your doctor before using herbal supplements.

- Educate yourself. Consult your doctor and gather information from herbal supplement manufacturers to learn everything you can about the herbs you're taking.

- If you use herbal remedies, carefully read the label and only take the specified dosage.

- Never exceed the indicated amount. It is a good idea to work with specialists and monitor for adverse outcomes. Reduce the dosage or discontinue use if symptoms such as nausea, headache, dizziness, or upset stomach arise.

- Be vigilant for any allergic reactions. A severe allergic reaction may cause difficulty in breathing. If this occurs, call 911 or your local emergency number for assistance.

- Research the company that produces the herbs you're using. Not all herbal remedies are created equal, so it is best to stick with a well-known brand.

Sourcing Herbs

Herbs come in various sizes and forms, including annuals, biennials, trees, shrubs, perennials, climbers, and grasses. They can survive in various climates and conditions, from the equator to the poles. They can be found at sea level, in the sea, in clean water, and even at the highest peaks' summits.

Despite their diversity, many of the most well-known herbs are grouped into several categories. One category consists of plants from the Lamiaceae family (mint family). They are distinguished by young stems with four angles, simple opposing leaves, and flowers with five more or less connected petals. These plants frequently contain volatile aromatic oils in their glands. They are mostly from Central Asia or the Mediterranean and are used as herbs, perfumes, and therapeutic substances. Well-known herbs in this family include basil, calamint, hyssop, bergamot, lavender, lemon balm, rosemary, mint, sage, savory, and thyme.

Apiaceae includes chervil, anise, coriander, angelica, caraway, cumin, dill, Gotu kola, lovage, fennel, and parsley (carrot family). These plants can be found in temperate climates all around the world. They feature hollow stems with dissected leaves grouped in spirals that are frequently joined by a base that sheathes the entire stem and is aromatic. The five-petaled flowers appear in umbels, followed by strongly scented fruits. The leaves of the majority of these plants contain substantial amounts of herbs, and their fruits are widely used as spices.

The Asteraceae family, also known as the daisy family, includes French tarragon, which primarily grows in temperate areas worldwide. This plant group is distinguished by simple or split leaves grouped in spirals. Flowers are little discs clustered in compact heads and surrounded by a ring of strap-like ray flowers. This family includes dandelion, burdock, chicory chamomile, dandelion, yarrow, marigolds, pyrethrum, wormwood, and safflower. Some herbs are used in cooking, while others are used medicinally. This category includes herbs used to kill and repel insects and produce colors.

The Lauraceae, or laurel family, comprises aromatic, evergreen shrubs, and trees native to northern South America and Southeast Asia. Plants and spices in this family include cinnamon, cassia, sweet bay, camphor, and sassafras.

Allspice, eucalyptus, cloves, cajuput oil, and myrtle are members of the Myrtaceae or myrtle family. These plants and shrubs grow in hot and humid regions. They have fragrant leaves that contain essential oils, and the majority of them have edible fruit.

Many useful root spices are found in the Zingiberaceae family, also known as the ginger family. These plants feature massive, upright, alternating leaves that sprout from fragrant rhizomes that have expanded. They are commonly found in tropical and subtropical regions of the world. This family includes galangal, cardamom, zedoary, Chinese keys, gingers, torch ginger, and turmeric.

Herbs for your home garden can be found in a variety of places. Some people buy herbs from the grocery store, while others prefer to visit a nursery or garden center. You'll want to choose an herb that is the proper size and color for your needs, as well as one that is reasonably priced because you'll need a lot of it. The difficulty is figuring out what kind of herb you want and where to find it!

Look no further for additional information about herb sourcing! We've compiled a comprehensive list of where you can locate these beneficial plants.

If you want to buy your herbs in a local store, you should start with your local grocery store. During the summer months, many larger stores have a significant range of herbs available, but they are frequently out of season.

If you live near a plant nursery, you can also find herbs there. You can always get your herbs online if you need one nearby. Several seed companies sell a variety of herb seeds that can be planted to produce these plants for culinary uses! Check out this list if you need help figuring out what to grow.

If you want to buy seeds and plants online, use this list to find the proper company to supply you with the required goods!

Herbs can be found in many places. These include:

- Garden Center: A garden center is where you can buy herbs like rosemary, oregano, and thyme. You'll want to ensure that the herb is easy to grow and maintain. Most garden stores require their herbs to be grown from seeds indoors before they can be sold. If the herb is produced from cuttings, it should be able to bloom and bear fruit without issue. If the herb is to be sold in a container, it should be clearly labeled.

- Plant stores: During the summer months, craft stores and garden centers frequently offer a selection of low-cost herbs for sale. Many plants can also be found at local grocery stores after being harvested from their containers.

- Nursery: A nursery is another option for getting herbs. Herbs like rosemary, lemon balm, and forsythia can be found at a nursery. You'll want to ensure that the herb develops well and blooms without issue. If it isn't labeled correctly

, make sure it's safe to take home with you if you intend to sell it to someone else.

Growing Herbs

Herbs have been used for culinary and medicinal purposes for years, and they are as popular as ever. Herbs add diverse flavors to a wide range of foods and beverages, which chefs appreciate. Certain flowers, leaves, and roots are prized by herbalists for their medicinal virtues.

Herbalists maintain the beauty and aroma of flowers and leaves by using potpourri, wreaths, sachets, and dried arrangements. Herbs are highly valued by gardeners for a multitude of reasons, including their vigor, low maintenance, and inherent insect resistance.

Herbs are commonly associated with well-known culinary components such as basil, rosemary, thyme, and sage. On the other hand, an herb is any plant regarded as beneficial. For example, an herb's leaves, roots, stems, seeds, or blossoms could be used as a flavoring, medicinal product, fragrance, dye, or other purposes. It is not only about functionality, and some gardeners grow herbs solely for their aesthetic value.

Where to Plant

Most herbs thrive in ordinary garden soil as long as it drains correctly. However, certain herbs, such as rosemary, lavender, and bay, are Mediterranean woody plants that thrive in rocky, well-drained soil. Because the roots of Mediterranean natives rot quickly in moist soil, drainage is critical. If your garden soil is heavy, grow these herbs in raised beds or pots. The majority of herbs thrive in direct sunlight (at least 6 hours per day). If you have a garden with limited sunshine, choose herbs that don't require as much sun. Here are some good options:

- Cilantro
- Shiso
- Tarragon
- Parsley
- Chives

Where to Get Plants

Some herbs germinate fast, while others take a little longer. Plants that grow slowly can be obtained from a nursery or divided from existing plants. In some cases, cuttings can be utilized to grow new plants. Read the seed packet before sowing any herb, whether in seed-starting trays or in the garden, as it contains important information. The following herbs are simple to grow from seed:

- Cilantro
- Calendula
- Parsley
- Sage
- Basil
- Borage
- Parsley
- Sage
- Chervil
- Dill

Perennial herbs are easily divided. With a garden fork, dig up your plant's root system and peel off the roots by hand (as with chives) or slice the root mass to separate pieces and transplant them elsewhere in the garden. Small divisions can also be grown indoors in containers over the winter. If the divisions will be used outside, the best time to divide and cut is in the fall when the plants begin to slow down for the season. Plants grow faster when divided and replanted in the fall. Perennial herbs that respond well to division include:

- Lovage
- Garlic chives
- Bee balm (monarda)
- Thyme
- Chives
- Marjoram
- Oregano

Herb stem cuttings are best acquired in the summer or spring when the plants are vigorous and growing quickly. Because rosemary and tarragon root well in the fall, take cuttings and grow them inside during the winter. Here are some suggested plants for cuttings:

- Lavender
- Thyme
- Sage
- Oregano
- Mint

Some of the cutting techniques are as follows:

- Select tender (usually green but not woody) stem segments 3 to 6 inches long with at least 5 leaves. Make an angled incision just above an outward-facing leaf node.

- Remove the bottom leaves from the stem, dip the cut end into rooting hormone powder, and plant it about

2" deep in a 4" container of moist potting soil. You can also use vermiculite or perlite.

- To create a humid environment, gently and loosely cover the cuttings with a plastic bag and keep them out of direct sunlight.

- Remove the protective plastic bag and water the plants again if there is excessive moisture. After a few weeks, look for new leaf development to verify that the plants are properly rooted. Plants should be repotted into larger containers using regular potting soil and gradually exposed to full sunlight.

Planting Herbs in Pots

Planting herbs in planters and pots allows you to grow sensitive perennials like rosemary and blooming sages all year. Bring them inside in the fall. Furthermore, container gardening is a great option for gardeners with limited space or soil that does not drain well.

To ensure good drainage, start with high-quality potting soil. Avoid using ordinary garden soil that does not drain well when used in a container. Like other container plants, herbs require frequent watering and fertilization during the growing season. Rosemary, a Mediterranean native, can tolerate very dry soil when watered. Watering is especially critical for plants with larger leaves. During the outdoor growing season, apply liquid fertilizer at the rate recommended on the packaging. If you bring them indoors for the winter, you only need to fertilize your plants once or twice a month. Herbs that can be grown in pots for a long time include:

- Rosemary
- Chervil
- Chives
- Basil
- Parsley
- Thyme

- Oregano
- Bay laurel
- Mint
- Scented geranium

Growing herbs is a terrific

way to add something beautiful and flavorful to your garden, and it can also be simple and uncomplicated if done correctly. Many herbs can be grown indoors in pots on your windowsill, but some require a little more effort to thrive. However, regardless of the type of herb you want to cultivate, there are some things that make life easier when grown inside, and others that don't.

The first step should be to plant your herbs. It's simple to grow them in containers, but if you want to get the most out of them, choose herbs that require more water or humidity. You can also use larger pots, but they should be at least 4 inches deep (or more) and 9 inches wide (or more).

Keep your herbs away from direct sunlight; if you can leave them on the ground for part of the day, that's even better. If you don't have a sunny windowsill, place pots on a table or shelf near a south-facing window.

Consider what it is excellent for and, of course, the smell when deciding which herb to cultivate. For example, you can grow basil and cilantro to enhance the flavor of your food, repel odors and flies, and promote your well-being. You should consider having at least one of each type of plant.

Some herbs require more water than others, so it's wise to be aware of their needs before growing them. For example, chives do not require as much water as parsley or mint (this depends on the variety you choose), and they will wilt or rot if they receive too much water.

It's also important to grow the same type of herb year after year, but you can use different pots and containers and keep some herbs in smaller pots and others in larger ones.

To grow herbs indoors, you'll need either a herb pot for each plant or a pot large enough to accommodate all of your plants (or you can buy 4-10). You should also drill drainage holes in the bottom of the pot. The holes should be about 1/4" wide and 1/4" deep to ensure proper drainage.

Before placing your plants in their containers, soak them in water (if necessary) and ensure they're completely dry; this eliminates the possibility of them molding or withering.

If your herbs are in pots, make sure to water them every day (or every other day), and if you keep them in their final pots, ensure they receive enough water (enough to fill the entire pot). Also, make sure that the soil is adequately irrigated."

Preparation

Natural therapeutic products can be obtained naturally or through cultivation, cell or organ culture, fermentation, microbial transformation, and biologics. Choosing the proper medicinal plant source and harvesting at the right time is crucial for improving the output of the required phytochemical content. Roots and rhizomes are collected at the end of the vegetative stage, bark in the spring, leaflets and herbs at bloom, flowers at anthesis or soon after opening, and fruits and seeds after maturity or ripeness.

Hand gathering is preferred for wild sources. Garbling, washing, air drying, oven drying, sieving, milling, re-milling, storage, and labeling with the plant's name, location, and harvest date are all important procedures in traditional herbal preparation. The active compounds in the obtained plant material should be safeguarded during transportation and storage. Freeze-drying, drying or lyophilization, stabilization, fermentation, and other preservation methods are popular.

Herbal preparations are made utilizing various techniques such as infusion, maceration, distillation, expression, decoction, fractionation, purification, concentration, and fermentation to extract from dried or fresh herbal medications.

- Infusions are formed by steeping fresh or dried herbs, primarily aerial sections, in boiling water.

- Decoctions are made from tougher plant material cooked for longer periods on the stovetop than infusions.

- Syrups are herbal poultices that are moist and held in place by a towel or cloth for localized healing.

- Lotions are infusions or decoctions delivered in a smooth liquid solution.

- Compresses are soft cloths squeezed from a cold or hot infusion/decoction and applied to the affected area.

- Tinctures are alcohol-based remedies that are also known as tinctures.

Non-alcoholic substitutes, such as vinegar or glycerites, can be consumed similarly. Oil-based products, such as ointments and infused oils, are used externally.

Herbal preparations serve as the base for finished herbal products. Pharmaceuticals that only contain herbal remedies (active ingredients) and herbal drug preparations are referred to as finished herbal goods. Herbal preparations are also formed by steeping and boiling herbal substances in alcoholic beverages, honey, or other materials, and they can be made from one or more herbs. In addition to the active compounds, they may contain excipients or natural organic or inorganic active components that are not derived from plants.

Synthetic compounds and/or separated herbal components, as well as completed or blended products containing chemically determined active substances, are not considered herbal. According to the binomial approach, herbal drugs are explicitly specified by their botanical scientific name. Herbal remedies include herbs, components, preparations, and finished herbal products. Crude medications must be stored in a dry, airtight container in a dry, dark environment to maintain stability and quality.

Crude drugs are ground to a powder with a desired particle size using a hammer, knife, or teeth mill to isolate a pure ingredient or manufacture a simple preparation. Cold grinding is preferred for crude medicines containing heat-labile components. Blast sifting and sieving procedures can be used to ensure particle size (2.00 mm to 0.18 mm). Extracts are natural medicine preparations that contain all of the solvent-soluble components. Tinctures are created by extracting the crude medicament with 5 to 10 parts ethanol of varying concentrations and leaving the end product unconcentrated.

A variety of factors influence the overall quality of herbal medications. Quality control and standardization of herbal medicines entail many methods. The stability and quality of herbal medicines depend on the quality and source of raw materials, as well as correct farming practices and production procedures. Because pharmaceuticals in commerce are frequently contaminated and fail to fulfill the standards set for authorized drugs, source herbal components should be thoroughly researched in terms of quality, efficacy, performance, and safety for standard herbal drug synthesis at the industrial level.

Infusion

Infusions are one of the simplest and least expensive methods of extracting taste and therapeutic properties from herbs. Herbs in infusions have varying health advantages, but each infusion has a distinct flavor, so try them all until you find your favorite. Infusions are also a great method to use herbs that may be more difficult to find or expensive than less flavorful alternatives.

Infusions are herb-infused drinks made by steeping herbs in water for up to an hour. After straining off the herbs, the infusion can be served hot or cold. Infusions should be consumed within two hours of preparation time, or they lose their potency. Infusions can also be used in cooking and baking recipes to enhance your meal's flavors while adding your own creative touches.

Making Herbal Oils

Essential oils are preferred by some people for their medical and therapeutic properties. These oils frequently need to be properly processed before they can be utilized in therapy or products, such as massage oil. An herbalist will make oil to the specifications of the individual who requests it. Other times, professional businesses do the preparations, but the individual or company must still perform some work before selling or using them. This article explains three ways to prepare essential oils: cold pressing, extraction, and self-titrating (gradually increasing and decreasing the amount of time spent extracting).

Using a cold press

Cold extraction is performed in a film evaporator, a basic glass or metal equipment in which oils are agitated at room temperature to extract the oil. It holds approximately 10 liters of oil. The operator inserts various cheesecloth bags into the evaporator to filter any silt that may accumulate throughout the operation. This entails wrapping the cheesecloth around the mixing bottle and squeezing it for 15 to 30 minutes. Following that, the cheesecloth bags are hand-washed.

Making use of an extractor

An extractor works by chilling essential oils with water vapor, which may or may not be present in all essential oils or individual oils. The mixture is then forced out of the extractor, a piston-operated apparatus made up of a pipe and a water-filled cylinder. Inside the cylinder, a small fan blows heated air over the coil and tube, extracting the oil through a small hole. It may generate 30 to 45 liters of essential oils each hour, depending on how fast you use it.

Self-titrating

Self-titration entails heating an essential oil and allowing it to cool without any external heat source. In other words, you'd warm up three drops of oil to body temperature and dab them all over your arm or wherever else you want them to go. Continue to take 3 drops for 3 days, then 6 drops for 3 days, 9 or 12 drops for another three days, and finally, you can use the entire amount without feeling any pain. This is known as self-titration. It can also be done by a herbalist who understands how much to take daily.

You may wonder what equipment is utilized to manufacture herbal oils and how they achieve maximum potency. Here's a list of everything you'll need to get started.

- A glass bowl or jar

- A food processor or coffee grinder (to make herbs into a powder)

- A plastic dropper or eyedropper (if using a glass bowl or jar)

- Vegetable oil - essential oil of lavender

You'll also need high-quality alcohol to extract the herbal oils and cotton balls if you're using an eyedropper. There are various methods for making high-proof alcohol; you can buy it already prepared or make it yourself. Combine if you have purchased it.

5g herbal oil dissolved in 2mL of high-proof alcohol. The ratio depends on the amount of oil to alcohol used; however, remember that too much strong alcohol might kill the herb before extraction; therefore, no more than 1mL per 0.5g is recommended.

EXTRACTION

Extraction involves the separation of medicinally active components from plant or animal tissues using specific solvents and recognized procedures. These extraction processes effectively separate the soluble plant constituents from the insoluble cellular material. Plant-derived products are typically complex mixtures of metabolites available in liquid, semisolid, or dry powder form, designed for oral or topical administration.

The purpose of standardized crude pharmaceutical extraction methods is to obtain therapeutically acceptable portions while eliminating undesirable material through treatment with a selective solvent known as a menstruum. Once standardized, the resulting extract can be used as a medicinal agent in the form of fluid extracts or tinctures, and further processed into various dosage forms such as tablets and capsules. Among the numerous medicinal plant metabolites identified in these products are alkaloids, glycosides, terpenoids, flavonoids, and lignans.

The quality and grade of an extract are primarily influenced by several factors, including the plant components used as raw materials, the solvent employed for extraction, the manufacturing method (extraction technique) along with the equipment utilized, and the ratio of crude drug to extract. Extraction technology, manufacturing equipment, plant materials, the extraction process, solvent, and adherence to good manufacturing practices all contribute to the production of high-quality extracts. From laboratory to pilot scale, all circumstances and factors can be accurately represented through process simulation for effective industrial-scale manufacturing.

Why do we extract herbs? To enhance the quality, aroma, and flavor of herbal medicines. Herbal preparations often involve the extraction of one or more constituents from plants for use in teas, tinctures, cooking oils, and other products. These methods make them easier to use as medications and allow for more precise dosage, which is crucial for certain plants that can be harmful if used incorrectly or in large doses, such as skullcap and valerian root.

Tools and Equipment

Active compounds are extracted from medicinal plants or herbs using extraction equipment. In the food industry, extraction is used to recover essential oils, oleoresins, perfumes, natural extracts, and proteins.

- Mortar and pestle are used for grinding.

- Fine mesh sieves are one of my favorite herbal tools.

- Funnels are used for pouring.

- Sprouting screens are used for making herbal infusions.

- A double boiler is useful for any recipe that requires melting.

- Cheesecloth can be used to strain many herbal mixtures. When producing herbal-infused oils, it facilitates the removal of every last droplet of botanical nectar. It is also used for straining tinctures, vinegar, and helpful herbal infusions.

- Dark glass dropper vials are excellent for storing light-sensitive chemicals as they can withstand certain levels of UV contamination.

Herbs are undoubtedly one of the most versatile resources available to humans today. They have a wide range of medical and culinary applications, but extraction is a different process. Using the right tools for this procedure can help you complete it quickly and easily, giving you an advantage over your competitors.

Here is the essential equipment you can use:

- Simple herb extractor (available for purchase on amazon.com or ebay.com).

- Olive oil or any other carrier oil (choose one that can withstand heat without being destroyed).

- A filter (choose one with larger holes for easier handling).

- A slow cooker or a coffee maker (this is optional).

- A chopper (a handheld one will suffice).

- A straining device (a metal one will work here).

- Lemon juice (optional; it helps ensure the freshness of your product for a longer period).

Extraction Techniques

There are two basic types of extraction techniques: water-based and solvent-based.

Water-based extraction is arguably the most prevalent and is used for extracting most medicinal plants. This method involves extracting plant material, such as roots or leaves, into water. The herb can then be extracted as a tincture (a liquid extract) using alcohol, glycerin, or alcohol-glycerin blends.

Water-based Extraction: This method utilizes maceration and alcohol extraction to create an oil-free tincture of your herb. In this procedure, finely chip your plant material and place it in a container with pure water. Ensure that the bottle is properly sealed and stored in a cool and dark place. You can leave it for weeks or months, but three weeks is usually sufficient. The longer the ingredients mix (soak) together, the stronger the tincture! Afterward, filter the liquid into another container using an eyedropper or connected syringe. Carefully extract the liquid with the dropper until all the plant material has been extracted. Depending on the size of your herb, this should take approximately 5-8 drops. This procedure can be repeated multiple times.

Solvent-based Extraction: This method is less common than water extraction but can be highly effective for extracting high concentrations of herbaceous material and specific oils and essences from plants. This method is known as "aqueous phase" extraction. The herbal material is placed in water and stirred to release certain elements from the plant. Then, a solvent such as alcohol or acetone is added to aid in the dissolution of your herb. The solution can be extracted several times until no more oil is recovered from the plant material.

For this approach, you'll need an extraction container (a blender or a coffee grinder), an alcohol tincture, and an eyedropper for dosing. If you're using alcohol tincture, make sure it's 100% pure ethanol (also known as grain alcohol). If you're not using ethanol, any other form of pure grain alcohol will suffice. In a blender, combine 2-4 grams of plant material and blend on high speed until the plant material is very fine. Most herbs will release their entire amount of oil within 1-2 minutes. At this point, the plant material should be completely pulverized. Blend for a few more seconds and watch it work its magic! After grinding the plant debris into a fine powder, add 4-5 ounces of alcohol to the mix and blend at high speed again. The solvent should extract the oil from the plant mixture in about 2-3 minutes. After a few minutes, transfer the oily solution to something like a coffee grinder or an old-fashioned coffee press and place it in a dark area to evaporate. This procedure can be repeated multiple times. After multiple extraction cycles, you'll have a tincture with all the medicinal characteristics of your herb.

Herbs and medicinal plants, in general, are used in the following ways:

1. **Infusion**: Fresh infusions are created by macerating raw medication in either boiling or cold water for a brief period. These are typically dilute solutions of easily soluble crude medicinal components.

2. **Decoction**: The crude medicament is boiled in a set volume of water for a predetermined time before being cooled and filtered. This approach can be used to extract water-soluble and heat-stable components. It is often used in preparing Ayurvedic extracts known as "quath" or "kawath." The initial ratio of crude extracts to water is fixed, for example, at 1:4, and the volume is then reduced to one-fourth of its original volume by boiling during the extraction process. The concentrated extract is then filtered and used directly or further processed.

3. **Maceration:** The full or roughly powdered crude herb is placed in a jar with a stopper along with the solvent and allowed to stand at room temperature for at least 3 days with constant and frequent stirring until the soluble components have dissolved. After standing, the mixture is filtered, the damp solid known as the marc is pressed, and the blended liquids are clarified using filtration or decantation.

4. **Digestion**: This is a type of maceration where the extraction process is aided by applying gentle heat. It is used when moderately high temperature is not a concern, as it improves the solvent efficiency of the menstruum.

5. **Continuous Hot Extraction**: The crude drug is finely ground and placed in a porous bag or "thimble" made of strong and thick filter paper, which is then inserted in the chamber of the Soxhlet device. Heat is supplied to the flask to extract the solvent, and the vapors condense in the condenser. The condensed extractant drops into a thimble of crude medication and is extracted through contact. When the liquid volume in the chamber reaches the top of the siphon tube, the liquid contents of the

chamber siphon into the flask. This operation is repeated until a solvent droplet from the siphon tube evaporates without leaving a residue. This approach can extract considerable amounts of medication with significantly less solvent, saving time, energy, and financial inputs. It is typically used in small batches as a batch system.

6. **Extraction by Counter Current**: In counter-current extraction, wet input material is crushed using toothed disc disintegrators to produce a fine slurry (CCE). The extracted material is carried in a single direction within a cylindrical extractor, where it comes into contact with the extraction solvent. As the initial material moves further away, the extract becomes more concentrated. Complete extraction is possible when the amounts of solvent and material and their flow rates are regulated.

7. **Percolation:** This is the most common method for extracting active ingredients to produce fluid extracts and tinctures. A percolator (a narrow, cone-shaped jar with openings on both ends) is typically used. The solid components are moistened with an appropriate amount of the prescribed menstruum and left to stand for approximately 4 hours in a well-closed container before being packed, and the percolator's top is closed. A shallow layer of menstruum is placed on top of the bulk, and the mixture is allowed to macerate for around 24 hours within the closed percolator. The outlet of the percolator is then opened, allowing the liquid to flow gradually. More menstruum is added as needed until the percolate is three-quarters the volume of the final product. After pressing the marc, the liquid is transferred into the percolate. Additional menstruum is added to achieve the desired volume, and the mixed liquid is purified through filtration or standing after decantation.

8. **Fermentation of Aqueous Alcoholic Extraction:** Several Ayurvedic medical preparations involve fermentation to extract active components (such as cassava and arista). The extraction method involves soaking the crude drug, which can be in the form of a powder or a decoction known as kasaya, for a specified amount of time, during which it ferments and creates alcohol in situ, allowing the active chemicals in the plant material to be extracted more easily. The resulting alcohol also serves as a preservative.

9. **Extraction via Ultrasound:** This procedure uses ultrasound pulses with frequencies ranging from 20 kHz to 2000 kHz, which increases the permeability of the cell walls and induces cavitation. Although the process is useful in certain cases, such as rauwolfia root extraction, its large-scale use is limited due to higher costs.

10. **Extraction of Supercritical Fluid:** SFE (supercritical fluid extraction) is a sample preparation method that uses no organic solvents while increasing sample throughput. Consider factors such as temperature, pressure, analyte collection, sample volume, modifier (cosolvent) addition, restrictors, and flow and pressure control. Cylindrical extraction containers are often used for SFE, and their functionality is highly efficient.

Flower Essences and Aromatherapy

Aromatherapy can be a highly personal experience at times. You close your eyes, inhale the scent, and feel yourself relax. The aroma might evoke memories that have been buried for years. What makes it work?

Could our sense of smell be more closely linked to our memory and emotions than we previously realized? Perhaps there is something refreshing about these scents that can reduce tension and anxiety in minutes.

The fragrances in essential oils and aromatherapy blends can assist us in various ways. The good news is that we can enjoy the benefits of aromatherapy and floral essences without spending a fortune on faraway spa visits.

You can replicate the fragrance of your favorite rose with just a few drops of rose essential oil without having to grow one yourself. You can create your own aromatherapy blend or floral essence with just a few flowers from your yard.

TOPICAL PREPARATION

List of plants and their various topical applications:

Ginger: Ginger is an excellent muscle relaxant and a powerful nausea reliever. It acts as both an antihistamine and a digestive liver stimulant.

Valerian: This herb is a natural sedative and can be applied to pressure points to treat headaches and neck discomfort, alleviate sleeplessness, and reduce convulsive seizures.

Peppermint: It is commonly used to treat indigestion, nausea, sore throats, migraines, and muscle aches. It has such a wide range of applications that it is often referred to as nature's medicine cabinet. The leaves can disinfect cuts, reduce inflammation and pain in muscles and joints, and even relieve stomachaches caused by gas or bloating.

Marjoram: It is commonly used in cooking but has various additional applications due to its antibacterial properties. It can be applied to cuts or wounds to kill germs or fungi that may have entered the injury while promoting healing. It can also be used as a poultice to reduce pain and swelling. It has also been shown to alleviate muscle tension and spasms.

Chamomile: Chamomile is an herb with anti-inflammatory, antispasmodic, antiseptic, and relaxing properties. It can be used for burns or wounds to prevent infection and aid in healing; it is also effective for headaches, sore throats, coughs, and toothaches. There is also evidence that chamomile has anti-cancer effects.

Lavender: One of the most commonly used herbs in aromatherapy.

Lemon balm: This plant has long been used as an antidepressant (it also helps with anxiety). It is a natural insect repellent that can also help you relax, and it's also useful for headaches and acts as a sedative.

Cayenne pepper: This herb is commonly used as a pain reliever and muscle relaxant (such as alleviating cramping after a workout). It can also be used to treat inflammation.

You can incorporate any of these herbs into your bath, compress, balm, or topical preparation by chopping the herbs into small pieces and brewing a tea with warm water. Massage into your skin as needed or apply by rubbing the herb into the affected area after thoroughly rinsing it off. If possible, use this instead of an over-the-counter medication. Remember to be mindful of the amount of each herb you use to avoid overdoing it; these herbs are beneficial to the immune system and should not be overused.

Exercise caution when using any topical medication containing herbs and/or essential oils. Always consult a physician before starting a course of herbal supplementation or trying new methods or products. The information in this guide is provided for educational purposes only and does not constitute medical advice; it is your responsibility to ensure that you purchase from a reputable source and meet all health criteria.

Oil Based Extractions

Because oil can dissolve plant fats, waxes, and other lipids, it is a natural carrier for herbal compounds. When working with oil-soluble herbs, the practitioner can infuse them into oils either slowly or quickly to achieve complete extraction.

Why Do Oil-Based Herb Extracts Work Better?

Herbal plants use oils to store nutrients, which means that oil-based extractions preserve more nutrients, calories, and flavor in the plant. This is beneficial because herbs are highly potent medicines that should be taken with caution. To ensure maximum effectiveness, most herbalists begin drying herbs as soon as they are cut from the plant. Herbs can be dried and stored in an airtight container for later use.

There are several important reasons why oil is used for this form of extraction:

1. Oil dissolves plant lipids.

2. Herbal waxes dissolve in oil.

3. Oil dissolves therapeutic components that are either fat-soluble (e.g., turmeric) or insoluble in water (e.g., tinctures).

4. Oils contain compounds that can enhance the extraction process by improving the organic structure of the substance being extracted (e.g., turpentine found in pine trees is an effective solvent).

5. The process of infusing oil with herbs is straightforward. The herbal material is chopped, soaked in oil, and then filtered. The resulting herbal oil can be used to treat common ailments, added to foods, or applied topically to address various conditions. This extraction method works best with soft herbs that are easily broken down, as opposed to hard herbs that are more difficult to process. Examples of soft herbs include rosemary, lavender, thyme, sage, and thyme.

How Does Oil Extraction Work?

The extraction of oil-soluble plants is fairly simple. The practitioner first chops the plant into small pieces using a knife or other tool. Then, the herb bits are placed in a jar.

Next, a few drops of oil are added to the herb, allowing it to absorb the oil. This process essentially incorporates the herbal material into the oil. This method extracts more of the herb's medicinal compounds while allowing fresh air to reach them for drying. The herbs are typically left in this state until no more liquid remains or until it is clear that they have absorbed all the remaining liquid.

After extraction, herbed oils can be used in two ways: they can be maintained as-is, infused into food, or applied topically for treatment. If the herbal oil is to be infused into dishes, it is often mixed with a neutral oil such as olive oil, corn oil, or sesame seed oil to allow the herbs' flavor to come through.

Preserving Herb Oils

For those who intend to use their herbed oils topically or in food, proper preservation is essential to maintain their effectiveness. It is recommended to keep herbed oils in an airtight container with an attached eyedropper for easy dispensing. If the oils are not stored in an airtight container, they will evaporate and lose potency over time. Herbal oils can be stored for approximately six months before needing to be replenished.

Lozenges

For their calming qualities, ginger, mint, fennel, and other aromatic plants are frequently given. However, few people realize that these herbs can also help with dry mouth. Though there are other ways to alleviate mouth dryness, such as rinsing your mouth with water after brushing your teeth or staying hydrated by drinking water throughout the day, many people find these methods too time-consuming. Fortunately, a new option is now available! Herbal lozenges are widely accessible at any nearby drugstore and provide a simple and efficient way to alleviate dry mouth. They come in various flavors, ranging from minty to spicy, and their natural ingredients make them safe for daily consumption.

Sage Mouth Lozenges by Natura Herbs

Natura Herbs Sage Mouth Lozenges contain no artificial colors or preservatives and are free of any harsh substances that may cause adverse effects. With 500 mg of sage extract in each lozenge, these are ideal for individuals who want to relieve dry mouth but dislike the taste of sage.

Herb Pharm H-5 Lozenges

H-5 Herb Pharm Lozenges offer a variety of benefits that may help prevent or relieve dry mouth. They contain pure mallow extract, an expectorant that loosens mucus in the lungs, throat, and sinuses. Additionally, mallow contains mucilage, which helps relieve dry tissues by forming a protective layer on their surface. Moreover, the lozenges include honey, a natural antibacterial that aids in preventing infections by inhibiting the growth of harmful microbes.

Bioticare Mouthwash Lozenges

Bioticare mouthwash lozenges offer a convenient solution for dry mouth. These lozenges contain a unique blend of over-the-counter herbs with anti-inflammatory, antiviral, and calming properties. The product includes extracts of blue daisy, peppermint, licorice root, and aloe vera gel, which acts as an expectorant by loosening mucus in the airways and potentially aiding in the clearance of phlegm from the lungs. Moreover, these lozenges incorporate xylitol, a natural sweetener that has been shown to inhibit the growth of potentially harmful bacteria.

Licorice Lozenges by NOW Foods

Licorice has been used for millennia to relieve dry mouth by reducing saliva production. It's no surprise that licorice extracts are frequently used in lozenges designed for dry mouth relief. NOW Foods licorice lozenges contain 1,000 mg of licorice flavonoids per dose, making them an effective yet gentle treatment for dry mouth.

Delsym Cough Relief Herbal Lozenges

Delsym cough relief lozenges are an excellent method for treating dry mouth caused by coughing. The constituents of these lozenges include dextromethorphan, guaifenesin, and honey. Dextromethorphan is an antitussive that works by inhibiting nerve signals in the brain that trigger coughing. Guaifenesin is a mucolytic that helps loosen mucus in the respiratory tract, making it easier to expel. Additionally, guaifenesin has expectorant properties that help break down thick mucus in the airways, facilitating its expulsion during coughing. On the other hand, honey is a natural antibacterial that can prevent or treat bacterial infections in the mouth.

HERBAL FORMULAS AND EFFECTIVE HERB USE

Herbal formula design is relatively similar to normal formula design, but there are key differences to be aware of before you begin. It's also critical to understand the types of herbs you're utilizing when creating formulas or deciding which ones to buy.

High-molecular plants, which tend to stay put in a different formula, are best distilled, tinctured, or frozen. For medium-molecular plants, steaming is ideal. If you're using low-molecular-weight herbs (like alfalfa or hibiscus blossoms), eating them raw is best. Raw is preferable to cooked, but if you must cook with them, steam them for 10 minutes first to retain their nutritional essence.

During the formulation process, to ensure adequate nutrient supply, many herbal formulas begin with a nutritional base-usually bone meal or pancreatic enzymes.

When constructing your formulas, remember that the body only works with what it requires; thus, you need more than simply complicating your formulas to make them work properly. Determining the appropriate amount of each herb to use in a blend might require some work. When you're almost finished, use the same proportions as you would for a food supplement. Taking this approach will make it easier to consume these herbs without feeling ill, gassy, or experiencing any other adverse reactions. You will also notice that you achieve better outcomes than if you followed an overly complex formula.

Chickweed contains bisabolol, a plant compound that is highly anti-inflammatory and is often used to treat rheumatic pain, arthritis, and gout. The fresh plant can be made into tea or medicine. To make tea, mix two teaspoons of dried chickweed with two cups of boiling water. Steep for 5–10 minutes and drink three times per day. To prepare a tincture, combine one tablespoon of dried chickweed with one cup of grain alcohol (100 proof is best). Simmer for 45 minutes on low heat, cool, strain, and use within eight weeks.

To create a compress, fill a bowl with boiling water and add three to four chickweed leaves. After 10 minutes, drain the water and pat the leaves dry. Place them on the affected area for 15 minutes and cover with a warm cloth.

Milky oats are an emollient and anti-inflammatory plant that can be used as a salve or poultice to treat swollen joints or injured skin.

To make a poultice out of milky oats, combine 3 tablespoons of powdered milky oats with enough hot water to make a paste. Apply this to inflamed areas as needed.

Milky oats can also be used to help repair injured skin.

Making your own herbal remedies can be a fun and rewarding activity. Here are some fundamental stages for creating a successful herbal formula:

- Look for herbs that will address the individual's specific health issues.

- Select one or two herbs that can be used as a general tonic, meaning herbs that can tone the body's essential organs, boost immunity, etc.

- Select one or two remedies for the current problem (e.g., a specific pain reliever for pain-related complaints).

- Include any additional desired benefits (e.g., tonics, liver support, etc.).

- If desired, add herbs with additional advantages, such as anti-aging qualities, to create a comprehensive formula.

- Follow all usage instructions.

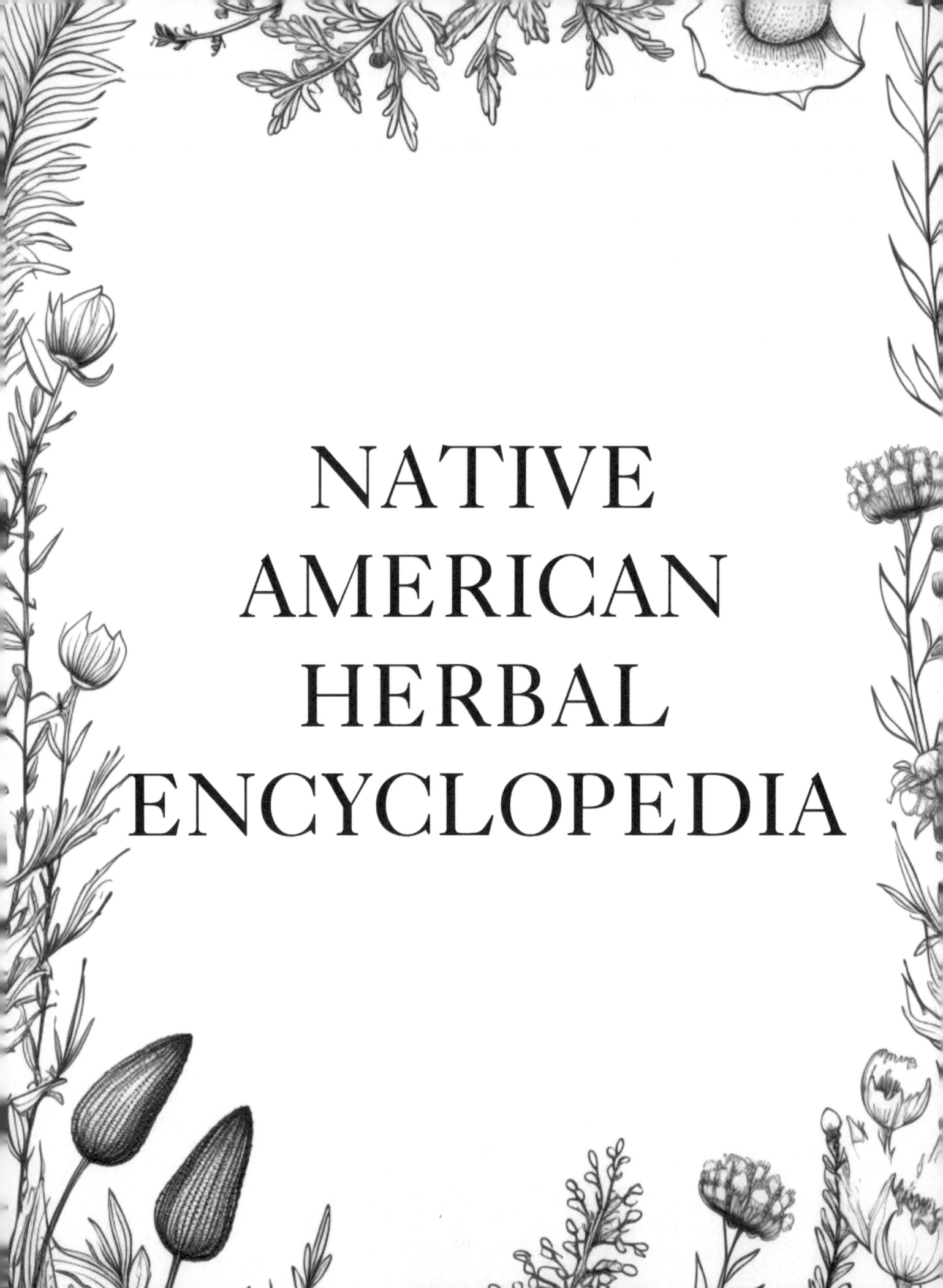

NATIVE AMERICAN HERBAL ENCYCLOPEDIA

INTRODUCTION

Native Americans in the United States developed substantial knowledge of herbalism that was passed down over multiple generations. Society has largely lost this rich legacy and the many medical benefits found in our natural world. However, there is hope: we can regain some of these lost treatments with more knowledge and investigation.

I have created this book for inexperienced individuals interested in Native American herbalism. You will learn about its history as well as its numerous benefits. It is a form of herbalism that stands in stark contrast to modern Western medicine, and many still practice it.

In addition to healing diseases, Native American herbalists used herbs in their religious rites, daily routines, and even clothing. They possessed a thorough understanding of all aspects of plants, from proper plant care and harvesting to how plants absorbed the sun's energy and utilized nutrients for bloom development.

Estimates suggest that Native Americans used between 700 and 2,000 plants for medicinal purposes. Those who did not grow their own plants relied on plants obtained from neighboring tribes. Herb knowledge was passed down through various methods. It was sometimes transmitted orally, while in other cases, a healer would memorize and write it down or preserve it in a scroll. There were often crucial times when this knowledge was essential, such as during harvest or drought seasons.

Native American culture placed great value on hunting and gathering plant knowledge. Misuse was frowned upon within tribal groups, as misinterpretation or mismanagement of a patient's ailment—whether physical, mental, or spiritual—could lead to death and, worse, spiritual punishment from the offending spirit. The Native American Herbalism Bible serves as a reference book on North American plants and their use in herbal therapy. It is an excellent resource for anyone interested in learning about the ancient healing practices of Native American tribes.

The Native American Herbalism Bible delves deeply into Native American ethnobotany. Its purpose is to help readers learn more about their own or other cultures by providing knowledge about plants and their uses, as well as a historical perspective on how indigenous peoples have employed traditional medicine. This book is an excellent reference for anyone interested in alternative healing approaches, particularly in North America.

HISTORY OF HERBAL MEDICINE

Since the dawn of time, humans have utilized natural ingredients for healing, often referred to as herbs. While some herbs are specifically cultivated for medicinal purposes, many are grown for culinary uses.

Due to increased awareness of environmental hazards and their impact on human health, herbal treatments are currently experiencing a resurgence of interest. Furthermore, the proliferation of ineffective drugs or those with alarming side effects has contributed to this heightened interest.

The origins of herbal medicine remain unknown, but the widespread use of herbs can be traced back to prehistoric times. According to several authors, early humans primarily used many herbs, particularly those mixed with water, for cleansing purposes. There is also evidence that early humans knew how to utilize specific plants for seasoning, flavoring, and producing fragrances. The earliest documented evidence of plant usage dates back to 3000 B.C. in Egyptian writings.

A significant development in phytotherapy occurred during the medieval period when people began incorporating plants into religious ceremonies. Some modern medicines, such as teas and tinctures, are derived from prescribed herbs. These medicines were primarily employed to address medical issues such as lice, body odor, and dysentery. During this period, herbalists began utilizing plants exclusively for medicinal purposes, leading to the discovery of a vast array of plants with medicinal properties.

Herbalism has been intertwined with the history of medicine since the 11th century, as evidenced by Arabic literature detailing plant-based remedies. In 1234, Cosmas Indicopleustes described medicinal practices employed by Indian physicians to treat ailments that were uncommon in Europe. Li Shih-Chen's 1653 publication marked the advent of the modern era of herbal medicine, providing comprehensive information on the usage of various plants. This book piqued the curiosity of readers in China and Europe, eventually being translated into English nearly 250 years later. Another notable herbalist, Nicholas Culpeper, authored the renowned book "Culpeper's Complete Herbal" two centuries later, which extensively covered the practical applications of numerous common herbs.

Phytotherapy gained widespread popularity in America during the colonial period when settlers were introduced to various herbs, spices, and fruits. Native Americans also shared their herbal remedies with the settlers, leading to the emergence of the first American herbalists.

Influential figures such as Benjamin Franklin suggested the consumption of sage to enhance memory, George Washington Carver proposed the use of peanuts to boost agricultural revenue, and Euell Gibbons advocated for the consumption of wild vegetables.

In 1805, Columbia Hospital in Philadelphia inaugurated the first hospital pharmacy in America, offering herbs and other remedies.

During the early 1900s, herbal medicines and practices remained popular, thanks to herbalists like John Uri Lloyd, who authored numerous volumes on plant-based cures, including books on herbal care. Another prominent early herbalist, Louis Kuhne, began commercially selling herbs in 1820 and is regarded as one of the most influential herbalists of all time.

Herbal Medicine's Benefits

If you're seeking herbal medicine, you might be asking yourself, "What are the benefits of herbal medicine?" This is an excellent question and one that many individuals ponder before considering any alternative treatment.

Herbal medicines have been utilized for centuries to treat various health conditions, tracing back to ancient times when all healing was accomplished naturally through plant or animal-based remedies. Herbal practices continue to be widely employed in modern societies worldwide. In addition to other medications or therapies, Western doctors and medical experts often prescribe herbs.

Herbal medicine offers numerous advantages, including but not limited to:
- Pain and inflammation relief
- Reduction of stress and fatigue
- Disease prevention
- Increased energy and performance
- Boosting the immune system
- Relief from anxiety and depression

Gathering Times

Preparation of the Soil

The soil must be properly aerated, nutrient-rich, and sufficiently acidic to support healthy plants. Directly planting into soil that has been fertilized with highly acidic chemicals will not yield optimal results! Fortunately, the resource explains everything in great detail, so let's review:

"Choosing a Healthy Seedbed: Planting too deeply will prevent your plant from reaching crucial root cells that it relies on for nutrients. Planting too shallowly can result in roots spreading out randomly. Dig into the soil, avoiding rocks and any hard or woody materials, or lightly scratch the surface with a hand cultivator or rake to loosen it. The goal is to prevent topsoil compaction and deepening."

"What not to do when selecting a seedbed: Never plant in a bed enriched with manure, as it can lead to beautiful carrot tops while the roots decay."

"How to Loosen Compact Soil: Add compost, rotted manure, well-rotted farm animal bedding, or peat moss. Incorporate organic matter such as seaweed, alfalfa meal, and perlite (tiny volcanic glass pieces that expand to about 1/8 inch thickness) to help retain moisture – an organic 'grow-stone'."

Overall, the text appears to be well-written and aligned with the given style and target market.

Cultivation Methods

Cultivating Techniques of Native Americans is a valuable resource for learning about practical living techniques that have been passed down from generation to generation. It provides guidance on vegetable and fish cultivation, deer or fox hunting, finding shelter in diverse terrains, and more.

The study also covers methods of making fire using natural ingredients, such as rubbing sticks together or using flint and steel. In today's complex society, these tactics are often forgotten or not discussed as frequently.

First, ensure that your soil has been properly composted to facilitate adequate nitrogen absorption and aeration. The resource will demonstrate how to create compost using a convenient container without the need for expensive store-bought items. Second, plant seeds and bulbs early in the spring (March or April) so they have sufficient time to mature before the arrival of summer heat. Last but not least, allow nature to take its course! Water plants when necessary in the morning and leave them undisturbed for the remainder of the day. Plants will grow and flourish according to their natural patterns.

Microclimates

Some plants can be started earlier and grown later during the growing season due to microclimates within a given place. The majority of microclimates occur naturally within protected locations. However, humans can also contribute to their formation.

Historically, rocks were placed around struggling plants in areas with abundant sunlight to absorb daily heat and reflect it back at night, evening out temperature variations. Alternatively, warm stones from the fire pit could be used to protect delicate crops in fields and orchards from frost.

Selection of the Plants

It is crucial to consider the growing requirements of your plants.

Variety is important in creating a wildlife-friendly garden as it breaks up what could otherwise be a monotonous environment and provides a more interesting landscape.

Choosing "naturally diverse" plants will help maintain the health and productivity of your garden. Look for plants that have been selected for their ability to thrive in your area and are well-suited to specific conditions. You could even choose a few tree or shrub species that are suitable for the climate in which you plan to establish a small grove."

Gourds, beans, and peppers were cultivated in Mexico around 5,500 BC, and maize and potatoes were grown in Mesoamerica and South America by 5,000 BC. The success or failure of these crops had a significant impact on human survival. It was crucial that the land not only provided nutrition but also sustained them season after season, which required knowledge of long-term farming practices to preserve the land for future generations.

Many techniques described below are considered "new" in the cultivation industry, even though they have been around for a long time. They have all been used by Native Americans in the past, but it doesn't mean they were used by all Native American societies. Similarly, different countries have diverse cultivation theories and methods, and indigenous tribes have different cultivation philosophies and practices. Here are a few eco-friendly landscaping ideas to consider.

According to a time-honored gardening philosophy, growing specific plants together improves their health and productivity. For example, some plants attract beneficial insects that protect their neighbors, while others (particularly herbs) repel them.

A well-known example is the Three Sisters garden cultivated by the Wampanoag inhabitants of what later became the northeastern United States. Corn provides a structure for pole beans to climb, beans add nitrogen to the soil for future crops to utilize, and squash leaves act as a living mulch, shading the soil around taller plants. Squash's prickly leaves also deter invading animal pests.

Companion planting (intercropping/polyculture of plants with mutual benefits) mimics the way different species grow together in nature. Monoculture, on the other hand, depletes soil nutrients. Indigenous peoples recognized that plant diversity meant a diverse range of foods. If one crop fails, others may make a difference.

Try "intercropping" in your vegetable garden. Small crops can be nestled between larger ones and harvested well before the larger plants require the space.

Phenology

Phenology studies natural signals that indicate whether or not a plant is suitable for cultivation. Before planting specific crops, native peoples waited for migrating birds and animals to return and for trees and plants to leaf out and flower, which signified the arrival of spring.

The Old Farmer's Almanac is famous for sowing maize, beans, squash, and other crops based on natural treatments. It may sound like an old wives' tale, but environmental monitoring is essential in unpredictable weather and climate.

Furthermore, typical frost dates are only estimates. It is important to take Mother Nature's warnings seriously to avoid a late spring or early fall frost surprise.

Terracing

Terracing generates flat planting plots in steep terrain, which reduces erosion by slowing the flow of water and allowing it to sink into the beds.

Creating terraces is an exceptionally effective cultivation method in areas where rain is seasonal, sporadic, or often occurs in heavy downpours. In the southwestern United States, for instance, terracing was essential to the Anasazis and their descendants, the Hopi, who continue to utilize terraced gardens to this day. An example can be seen in Hotevilla-Bacavi, a northern Arizona hamlet where old terraced gardens were reconstructed in the 1990s. If you plan to farm on sloping terrain in the future, terracing is crucial for preventing soil erosion that can wash away your valuable topsoil.

Terracing can be implemented in various shapes and sizes. If you have a slope, consider using rocks or retaining structures to create a series of level zones and prevent runoff.

The text appears to be well-written and aligned with the given style and target market.

Irrigation

The Anasazi people lived hundreds of years ago in what is now known as the Four Corners region of the United States, which is renowned for its minimal annual rainfall. They historically constructed catchments to capture rare stormwater, check dams (rock dams that hold soil in place but allow water to flow through), and reservoirs. Despite advancements in modern technology that have facilitated stronger water conservation techniques, the Hopi people of northern Arizona continue to employ these ancient practices for irrigating their lands in this arid region.

If you reside in a dry area, it is wise to store water in ponds, cisterns, or even rain barrels, as this water can be utilized for irrigation when needed.

Conversely, individuals in flood-prone areas have learned how to turn what could be disastrous into a source of income. One strategy, for example, involves excavating small depressions to retain water during periods of increased flooding. Another option is to utilize canals near rivers to direct water to adjacent areas.

Rain gardening is a growing trend where individuals create spaces that absorb rainfall runoff from roofs, roads, patios, and lawns. To temporarily control and absorb the excess water flow, a small depression is planted with native shrubs, perennials, and flowers.

The text appears to be well-written and aligned with the given style and target market.

Fertilization

Farmers learned that if you benefit from nature, you must give back. Therefore, crop leftovers were routinely returned to the land. Since there was an abundance of fish, they were buried in the earth to decompose.

By burning bones and other leftovers in the fire, ashes were formed and spread on the gardens or fields. This eradicated weeds and brush while also delivering phosphate and potash to the soil.

Soil fertility can be preserved without fertilizer by growing beans with other crops on the same hills. The legumes recharge the nitrogen levels in the soil, allowing corn and squash to thrive.

Growing Healing Plants

Plants can be used for more than just food. Many ancient communities used plants for fuel, building, tools, fabrics, dye, glue, and medicine in the past and continue to do so now. For example, the serviceberry provided excellent berries and raw materials for arrows, bows, canoes, shelters, baskets, and containers made from western red cedar trees.

The ability of plants to heal is arguably the most basic way to understand their power today. For instance, crushed mint leaves can be applied to the temples to relieve headaches. Inhaling the vapor of crushed eucalyptus leaves may aid in mental cleansing. The majority of herbal treatments are brewed into a tea and consumed.

Rotation of Crops

Crop rotation is another concept that has been used for hundreds of years. It reduces soil nutrient depletion and the accumulation of pests and diseases that can arise when one crop is planted in the same location year after year.

If you plant your tomatoes in the same garden bed year after year, you'll notice an increase in pests and illnesses.

Seed-Saving

Seed preservation has helped gardeners select and breed the best plants to continuously improve their crops. For example, maize evolved from the wild grain teosinte, native to Mexico and Central America, into the hardy corn we know today!

Even before the numerous seed companies of today existed, people methodically selected seeds for desired characteristics. They ensured species integrity by planting varied seeds sufficiently apart to minimize cross-pollination. If it hadn't been for this project, corn would have remained a weedy grass.

Using No-Dig Cultivation

No-till gardening, also known as no-dig gardening or layer gardening, is a soil-turning-free approach. Instead, you simply add a fresh layer of compost on top.

Although tilling removes weeds and soil clods and creates a level surface, no-till gardening is a great way to save your back while enhancing the health of your soil!

Foraging and Harvesting

Native Americans in the Pacific Northwest sustain themselves through foraging and harvesting. They have embraced this way of life as they understand the importance of self-sufficiency while honoring the natural world.

Foraging and harvesting are integral components of Native American culture in this region. They skillfully choose which plants to gather, identifying them based on taste, smell, and appearance. These plants are often cooked alongside other ingredients like wild game or fish. To begin your exploration and gain insight into the lifestyle of the local communities, here are some guidelines for plant identification.

Foraging

It is a skill that all Native Americans should possess. Foraging can entail certain risks, which is why it is advisable to always go foraging on a full stomach. If you find yourself lost or encounter any unfortunate circumstances, it is important to be accompanied by someone knowledgeable on how to handle such situations.

Foraging also served as a means for Native Americans to familiarize themselves with their surroundings and establish a spiritual connection. Plants played a crucial role in every aspect of life in the region. Cedar and spruce were utilized in creating baskets, mats, garments, clothing, and blankets. Tree bark was employed for constructing shelters or providing cover during the night. Berries served as both sustenance and medicine, possessing properties that acted as a deterrent to animals and parasites. Even in the Pacific Northwest, understanding how to utilize the resources provided by nature was vital for survival.

Harvesting

Gathering plants for food, medicine, and other purposes is one of the most important and sacred tasks for Native Americans. Spring through September are the main seasons for collecting various plants, and plant gathering involves people of all ages and is often a family project.

Like many other societies around the world, Native Americans relied on seasonal harvests of wild foods such as berries, roots, and furs for sustenance. They also hunted specific animals at certain times of the year, such as salmon, when they traveled upstream to their spawning grounds.

In the Pacific Northwest, Native Americans frequently harvested salmon to feed their families or trade with others. To preserve the fish, they would smoke, dry, or prepare a dry food product called pemmican.

Every day, we witness miracles. Our animal and plant brethren have always called out to us, giving us the courage to live in and explore the wilderness—a place filled with various natural and nutritious superfoods, not just a barren land. Even the smallest plants, fungi, animals, and natural protists contribute to the stability and security of the world. The cactus invokes rain and helps regulate the climate.

Our desert is a rich landscape of plant crops, familiar and new to Western agriculture. Anyone who has ever eaten strawberries, beans, potatoes, cocoa, tomatoes, or vanilla has consumed Native American foods.

Turkeys, sunflowers, pitahaya (related to goji and dragonfruit), cacti rich in betalain and calcium (such as prickly pear and cholla), antidiabetic mesquite with a chemistry similar to that of beets and beet greens, and arugula were all raised, produced, and supplied to the people of Arizona.

Corn has been cultivated in Arizona for about 4,100 years. Plants such as saiya, pepper grass, amaranth, and wild mustard produce more when harvested carefully. When relocating agaves and palms, the People have utilized terracing, the exploitation of Charco/akachin topography, and rock mulching to improve and work in harmony with natural desert soils.

A teaspoon of healthy soil contains a billion creatures, including mammals, actinomycetes, plants, protists, and mycorrhizal fungi. In our sustainable desert soils, there is also a 4-mm surface layer that includes cryptogamic soil—a population of lichens, bacteria, algae, fungi, mosses, and liverworts. This layer creates a nutrient-rich seedbed and helps protect larger plants from wind and solar desiccation. Caring for the land is a vital aspect of sustainability.

Sustaining foraging practices also involves restoring the 8,000-year-old cactus and bean forests of the Sonoran Desert, including their somewhat counterintuitive effects on climate, as the cactus has the power to call the rain.

Displaced from Land

When European Americans permanently settled on the most fertile territories in North America and acquired seeds that Native farmers had carefully nurtured, they enacted laws that rendered Native agricultural techniques unsustainable. In 1830, President Andrew Jackson signed the Indian Removal Act, making it official US policy to expel Native Americans from their homes and relocate them to less desirable territories.

On reservations, Native women were prohibited from cultivating anything larger than small garden plots, while Native men were compelled to adopt Euro-American monoculture. Through allotment restrictions, small parcels of land were allocated to nuclear families, severely limiting Native Americans' land rights and prohibiting communal farming practices.

Native children were forced to attend boarding schools, where they had limited opportunities to learn traditional farming skills or the preservation and preparation of Indigenous foods. Instead, they were raised on Western meals, which altered their palates and deviated from their natural flavors. By the 1930s, these practices had nearly eradicated three sisters' agriculture from Native American communities in the Midwest.

Rich Harvests

Throughout the Americas, indigenous plant varieties adapted to the growing conditions of their homelands. They selected seeds based on various factors, including flavor, texture, and color.

Native farmers grew corn, squash, beans, and sunflowers together, which provided mutual benefits. Corn stalks served as trellises for the beans to climb, and the twining vines of the beans protected the corn from strong winds. They also discovered that growing bean plants and corn together was often healthier than growing them separately. Bacteria living on the bean plant roots absorbed nitrogen, a critical plant element, from the air and converted it into a form that both maize and beans could use, as we now know.

Squash plants supported the cause by shielding the ground with their large leaves, limiting weed growth, and retaining water in the soil. The spines on heritage squash cultivars kept deer and raccoons from entering the garden for a feast. Sunflowers planted around the garden's perimeter acted as a natural fence, protecting other plants from wind and animals while also attracting pollinators.

The interplanting of these agricultural sisters resulted in bountiful harvests that fed large Native communities and supported prosperous trading economies.

The abundance of food crops discovered in the Americas astonished the first Europeans..

Reviving Native Agriculture

Native Americans across the country are diligently working to reintroduce indigenous squash, corn, sunflowers, beans, and other crops. This work is crucial for several reasons. Improving Native Americans' access to nutritious, culturally appropriate foods can help reduce the disproportionate rates of diabetes and obesity that affect Native American communities. Elders can pass down cultural knowledge to younger generations by imparting traditional farming practices. Indigenous farming techniques also contribute to the preservation of Native American lands and the surrounding ecosystems.

Wildcrafting

Many people who are new to herbalism or specifically interested in Native American Herbalism are certainly curious about wildcrafting. And the answer is straightforward: it is a method of obtaining therapeutic herbs from areas that have not been cleared or cultivated by people.

Gathering plants from the Earth's wilderness is referred to as wildcrafting. This practice is often associated with Native Americans who had to adapt to the natural conditions of their homeland.

Gathering plant seeds and berries for nutritional and therapeutic purposes is also referred to as wildcrafting. Native Americans introduced this technique to the world, using it as a food source and medicine for their families.

Wildcrafting can be challenging to master. It involves locating plant patches deep within forests or on slopes, far away from highways, trails, and other disturbances such as hikers and campfires. Foragers must be well-versed in native flora before venturing into such areas, as some plants can be toxic if mistakenly consumed. Before attempting to harvest from a certain plant species, one must first understand how to identify it and its distinct parts.

For those interested in wildcrafting, many people walk outside into their local environment, go hiking through different natural areas, or search for herbs in their own backyards. This helps them become acquainted with the plants growing there and learn which ones may be beneficial for therapeutic purposes. Many people who desire to learn about wildcrafting have discovered that it is easier than they imagined. There are numerous resources available, including maps of various regions that show where specific plants thrive.

Nowadays, wildcrafting is a popular pastime. It may interest Wiccans or Pagans who enjoy working with herbs. Like any other natural resource, herbs must be harvested correctly; otherwise, a once-abundant plant may soon be added to the endangered species list! A responsible wildcrafter will never cause harm to another person or deplete a resource. Here's how Native Americans should conduct themselves as responsible wildcrafters:

1. Obtain Permission: First, make sure that wildcrafting is legal in the area you're visiting. Permission is required before harvesting any plants on public property. When on private property, seek permission from the landowner. Also, check with your local Agriculture department extension to see if any plants in your area are currently listed as endangered. If wild ginger is scarce in your area, it is best to avoid harvesting it.

2. Choose a Location: When searching for herbs to harvest, avoid taking the first bunch you come across. The first patch you encounter along a trail is usually the one that catches everyone's attention. Instead, venture further and look for another patch, perhaps off the trail if it's safe to do so. This way, you can harvest from a location that won't be easily destroyed by subsequent visitors. Some public parks may have regulations specifying a distance from paths where harvesting is allowed, so check with local authorities.

3. What to Consider: Start by collecting plants that are more resilient before moving on to the more delicate ones. For example, plants like dandelion, yarrow, and blackberry can withstand regular harvesting as they regenerate regularly. When selecting a plant, only take what you can use within a short period. Many wildcrafters follow a one-in-four or one-in-five ratio, which means that for every plant harvested, four to five plants must remain in the same patch.

While out in the wild, make sure you are familiar with the herbs you seek. Some plants may appear enticing, but if you have no plans to use them, it's best to pass them up and leave them for the next visitor. Prior knowledge of magical plants can help you identify valuable finds.

4. Appreciation: When gathering wild herbs, it is customary in many magical traditions to offer a blessing or even a prayer of thanks. You may even scatter seeds as an offering to ensure the growth of new plants to replace the ones you've harvested. While wildcrafting, always double-check state and municipal laws to ensure you are legally and respectfully harvesting herbs.

Wildcrafting that Benefits Everyone:

Developing harvesting procedures that promote plant growth and sustainability will ensure the availability of these medicinal herbs for future generations. For example, when harvesting from shrubby plants, cutting above the leaf node facing out of the center can promote a bushier growth pattern, resulting in larger and lusher plants. Cut the stem or branch at a 45-degree angle about 1/4 inch above the leaf node. For plants with opposing leaves, cut straight through. Cutting the plant at the right angle point from the node prevents severe damage.

When possible, replant root crowns, leaving a portion of the root with visible root hairs. For herbaceous perennials, bury only the back end of the roots or rhizomes, leaving the front end with the next year's bud to bloom in the spring. When digging up the entire plant, snip off the back end and replant the front end.

Dig roots in summer or autumn after the seeds have matured and the leaves have started to fall back, as the plant's energy has shifted to the roots during this phase of its life cycle. At this point, the roots are filled with accumulated life energy and therapeutic components from the growing season. Timing is more crucial for fleshy perennials with thick, firm roots, such as sharp teeth angelica or Gray's lovage, compared to woody perennials with dense, hard roots, such as redroot or California bayberry.

Traditionally, only the roots of various plants have been used, not because they are the only medicinal part, but because they are easier to transport and preserve their freshness and efficacy for longer periods, making them ideal for commerce and business. However, there are cases, like Western aralia, where the leaves have been found to be therapeutic as well. Harvesting and utilizing leaves for medicinal purposes is becoming more common, as it is gentler and has a milder impact compared to digging up roots in the fall.

Drying Out

What is Drying?

Food drying, also known as desiccation or dehydration, removes water from food to extend its shelf life. Drying prevents the growth of germs and fungi that could otherwise degrade food by causing the water inside cells to evaporate. Sun/wind drying, air drying, direct heat drying, and freeze-drying are the many methods of drying. Most Native Americans would use sun/wind drying to preserve their food.

Drying is one of the oldest preservation methods utilized by Native Americans. Sun drying and salt curing would remove moisture from berries, roots, and meat.

Drying as a Preservation Method

Native Americans dried food not only for preservation purposes but also to provide nutrients. When water is removed from food, the nutrients in the food are exposed to the air. The food can then be consumed either cooked or raw. When grasses and grains like maize are dried, they can be eaten whole. Other items such as nuts and fruits were dried whole or ground into a meal. Flour was prepared from roots and tubers. Additionally, drying extended the shelf life of items for longer journeys.

Methods of Drying Food Used by Native Americans:

1. Air drying

The foods were dried by exposing them to the elements. Foods that were consumed as snacks or on their own could be left out to dry for 6-12 hours. When the time came, they would be brought inside and either eaten or further dried.

2. Sun/wind drying

Dried foods made from berries, roots, or meat provided essential nutrients such as vitamin C and protein. The dried items were combined with different meats and included in stews and soups. Dried berries were incorporated into pies with fruits, nuts, and hearts. When eaten as a snack, they could be sweetened with honey, maple syrup, or raisins.

3. Drying with heat

When food was dried over direct heat, beeswax was used to seal it. Applying beeswax to food dried with direct heat accelerated the drying process and reduced the chance of microorganisms forming on the food. Salmon skin was also utilized to wrap the food. Salmon skin, rich in protein and fat, was ideal for binding food together.

4. Freeze-drying

Freeze-drying was one of the first preservation methods employed by Native Americans. It preserves food by removing moisture. Freeze-drying involves freezing the food at low temperatures before removing moisture through vacuum chambers and heat. Freeze-drying can keep food fresh for months, years, or even decades. Frozen fruits, when combined with honey, can have a texture similar to dried apples or raisins.

Dried fruits and vegetables were preserved using these methods, often by wrapping them in leaves, wood, or bark. Desserts resembling pies were made with dried fruits, nuts, and seeds.

Herb Storage/Purchasing and Storing Herbs

Many factors influence how long fresh herbs last. However, there are a few fundamental rules to follow:

Fresh herbs can be stored and handled properly for 4-6 weeks. However, they can be stored properly for up to a year.

If possible, avoid storing your herbs in plastic containers. Instead, use glass or heavy-duty freezer bags for the best results. Some plastics emit compounds that can cause your herbs to spoil, even if you store them in the refrigerator! However, certain plastics are suitable for preserving herbs. Make sure that any container you choose has an FDA-approved recycling code of #1 (HDPE), #2 (LDPE), or #4 (LLDPE).

Herbs will last longer when stored in a cool, dark room away from direct sunlight.

Keep your herbs in the plastic bags they came in. This makes it easy to see and identify their contents when searching for them, saving time during cooking!

Remember that freezing herbs is acceptable. Most herbs retain their flavor well after being frozen in the freezer for up to six months. If frozen for more than six months, their flavors may begin to fade.

Keep in mind that herbs generally do not last very long. Even if you store them in the best available containers, they will usually deteriorate before their expected shelf life. This is particularly true when using fresh herbs instead of dried ones.

The good thing is that herbs can be expensive, so you don't have to worry about wasting small amounts that have gone bad. They are used to treat a wide range of ailments and diseases.

Essential Tools

Herbs

It goes without saying that every herbalist requires herbs to work with. You can grow them in your own yard or buy them from local herbal stores or reliable online vendors. In either case, depending on your hobbies and wellness requirements, you'll need a range of herbs.

Saucepans and Mixing Bowls

A variety of sized bowls, from small to large, will be necessary whether you're weighing, storing, and measuring herbs or mixing ingredients. You'll also need a variety of pots and pans to infuse and dissolve ingredients. I recommend glass, stone, enamel, or stainless steel bowls and pans.

Utensils for Measuring

Glass measuring cups, spoons, dry measuring cups, and graduated cylinders are all essential for measuring varied amounts of herbs, solvents, waxes, and other ingredients for every recipe. Except for the graduated cylinder, which you will only need if you are measuring very accurate volumes of dye solvents, you most likely already have them in your kitchen.

Solvents

A variety of solvents will be beneficial in creating typical herbal remedies such as syrups, tinctures, and infused oils. Herbal tinctures are made with various alcohols with varying percentages of alcohol, such as vodka, gin, and high-proof alcohol. Herbal recipes frequently use apple cider or white wine vinegar, glycerin, and honey.

Utensils for the Kitchen

1. The Kitchen Scale

A kitchen scale will be helpful when it comes to weighing plants for herbal treatments that demand exact measures, such as weight-volume tinctures. Look for a scale that can weigh in both grams and ounces.

2. Pestle and Mortar

Native Americans frequently used a mortar in conjunction with a pestle. The pestle was often used for crushing and grinding food, such as converting wheat and corn into grain and flour, against the mortar. Mortar and pestle were also used in the creation of medicines and the production of paintings. This tool set comes in handy for making spice blends with aromatic seeds or crushing fresh black peppercorns.

3. Funnels

Funnels are necessary for moving liquids from one bottle to another to avoid losing even a single drop of the precious tincture you've been infusing and shaking daily. You should have a selection of funnel sizes available to accommodate a wide range of bottles. A stainless steel funnel is required to preserve herbal recipes in Mason jars.

4. Spice Mill

Store whole herbs for as long as possible before grinding them when ready to use. This maintains many of their therapeutic characteristics and keeps them fresher for longer. Herbal powders oxidize quickly and lose their efficacy. Maintain a spice grinder and process your herbs for the finest flavor and medicine. You can use an electric model, or a manual grinder will suffice.

5. Cheesecloth

Contrary to popular perception, cheesecloth is not only used to make cheese, and it acts as a filter for various herbal preparations. It aids in extracting every last drop of botanical goodness while producing herbal-infused oils. The same applies to straining tinctures, vinegar, or healthy herbal teas. Organic cotton that is 100% unbleached is ideal.

6. Potato Masher

A potato masher is probably the best tool you can own. Have you ever come across a potato ricer? A potato masher will do the same thing! When straining any infused tincture or oil, use this, and you will extract every last drop of liquid from your herbs.

Containers for Storage

Storage containers are essential for preserving herbs and any herbal products you make. Dry herbs can be kept in glass jars like Mason jars, while finished herbal products can be kept in various glass bottles, jars, and cans. These containers are ideal not only for storing goods and making preparations but also for gift-giving.

1. Preserving Jars

These glass jars, which come in various sizes, are used for canning food. They are long-lasting, easy to clean and disinfect, and affordable. Lids are offered in two styles: a two-piece metal ring and cap or a one-piece cover. These jars come in various sizes and can be used to prepare tinctures, infused oils, vinegar, and elixirs. They are also an effective and attractive way to store dried herbs, as long as they are stored in a dark cupboard to protect them from light exposure.

2. Metal Jars

Metal jars are made from a simple cylinder with a squat base and a lid that glides over or screws onto the base. They are commonly made of steel, and metal cans are commonly available in sizes ranging from 14 to 16 ounces. Metal cans are an excellent choice for herbal preparations that do not include liquid sauces, conditioners, dry tea, or spice blends.

3. Glass Jars

They are available in the same hues as the bottles, ranging from clear to amber, blue, and green. Jars are perfect for storing and dispensing skin and body care products like ointments, lip balms, lotions, body butter, and wet or dry scrubs.

Bag for Foraging

You'll need something to store the plants you pick when doing herbal work. A lightweight canvas or cotton bag with pockets is an excellent item to have on hand.

Dropper Bottles in Dark Glass

Dropper bottles in amber or cobalt colors make your herbal compositions convenient and straightforward. They are carefully constructed to withstand specified amounts of UV contamination, making them an excellent choice for keeping light-sensitive substances. Remember to label each bottle.

Gloves

There are numerous methods for protecting your hands from dirt and bacteria while gardening. Gardening gloves are an inexpensive way to keep yourself clean while also protecting yourself from infection or disease caused by soil or dirty hands.

Knife for the Soil

A soil knife is a tool for breaking up dirt while planting seeds. It's a cheap approach to getting the job done!

Scissors, Shears, Knives, and a Magnifying Glass

Forage shears are essential for cutting flowers, stems, and small branches.

More important stuff, including roots and larger branches, will require pruning shears, while picking up the bark will take a good sharp pocket knife. Finally, remember to bring a hand lens to get a better look at the plant you're collecting.

Shears for Pruning

These shears will be an essential component of your tool collection, whether you are cultivating fruit trees, shrubs, roses, brambles, or other species that require pruning. They're also excellent for herb collecting!

Sprayers

Sprayers come in a wide range of styles! They range in price from simple hand-pumped spray bottles to backpack sprayers, with a wide variety of pricing in between. Hand-pumped sprayers are the least expensive, while backpack sprayers are the most expensive.

Notebook

The first rule of any herbalist is to keep a variety of notebooks on hand to record ideas, recipes, lessons learned, and anything else that comes to mind. No matter how often we recall our most recent culinary success or failure, the truth is that if we don't write it down, we may lose it forever.

Writing Instruments

Pens, paper, colored pencils, and watercolors are excellent tools to have on hand when constructing your herbal materia medica or taking notes. You can use them to draw, sketch, and paint the plants you're learning about to supplement your herbal studies.

Use and Abuse of Herbs

Safety Tips

1. Ensure that any plant you consume is not toxic to humans.

2. Be aware that medicinal plants may interact with the prescriptions you're already taking (remember, an overdose can be fatal!).

3. If you have any allergies (plants, animals, mold, etc.), be cautious about potential allergic reactions to herbal medicines.

4. Never self-medicate with plants from a park or backyard without conducting thorough research!

5. Seek a recognized and trustworthy source.

6. Verify that you're using the correct plant!

7. Dry herbs before use (they contain fewer chemical constituents than fresh herbs).

8. Pay attention to dosage quantities, as the strength of each herb varies.

9. Differentiate between dangerous and poisonous-looking plants and edible, safe plants.

10. Avoid mixing wild and cultivated herbs.

11. Don't take risks with herbs you are unfamiliar with or cannot confirm as safe.

12. Some plants can produce lethal amounts of chemicals if crushed, chewed, or consumed in any other way.

13. Remember to teach a friend or family member how to safely prepare a herb if they are using it for the first time.

14. Make sure not to bring any plant (or natural substance) that is prohibited in another country and use it only in moderation.

15. Keep in mind that indigenous people have been practicing this for a long time, and it can be beneficial and effective if done correctly.

Herbal Preparation

Here is the revised text with the grammatical, punctuation, and syntax errors corrected:

Herbs are surprisingly simple to use for a variety of health-related purposes. Herbal preparation is often overlooked as a vital process that can result in greater health benefits than simply acquiring herbs. On the other hand, knowing how to prepare herbs is quite advantageous because it can help you use herbs more efficiently and effectively over time. This post will teach you how to make an herbal tisane or herbal infusion, which requires identical components and preparation procedures.

What You'll Need:

• Herbs of your choice

• An abundance of water (depends on the number of herbs)

• A strainer or metal strainer bag, such as a tea infuser, to filter the herbs from the liquid

• Water-boiling pot or pan

Directions:

Step 1: Prepare your herbs in stainless steel containers. Glass containers can create chemical reactions with certain herbal substances, resulting in flavor and color changes in your infusion. If you do not have a stainless steel utensil, utensils made of an alloy or pottery are allowed.

Step 2: Prepare and weigh the herbs you want to use in the infusion. This is the herb-to-water ratio you will employ.

Step 3: Use around an ounce of herb per cup of water to distribute your herbs.

Step 4: Bring the amount of water required for one cup of herbs to a boil for two to three minutes or until well infused. If you still don't think it's done after this time, reduce the heat and continue to cook until you're happy with the consistency and flavor. Begin checking after about one minute and finish after three minutes to allow the preparation time to attain its volume and temperature without overcooking or burning your ingredients.

Step 5: Strain the herbs from the liquid using a strainer or strainer bag.

Step 6: Allow the pot or pan to cool before boiling. This step applies when producing the infusion if you are steeping more than one herb at a time.

Step 7: Transfer the infusion to a glass container. A glass container is preferred since it holds heat effectively, preserving all of the aromas and benefits of the herbs in your drink.

Step 8: Refrigerate your herbal tea for up to two weeks in an airtight or sealable container. Wrap tea bags in aluminum foil for freshness and preservation if desired for prolonged storage.

Step 9: Sip your herbal tea and relax!

Benefits

Herbal tisanes are made the same way as herbal infusions, and the key distinction is that they are normally consumed immediately after brewing. It may take some time to get into the habit of brewing a fresh batch of herbal tea each morning, but it can be a terrific way to start your day while addressing various needs and enhancing your overall health.

Availability

In terms of availability, herbal tisanes differ from commercial tinctures. Because they are typically produced from herbs farmed by the individual, they are frequently only accessible in bulk sales or small retail outlets. Seven of the top ten best-selling botanicals in the United States were employed as cures by Native Americans. Most of the stated benefits of these supplements are based on what they were used for by these early Americans. However, according to Borchers, little is known about how they used these substances, including how they harvested plants, which plant components they used, and how they prepared them.

According to Borchers, the first North American residents' use of therapeutic herbs was "by no means haphazard but extremely selective." They made extensive use of some plant groups while avoiding others. They employed diverse plant components to treat various ailments, combined numerous botanicals for specific therapeutic purposes, and identified hazardous plants as poisons and medicines.

"The fact that Native Americans have traditionally used various botanicals so well suggests that some of the substances they used are highly promising. However, many of these compounds have received little scientific attention thus far," Borchers elaborates.

Both Echinacea (purple coneflower) and Urtica dioica (stinging nettle) have been investigated, and Borchers and colleagues feel there are hints that both have therapeutic characteristics.

Sage was another important herb to Native Americans since it was thought to treat a range of disorders affecting the stomach, kidneys, colon, skin, liver, lungs, and other organs, as well as to defend against bad spirits and draw them out of the body or soul.

Though the medicinal herbs carried inside a Healer's preparation bundle are numerous and varied, the most commonly used were commonly carried, such as preparations for common colds, such as American Ginseng / Boneset; aches and pains herbs, such as Pennyroyal, Wild Black Cherry, and Hops; and fever remedies, such as Feverwort, Dogwood, and Willow Bark.

Among the hundreds of herbal plants used in Native American medicines, tobacco is one of the most important. It was used to treat various diseases and in ceremonies and rites, and it was smoked as it is now, unfiltered and without additives

Convenience

Because no precise measurements or specific ingredients are required, you don't have to worry about how many herbs you'll need or which herb should be used for what reason most of the time. Furthermore, the procedures for creating herbal preparations are simple to follow if you have some familiarity with basic cooking skills. It is also far less expensive than producing commercial tinctures and can be created with any herbs you have on hand.

Drawbacks

Herbal tisanes can be time-consuming to make due to the preparation process, and they should be produced in small amounts to avoid dilution of flavor and benefits over time. This should be avoided if you want to continue receiving all the health benefits of drinking herbal tea.

Active ingredients and herbal preparation

Herbal preparations include active substances. The active ingredients in many herbal medicines are yet unknown. A single active component derived from plants is used in various medicinal formulations. Herbalists believe separating an active element from the rest of the plant reduces its effectiveness or makes it less safe.

Salicylic acid, for example, is a chemical found in the plant meadowsweet and used to make aspirin. Meadowsweet contains additional components that protect your stomach lining from the irritation of salicylic acid, whereas aspirin causes stomach bleeding.

Echinacea is a flowering plant often used to treat and prevent colds.

Ginseng is a Chinese herbal supplement that boosts immunity, cognitive function, and energy levels. Human research, on the other hand, is in short supply.

Elderberry is used to treat cough and cold symptoms, and some research indicates that it is at least marginally effective. Herbal medicine practitioners believe that the whole plant has a bigger impact than its constituents. According to critics, the essence of herbal preparations makes giving a precise amount of an active component difficult.

Herbal and conventional preparations have both been used for thousands of years. In reality, herbal preparation is the foundation of contemporary medicine. Unfortunately, herbal preparations are frequently disregarded in favor of conventional pharmacological therapy, which is unfortunate because herbal preparations offer numerous health benefits. In today's society, herbal remedies are most regularly used to treat severe and chronic ailments.

• Less expensive than standard medications

• Much easier to obtain than prescribed medications

• Stabilizes hormones and metabolism

• Natural remedies

• Strengthens the immune system

• Decreased side effects

• Cost-effective

Plant Infusions and Decoctions

Infusions are created by steeping herbs in hot water, while decoctions are created by boiling herbs before straining them.

Native Americans used plant life and tree bark as spices to enhance the flavor of their cuisine. They even substituted garlic or onion for salt in certain meals. These spices and herbs added a unique taste to their meals compared to previous civilizations and made them feel better about their food.

Decoctions:

Decoctions also have therapeutic properties and can be used to treat conditions such as fevers, psoriasis, and even cancer. They also aid in digestion. To prepare a decoction, boil fresh herbs in water for a few minutes and then strain the mixture. Serve it plain or with honey or lemon juice. One advantage of decoctions is that they can be made in large quantities and stored for extended periods since they have good shelf life.

The key thing to understand about decoctions is that they can be prepared from herbs that have been cooked to extract their active ingredients or from substances that have specific effects on the body, such as antibacterial properties.

Infusions:

Infusions are beneficial for purifying the blood and treating conditions such as headaches, common colds, and insomnia. To make an infusion, boil fresh herbs in water and then pour the mixture into a teacup, adding honey or lemon juice. Drink this mixture 2-3 times daily for the best results.

Herbal Balms and Slaves

Herbal balms are often the most useful form of homeopathy. Many recipes and ingredients are available online if you want to make some for yourself. What's crucial is that you understand the ingredients in your balm; otherwise, it could do more harm than good.

If you notice your health deteriorating rapidly, it may be due to a hazardous environment. This guide will provide advice on using herbal remedies to live a healthy life for yourself and those around you.

Herbal balms can be extremely beneficial to you and your loved ones. Many herbal balms can be used for various ailments, including muscle pain and skin problems.

There are numerous recipes and online resources available to help you create your own natural treatments and balms. However, before you start preparing these herbal balms, it's important to understand the ingredients and whether they will benefit or worsen your condition.

For example, lavender oil has been associated with headaches when directly applied to the head, but others find it effective as a sleep aid.

Herbal Bath

Taking a nice bath is one of the most calming methods to decompress. Nothing beats a herbal bath, whether it's been too long since your last soak or you want to try something new.

Herbal baths contain natural elements that leave your skin and hair looking and feeling great. They also improve general well-being and create a sensation of tranquility.

Don't worry; herbal baths are simple and can be performed at home. The herb is the most significant component (aside from water). Different herbs have different effects on the skin and hair. Choosing the perfect herb for your needs will result in a soothing and healthy bath.

The second most significant component is your oil selection, specifically essential oils. Essential oils enhance the fragrance of any herbal bath. More importantly, they have therapeutic characteristics that promote relaxation, healing, and healthy skin. The oils can be combined with warm water or applied directly to dry skin. Concentrated extracts are the most effective, while oils in smaller amounts are also recommended.

Here are some herbs that are beneficial for skin and hair health:

• Lavender

• Chamomile

• Rosemary

• St. John's Wort

And here are several oils that can help with relaxation and healing:

• Lavender

• Ylang Ylang

• Sandalwood

After you've decided on your herb and oil, you'll need to prepare the herbal bath. Start by filling your tub with four inches of warm water. Add your chosen herb to the water. You can also add oils directly to the bath if you're using them.

Sacred Medicine (Smudging – Sweat Lodge Ceremony – Sacred Pipe Ceremony)

A modern term for a Native American practice is the smudging ritual. Native American tribe members would cleanse, purify, and bless themselves by burning sacred herbs like sage to invite positive ideas and feelings into their lives. This ritual was often performed before entering specific areas or engaging in spiritually significant activities.

In Native American culture, smudging, or the sacred act of burning sage and other herbs, is common. Smudging was traditionally used to clear an area of negative energy and improve the environment. It was also incorporated into ceremonies to purify the soul, along with prayers and hymns. The smoke produced by burning plants can have spiritual, psychological, emotional, and physical cleansing effects on a person.

This will provide readers with a basic understanding of the traditional practice of smudging among Native Americans and why it is important for everyone, not just Native people. The author will also explore the technique further, discussing how smudging can be incorporated into everyday life to improve one's environment and spiritual journey.

Instructions and advice on using smudging as a powerful tool will be provided to readers. The author will also include information on the plants traditionally used in Native American culture and provide connections for further information.

Before we begin, it is crucial to know that while smudging is commonly associated with Native Americans, it is not solely a Native American custom. The use of incense and herbs is observed in many civilizations worldwide. These herbs and bundles are sometimes referred to as "smudge sticks" or "herbs."

Native American smudging has been practiced for many years and remains one of their most cherished traditions. They not only practice it themselves but also share it with individuals who may not have had the same spiritual upbringing. They welcome anyone who wishes to smudge, regardless of ethnicity or religion.

As Native American smudging is a practice that anyone can adopt, it has spread throughout America. Many people who were not raised in a Native American community or adopted into one are drawn to this practice because it resonates strongly with their spiritual way of life.

Native American smudging has become a topic of debate, as some believe it is a sacred ceremony that has been appropriated from their culture for public use and benefit. Some individuals believe it is being performed incorrectly or without proper respect, particularly in public settings.

The practice of smudging has sparked controversy, as some people find it disrespectful if performed by non-Native Americans. It is a sensitive and complex matter, as Native Americans feel their culture is being exploited when smudging becomes a public issue.

For this reason, Native American smudging was originally intended to be performed privately. It has been used as a spiritual practice by various cultures worldwide, including Christian groups. For some individuals, it remains a way to find peace of mind by connecting with nature and protecting their homes and sacred spaces from negative influences.

Some individuals become upset when they see smudging being practiced in public spaces, as they believe their cultural practices are being exploited for profit. This is where the disagreement arises. Some believe that smudging should only be practiced within one's own community or on tribal lands, while others argue that due to its long-standing history, it should be accessible to all. Each group feels that their rights are being violated if others practice smudging outside of their territory or community.

Native American smudging has become a contentious issue as some believe it is deeply rooted in their cultural traditions and should be considered sacred. Some studies have even been conducted to demonstrate the benefits of this practice in enhancing overall well-being. However, whether or not this ceremony will continue in the future is still uncertain. With so much controversy surrounding it, the longevity of this practice remains to be seen.

The Sacred Pipe and the Sacred Pipe Ceremony

The Sacred Pipe is a ceremonial instrument used to send people's prayers into the "Great Mystery" or express gratitude for blessings received.

Throughout history, the Sacred Pipe has played a significant role in Native American culture. Its ceremonies are elaborate, and its use is governed by strict rules. Its physical construction varies based on tradition and the intended user.

We will explore the process of making a Sacred Pipe and how its construction varies depending on the recipient (chiefs or other tribes) and the occasion or location of use (everyday life vs. general ceremonies). We will also delve into the sacred rules and ceremonies associated with the Sacred Pipe.

The Sacred Pipe can serve various purposes, such as hunting, ceremonial rituals, keeping track of time, or communicating with spirits. It is an essential component of traditional rites and rituals, often symbolizing a person's tribal identity and their connection to the past and future. It represents both tribal pride and affiliation (Cornell). Many tribes have been performing the Sacred Pipe Ceremony for generations. It is a ceremony that uplifts people's spirits and brings them closer to their creator. It serves as a means for individuals to connect through a spiritual ritual.

The Sweat Lodge

A sweat lodge is a dome-shaped structure constructed from natural materials such as bent saplings, animal hides, or blankets covered with clay. The dome shape resembles an inverted bowl. Its structure retains the heat generated by a fire, and the warm air circulates inside the lodge.

According to Native Americans, sweat lodges are essential for spiritual purification in healing rituals, such as before hunting or warfare, as well as for ceremonial initiations like birthdays or weddings. They believe that sweat lodges cleanse their souls and restore balance to their minds, bodies, and spirits by eliminating negative energy and evil spirits.

Sweat lodge traditions may have originated in Canada, where the Algonquian people built sweat lodges and referred to them as "abodes of the spirits." The construction is similar to that of steam baths. They were used before going to war or hunting. George Thornton Emmons' book "The Tlingit Indians: Part I and II" describes such a structure. This type of lodge is still used today in the lodges of Alaska Native communities. Although other tribes have similar structures, the sizes and shapes of sweat lodges may vary.

The smaller type is commonly referred to as a "little sweat lodge," while the larger one is known as a "big sweat lodge." Both are built by digging a circular hole in the ground, then excavating around the space to create a dirt or grass dome. Sweat lodges are also used for mourning, healing, and religious rituals. Sometimes, a sweat lodge is specifically built for the birth of a child. The medicine man would coordinate with the family of the newborn to determine the appropriate date and provide instructions on the required heat and construction methods.

The largest type, known as "wai," has a central fire pit and can accommodate forty or more people. Sweat lodges continue to be widely used in many native societies in the 21st century, including various Canadian First Nations. Indigenous peoples in Central America, such as the Maya and Aztecs, also used sweat lodges, referring to them as "baths" or "houses of heat."

While sweat lodges are primarily used for sacred rituals, they also have practical applications. The "little sweat lodge" is used for spiritual and physical cleansing. Participants heat stones in a fire pit to raise their body temperature and eliminate illness and negative energy. The stones are often placed on wooden frames or racks to allow for rotation as they heat up in the fire.

During the rituals, leaders may chant prayers and sing songs to increase positive energy, counteracting any negative effects. The "big lodge" can serve as a meeting space for community members to discuss issues and is often constructed specifically for this purpose by groups. It can also function as a ceremonial sweat lodge where people can spend the night.

The Four Main Ceremonies

The pipe aims to enhance communication between individuals and deities, ancestors, and spirits. When smoking the Sacred Pipe, one can spiritually connect with departed loved ones and strengthen their bond. Smoking the Sacred Pipe also helps individuals remember their place as members of their tribe and the community surrounding them. It assists in maintaining a connection to their roots, even if they have been adopted into another family or tribe (Berry).

Certain guidelines govern the construction and use of the pipe, with each pipe being uniquely crafted depending on the specific ceremony and the person creating it. In most cases, a particular pipe style is reserved for a specific clan or family. For example, only the Coyote Clan can use a pipe style known as "Loon" (Gayton).

The Sacred Pipe Ceremony is practiced differently among different tribes, depending on various factors. Some tribes carry their pipes with them during times of war or relocation. The pipe is considered sacred and represents their unity. It serves as a link between the people and the land, connecting them to the spirits of their ancestors (Cornell).

Native Americans believe that the Sacred Pipe has been in use for thousands of years, as it has been incorporated into birth and death rites. When a child is born, relatives from another community visit and smoke the Sacred Pipe with the new parents. During this ritual, they "see" in the child the kind of person they will become as they grow up, providing insights into how they should be guided (e.g., education or marriage) (Berry). The Sacred Pipe Ceremony has evolved into a sacred rite that is still practiced today.

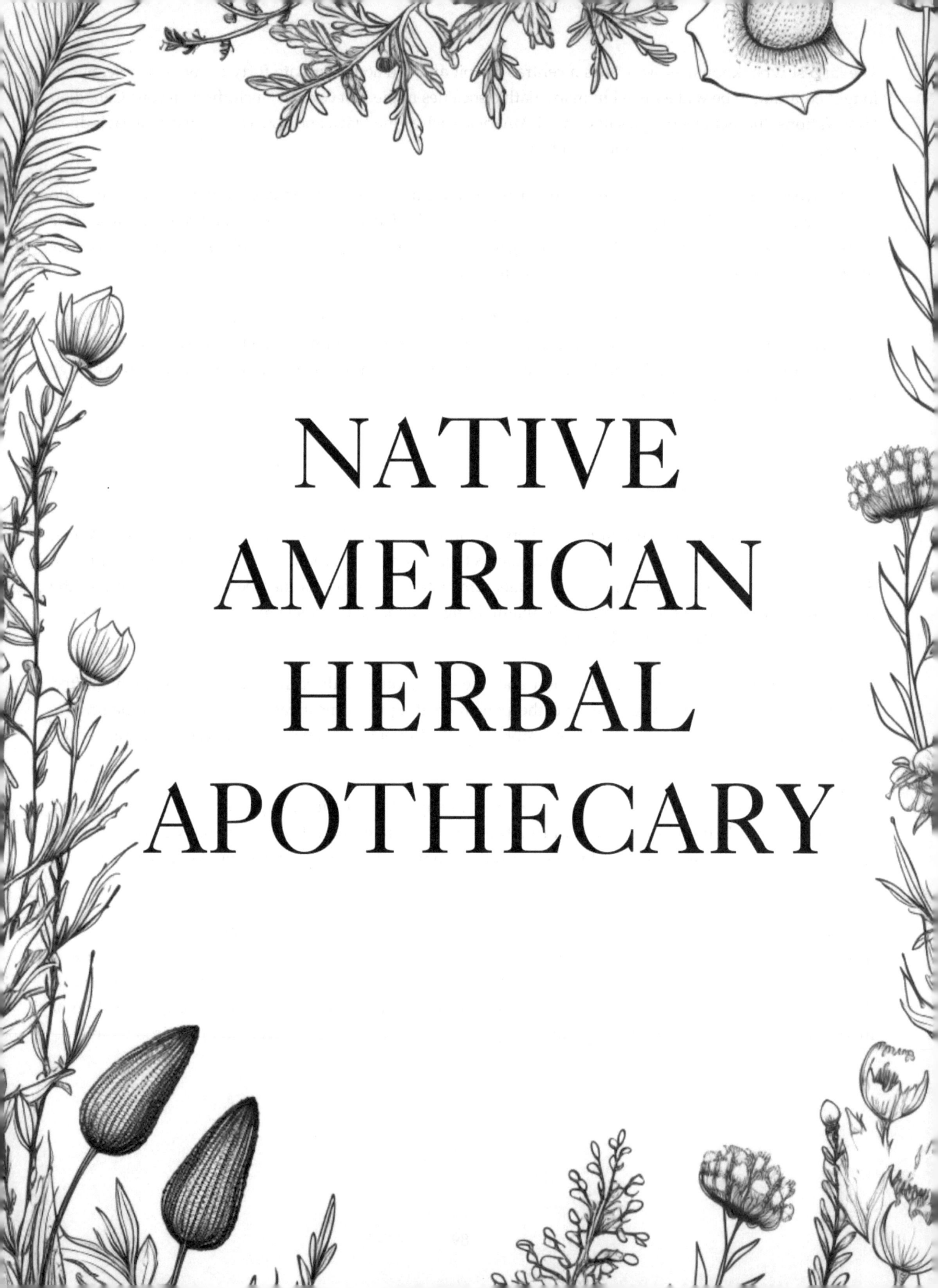

NATIVE AMERICAN HERBAL APOTHECARY

INTRODUCTION

Herbal medicine has been around since the dawn of time. It predates written and oral history, as well as the existence of humans. Herbalism uses plants to rebalance the body in the broadest sense. Herbalism is defined as the consumption of herbs in the form of vegetables and fruits. It is the world's oldest acknowledged medical school and the foundation for all subsequent medicinal approaches. It involves the scientific investigation of plants, including their energetics, flavors, activities, rhythms, and affinities.

Herbalism is the art of weaving numerous pearls of wisdom together with purpose and mindfulness to help bodies heal, balance, and rebalance discordant inclinations with plants and practical magic.

Herbalism is widely used to treat common ailments and promote overall health and well-being. It encompasses some of the oldest and most powerful therapeutic techniques, and its popularity is growing as people become more interested in natural recovery and wellness.

According to the WHO, medicinal plant preparations continue to be the primary source of healthcare for 80 percent of the world's population. Plants have been used for medicine and food for as long as humans have existed, and we have lived near or among them for decades. Unsurprisingly, this intimate relationship has resulted in a co-evolution in which people use plant remedies and consume wild food.

Most of us unknowingly incorporate herbalism into our normal routines, especially during the time of year when such plants - both wild and in gardens - are abundant.

History Of Native American Medicine

"Native American medicine has been built on commonly held ideas about healthy living, the potential consequences of disease-producing behavior, and spiritual concepts that restore balance," says Ken "Bear Hawk." All tribes share similar beliefs, although the techniques for diagnosis and treatment vary greatly from tribe to tribe and healer to healer.

Native American healing techniques have been practiced in North America for at least 12,000 years and possibly as long as 40,000 years. While Native American medicine implies a single healing system, there are over 500 indigenous peoples in North America, each with their own rituals, healing knowledge, and ceremonies.

Many aspects of Native American healing were kept secret and undocumented. Elders, vision quest spirits, and initiation have passed down the traditions through oral transmission. It is believed that freely or casually disseminating therapeutic knowledge reduces the spiritual power of the medicine.

On the other hand, several Native American healers recognize the importance of documenting these healing methods to preserve the traditions for future generations. Many people believe that sharing their healing beliefs and practices allows everyone to achieve greater harmony with nature and all forms of life.

Native American medicine can assist anyone who wishes to live a complete and balanced life. These benefits can be emotional, physical, or spiritual. However, there is an understanding that "civilizational infirmities" or illnesses commonly associated with Western society often require Western medical treatment. In some cases, Native American medicine may be a crucial component of an integrated approach to healing. For example, the most effective alcohol addiction treatment programs in Native communities combine Western psychology counseling, social services, and traditional Native American healing methods.

Inherited disorders such as congenital disabilities and retardation are challenging to treat using Native American medicine. Some illnesses, according to tribal healers, are believed to be caused by the actions of the afflicted individuals themselves. Occasionally, healers may refuse to treat a patient because they do not want to interfere with the patient's life lessons. Other illnesses are left untreated because they are considered "callings" or initiation diseases. "The calling can take the form of an accident, a dream, sickness, disease, injury, near-death experience, or even true death," explains Grizzly Bear Lake, a Native healer of medicine.

Understanding Native American Medicine

Native American medicine is based on a spiritual perspective of reality. A person who has a sense of purpose and follows the directions of the Great Spirit is in good health. This advice is ingrained in everyone's heart. To be healthy, one must commit to a path of harmony, beauty, and balance. Gratitude, respect, and kindness are essential for leading a fulfilling life. "Health means achieving balance and wholeness in your body, spirit, and mind," explains Ken Cohen. "This includes balancing life energy within the body, practicing ethical, reasonable, and just behavior, fostering family and community bonds, and interacting harmoniously with the environment."

Beliefs about the causes of illness and disease nomenclature vary among different tribes. Diseases may have external, internal, or both external and internal causes. According to Cherokee medicine man Rolling Thunder, negative thoughts are an important internal source of disease. Negative thinking encompasses guilt, blame, low self-esteem, greed, despair, worry, sadness, anger, jealousy, self-centeredness, and negative self-perception. "No sorcerer can cause as much harm to you as you can cause to yourself," says Johnny Moses, a Nootka healer.

External influences also contribute to the onset of diseases. "Germs are also spirits," says Shabari Bird of the Lakota Nation. If you live an imbalanced life, have a weak constitution, engage in negative thinking, and experience stress, you are more susceptible to harmful bacteria. Other individuals or spirits may also be responsible for an illness. Toxins in the environment, including alcohol, polluted air, water, and certain foods, are another external cause of sickness.

According to Native American healers, disease can be caused by physical, mental, or spiritual trauma. These traumatic incidents can lead to mental and emotional distress and a loss of soul and spiritual strength. In such cases, the healer must employ rituals and other techniques to physically restore the patient's soul and power. People who break the "rules of living" may also become ill, and these rules may involve considerations for individuals, animals, places, ritual items, events, or spirits.

Native American healers utilize a variety of techniques for diagnosing ailments. Some examples include discussing one's symptoms, examining family and personal history, observing nonverbal cues such as posture or voice tone, and employing medical divination. The healer's sensitivity, intuition, and spiritual strength are more important than the specific technique used.

Healing techniques encompass chanting, smudging (burning sage or aromatic woods), prayer, music, counseling, massage, laying on of hands, herbal remedies, dreaming, fasting, imagery, harmonizing with nature, taking hallucinogens (such as peyote), cultivating inner silence, sweat lodges, ceremonies, and embarking on shamanic journeys. Family and community play a significant role in many healing sessions.

Healing can occur rapidly in some cases, while in others, the healing process may take a longer time. The intensity of the therapy is considered more important than the duration of treatment. Even if recovery is swift, lifestyle changes are often necessary to ensure long-term healing.

A medicine bundle can also be utilized in Native American healing. Inside a bundle made of leather or animal skin, the healer carries various ritual artifacts, herbs, charms, stones, and other therapeutic tools. The bundle represents the physical manifestation of the healing power bestowed upon the healer by the spirits, whether for general healing or the treatment of a specific illness. Bundles vary among clans, tribes, and individuals.

Unless the practitioner is a highly certified healthcare professional, insurance does not typically cover Native American medicine. The majority of Native healers do not charge a fixed fee. It is said that healing comes as a "gift from the Great Spirit." However,

gifts to the healer are greatly appreciated. Giving a gift "ensures the success of the treatment since healing spirits value generosity." Gifts can be groceries, money, fabric, or another personalized expression of gratitude and admiration.

The Magic of Herbs

Native American healing practices and ceremonies have as many and varied roots as the hundreds of tribes that comprise the United States. Nature has bestowed treasures upon Native peoples, who have served as a vital link between spirituality and culture. The Four Sacred Medicines (cedar, tobacco, sage, and sweetgrass) have long been associated with the spiritual, physical, and emotional well-being of Indigenous peoples.

These four sacred medicines are as follows:

• Sage - Sage is commonly used for smudging and ceremonial preparation.

• Tobacco - Tobacco is offered as a gift to healers, elders, and the Creator.

• Cedar - Cedarwood has antioxidants, antibiotics, and anti-inflammatory properties, making it beneficial for purifying your home.

• Sweetgrass - Sweetgrass is considered the holy hair of Mother Earth. It can be used as a cleansing herb or as smudging incense.

Growing your Herbs

If you're ever at home because you're in self-quarantine and want to try out a new interest, here's the perfect at-home hobby: Plant some herbs in your garden. They grow well indoors and outdoors, are affordable, and will give you—and potentially the kids—something to do.

Dusting rosemary or fresh basil on spaghetti, poultry, roasted meats, and vegetables can also add flavor to any dish. Growing your own herbs is simple; you need the right materials, planting pots, and a sound approach. Here's what you need to do:

Step 1: Gather a couple of pots.

One of the most appealing aspects of a homegrown herb garden is that it's always ready to use. Want to season your spaghetti or roast chicken? Just a few leaves of basil, thyme, or sage will do. You can place your herbs in a pot anywhere you choose, such as on your deck, porch, or kitchen counter.

The material of your container may vary. There are numerous options to choose from, including wood, clay, resin, and metal. The most important aspect is that it has proper drainage. Any pot or planter you choose must be able to drain excess water, which is why most planting containers have holes at the bottom.

Although Mason jars may look appealing, they may not be the best choice for herb gardens. If you don't provide proper drainage for your herbs, they can eventually develop root rot.

Choose a container that is appropriate for the size of the herbs you intend to grow. If you choose something too large, your plants will spend too much energy developing their roots. Overcrowding the planter will cause your herbs to become root-bound, which will hinder their nutrition, induce stress, and kill them.

Step 2: Choose the herbs you want to grow.

If this is your first time growing herbs, start with the basics. Parsley, basil, and mint are excellent choices for container plants; they grow quickly and can withstand frequent harvesting. Here are a few examples of common herb types and their characteristics:

Rosemary: Rosemary has resinous leaves with a pungent aroma. It thrives in cool climates with ample light and moist (but not rainy) soil. It's also a good idea to keep rosemary indoors during the winter.

Thyme: This plant has intensely fragrant leaves and prefers to grow in a dry climate. Thyme needs full sunlight and well-drained soil to thrive.

Mint: Mint thrives well in its own pot and above ground due to its rapid growth rate. It can tolerate shade but prefers direct sunlight.

Basil: Basil is a sun-loving plant that is quite easy to grow. It also grows well in well-drained soil.

Parsley (flat-leaf): Chefs prefer flat-leaf parsley over curly parsley because it has more flavor. Parsley grows best in moist, well-drained soil but can tolerate light shade.

Oregano: The leaves of this herb are small and flavorful, requiring plenty of sunshine and good drainage. Greek oregano is a delicate perennial that needs to be brought indoors during the winter.

Step 3: Start with starter plants instead of seeds.

Unless you are an experienced gardener, it's recommended to use starter plants for the herbs. This will save you 2-3 weeks of growing time and provide you with more options for harvesting.

Step 4: Choose the appropriate soil.

When planting, use potting soil instead of garden soil. Potting soil drains better. It is porous and lighter, while garden soil is denser and retains moisture in containers. If you don't have one already, get a trowel. It can be used to dig holes, handle soil, and weed as needed.

Step 5: Harvesting and care.

Herbs require constant and consistent attention to thrive. That means you'll have to water them regularly, and you'll also need to harvest them frequently to promote new growth. Make sure that any treatment you give your herbs is suitable for their species.

Wild Crafting and Harvesting

Wildcrafting is the practice of gathering herbs and plants from the wild. If the name conjures up images of American frontier pioneers, you're not far off; for example, Daniel Boone earned and lost a bundle of ginseng.

Wildcrafting, however, has been carried out throughout North America for centuries before the arrival of the first Europeans, and it is closely connected to ancient Asian medicinal techniques. Ethical wildcrafting encompasses the gathering of food, medicine, and cosmetics. It is also known as foraging, and those who engage in it are referred to as wildcrafters, foragers, and herbalists.

Conservation of endangered species

Several plant species serve as cautionary tales about the dangers of unethical wildcrafting.

Ginseng has been excessively harvested in parts of the United States, putting the plant's survival at risk, leading many states to implement ginseng management plans. Ginseng has been used since ancient times for a variety of purposes, including boosting energy, reducing stress, and balancing blood sugar.

Arnica, known for its purported pain-relieving and anti-inflammatory properties, is listed as an endangered species in the United States and Canada and is dwindling in Europe, where several countries have made efforts to conserve it. Ramps, onion-like plants that cannot be cultivated on farms, have gained popularity among American chefs, particularly those who value locally sourced cuisine. As a result, certain wild ramp populations have declined over the past few decades.

The significance of ethical wildcrafting

At first glance, wildcrafting seems to be in perfect harmony with nature. What could be more resourceful, natural, and practical than foraging in the woods for your own herbal plants?

However, it's a bit more complex than that. It is important to gather only what the habitat can sustain, ensuring a sustainable harvest. Additionally, it is crucial to comply with all applicable laws and respect the property rights of both government and private landowners.

Make Your Own Healing Herb Lab

After speaking with Wendell Combest, Ph.D., a professor of pharmacology at Shenandoah University's Dunn Pharmacy School, and visiting his labs, it is evident how cooking, chemistry, and horticulture are interconnected.

He is a plant and medical expert, making him the person to consult if you want to create a garden full of plants that can be used for homemade medications and excellent meals.

He has designed medicinal gardens in Virginia and Vermont, as well as a garden with approximately 100 plant species in front of a pharmacy school on the Winchester Medical Center campus's Health Professions Building. Many plants in the garden are categorized as "at-risk" on the threatened/endangered medicinal plant list maintained by the United Plant Savers. He also plans to create a zen garden at the back of the building before certifying his medical garden as a recognized botanical sanctuary for researching and conserving endangered flora.

Dr. Combest showcases the dried plant materials he studies to determine their medicinal properties. Plants that work well in moisturizing salt scrubs and bug bite ointments can also be used for a tasty supper. The lab where plant materials are dried and researched resembles a storybook witch's house, with shelves filled with dried roots, bark, and leaves. Not surprisingly, a handwritten sign on the wall reads, "Wendell Combest, a Potions Master."

However, Combest's work is not fictional. He, a skilled gardener, identifies himself as an ethnopharmacologist, researching the traditional use of medicines by people and investigating the efficacy of folk remedies.

What plants should you grow if you want the most practical lab around?

Here is Combest's list:
- Catnip
- Sage
- Thyme
- Rosemary
- Oregano
- Basil
- Spearmint
- Chamomile
- Watercress
- Peppermint
- Calendula
- Dill

- Sorrel
- Tarragon
- Fennel

- Marjoram
- Horehound
- Lavandin

It is best to start small with herbs that can serve multiple functions. "You don't have to cultivate everything," said Combest, who purchases dried plant and herb products (such as wild cherry bark/kava), clay, essential oils, and other components from Mountain Rose Herbs to create a variety of plant-based items. While most of the plants he recommends for a medicinal lab can be used fresh in meals, it is advisable to dry them for use in ointments, scrubs, lip balms, and lotions. Plant drying is also easier than you might think. Place them on a towel and use a fan to circulate air around them. Rotate the leaves regularly. If the leaves continue to bend, they still contain too much moisture.

Healing aromas

The general rule is that the scent should be barely discernible for its benefits to be noticed — there is no need to exaggerate the aroma.

Investing in some excellent essential oils to create products you enjoy using is a great option. Combest creates perfumes in the same way perfumers do, combining a base note (something woody/earthy like cedar), a middle note (herbal or citrus), and a top note (floral, for example). Vanilla acts as a strong binder, holding everything together. As you experiment with different scents, you will discover which ones positively affect your mood.

Making remedies

Making cough drops and creams is simply a matter of boiling dry herbs and a few other ingredients. To make cough drops, heat certain components in an enameled/stainless steel skillet, then add sugar and cook until the syrup reaches the "hard crack" stage. Essentially, you are creating a nutritious treat. "Cough drops can be made in various ways," said Combest.

Tinctures can be made by infusing dry plants with oil or alcohol. Plants can also be infused with witch hazel (a shrub with medicinal properties available in drugstores and pharmacies). This process can also be used to create lotions, ointments, and creams. Most of the beeswax is used in ointments, while lotions contain less.

According to Combest, the only tools you will need to make a cream, lotion, or ointment are a double boiler, a whisk, and a small pan or skillet to extract the herbs.

Combest enjoys discussing the development of plant-based remedies and demonstrating how simple they are. He frequently hears people say, "If I had known it was this simple, I would have done it years ago." One of the most basic preparations is tea (a tisane), where dry plant material is steeped in hot water.

Use your common sense

When it comes to using plant-based products, common sense is essential. "You must exercise extreme caution and discernment. It's the same with food," explained Combest.

So, while Combest analyzes plants in the pharmacy garden, such as an Osage Orange tree (investigating the antifungal properties of its root and bark), you can utilize plants to your advantage by walking into your garden and plucking specific herbs with a variety of uses, just as your grandmother or great-grandmother did.

A word of warning

All of this indicates that plants, even if they appear harmless, are not. He noted that someone might use so much lavender essential oil in a bath that they become sleepy and injure themselves by slipping. According to him, lavender quickly enters the skin, bloodstream, and brain. Many plants are also highly toxic. When planning a healing garden, it is crucial to stick to plants that have been thoroughly researched or consistently and effectively used.

When Do Scented Plants Bloom?

If you want to fill your house and yard with fragrance all year, choose plants that bloom at different times during the growing season.
• January – jasmine, paperwhites, freesia

• February – jasmine, winter daphne, sweet box, witch hazel, freesia

• March – hyacinths, forced Muscari, and daffodils

• April – hyacinths, daffodils, Muscari

• May – tulips, creeping phlox, lily of the valley, lilacs, wallflowers, bearded iris, wisteria, azaleas, citrus, sweetshrub

• June – rhododendron, mock orange, daphne, peony, sweet alyssum, roses, sweet peas, fringe tree dianthus, stock

• July – Oriental lilies, petunias, heliotrope, garden phlox, daylilies, sweet alyssum, lavender, yucca

• August – Oriental-Trumpet lilies, Nicotiana, four o'clocks, mignonette, gardenia, clethra, butterfly bush, tuberose, freesia, Brugmansia, acidanthera

• September – snakeroot, autumn clematis, Brugmansia, tuberose, acidanthera gardenia, glossy abelia, roses, ginger lilies

• October – variegated silverberry, sweet olive

• November – balsam fir

• December – balsam fir, paperwhites

Growing Herbs in the Kitchen

It's a straightforward process to start an indoor herb garden by rooting cuttings from outdoor plants in the fall when the weather cools. Most people begin displaying their indoor herb garden using purchased seeds several weeks before the season's first frost is predicted. Most herbs may be harvested in a few weeks, and there's no need to plant them too far ahead.

Before You Begin

Much debate is on which herbs are best for growing indoors. Sellers of prepared herb gardens spread misinformation, causing you to believe that practically any herb may be grown in their kits. However, only some herbs are appropriate for indoor cultivation. For example, standard rosemary has a woody, bushy form that is too huge and unmanageable for indoor use. Many herbs, instead, are widely regarded as great choices for indoor growth, including oregano, chives, thyme, mint, dill, coriander, basil, sage, and creeping savory.

It's important to mind each plant has different growing requirements, so do some research to ensure you have the proper amount of light, humidity, and air movement. It's also foolish to commit a lot of space to herbs you will use sparingly. Instead, use your window space to grow many herbs you regularly use in your cooking.

What You'll Need
- Tools / Equipment
- Scissors
- Trowel for the garden
- Plant grow lights
- Potting soil

- Materials
- Pot trays
- Planting pots
- Herb seedlings

Instructions

- **Choose a Location**

Your indoor herb garden will grow if you provide it with a sunny location (or equivalent artificial light), coolish conditions with slightly elevated humidity, and appropriate air movement.

The best position will provide at least six hours of direct sunshine through a window facing west or south. Herbs are cultivated under grow lights, which require 14-16 hours of supplemental light each day from fluorescent lamps placed 6-12 inches above the plant. Because artificial lighting does not have the same intensity as natural sunshine, plants will require additional exposure time to receive adequate light energy.

Herbs thrive best at temperatures between 65 and 70 degrees Fahrenheit during the day and 55 and 60 degrees Fahrenheit at night. Avoid placing your herb pots near radiators or other heat ducts, as they will

grow overheated and dry quickly. Herbs grow in an area with good air circulation but no drafts.

• Pots to Select and Prepare

To cultivate any herb in a container garden, you must first choose and prepare the proper pot. Herbs grow quickly and can fill a pot mostly with roots in less than a growing season, so select solid, roomy pots with plenty of depth for root development. Choose pots with adequate drainage.

• Plant the Herbs

After sowing herb seeds or transplanting herb plants, thoroughly water them. Allow the pot to drain completely before positioning it on a ledge or beneath grow lights, with a tray beneath to catch dripping water.

If the interior air is very dry — as it often is in locations with harsh winters — arrange the herb pots on stone trays. Fill the trays halfway with water, but keep the level below the drainage holes on the pots.

• Garden Tenderization

Most herbs require regular watering; however, the soil must be allowed to dry slightly before being watered again. Indoor herbs, like other potted plants, require a little more attention than those cultivated outside. Every two weeks, give the indoor herb garden one dose of water-soluble fertilizer. Too much food would dilute the flavor of the herbs, so keep it diluted. To ensure even sunlight and constant growth, turn the pots regularly.

Maintain vigilance over your herb garden. When plants are stressed and thirsty, they change their appearance. If you know how your plants look when they're healthy, you'll be able to notice problems before they get out of hand.

• Harvest as Needed

When most herbs are only a few inches tall, you can begin harvesting them. Herbs that are trimmed provide a larger, longer crop. Even if you're not using the herbs for cooking, try to cut back the new growth at least once a week. Long stems with flower buds should be cut as soon as they appear.

• Take your herb garden outside

When the weather warms up in the spring, many people choose to move their potted herbs outside onto the patio/deck. Herbs almost always appreciate the extra sunlight that comes with spending a few months outside.

Some of them can be rotated between outdoor and indoor growing spaces for years, while others must be removed when the stems become woody and thick and replaced with new seeds or seedlings. The organic material within the potting mix (usually peat moss) breaks down over time, necessitating the addition of new potting mix or the complete repotting of the plants.

• **Grow the herbs you eat the most**

"Parsley? Pah! What do I resemble, a hayseed? I'm going to grow some savory and marjoram." I've been there, believe me. It's appealing to grow something new or distinctive rather than the conventional candidates. But how many recipes actually call for savory ingredients? If you prioritize the herbs you use the most, you'll get much more usage out of your kitchen herb garden.

Find out which plants complement each other.

Some herbs - like lavender, rosemary, and thyme - prefer drier soil, while others - like chives, mint, and basil - need more water. Joey has observed that novice herb gardeners sometimes make the error of attempting to nurture plants with different wagering requirements in the same box, resulting in erratic growth. Rather, group plants that require similar growing conditions together and buy separate pots for those that do not. Remember that plants have invasive tendencies, especially when planted in the ground. Anything in the mint family will take over and reseed itself in whatever you plant it in.

Magic of Herbs in Cooking

Here are some tips on how to use herbs for your recipes:

• Only the twiggy, wiry, or woody components of herbs must be removed. Soft stems can be cut and chopped.

• Avoid chopping herbs too finely. According to Traunfeld, a "chopped" herb should be 1/8 to 1/4 inch across.

• Use stiff rosemary branches as skewers. Remove the lowest leaves and cut the lower tip at an angle to make piercing the food simpler.

• To cook spaghetti, add a handful of teaspoons of minced flat-leaf parsley.

• If you're only going to cultivate one type of mint, consider spearmint. It complements both savory and sweet foods.

• Finely chopped dill can be sprinkled on cooked or roasted cauliflower.

• When only one type of thyme is available, Traunfeld recommends English thyme. Spring vegetables and shellfish go well with lemon thyme.

• To avoid bruising, cut the basil with a sharp knife. When incorporating fresh basil into a cooked recipe, do so near the end.

• If a recipe calls for basil, it usually means sweet basil unless otherwise indicated.

Making Magical Seasoning Salts:

• First and foremost, the most important part is gathering oneself, ingredients, and equipment. You could always go to the Food Coop and buy fresh whole spices and herbs in the bulk section, which is a nice start, but if you truly want them to keep their magical properties, follow this three-step procedure.

• Use your imagination to be inventive. Allow yourself to be transported into the realms of legend. Learn about the history and uses of each spice or herb you buy. Discover where it grows and what it looks like in its natural environment. What is the point of it? What are some instances of its uses? Is it related to any mythology or folklore? Is it medical or magical in some way? Do they have any?

• Touch, smell, taste. Take in the aromas. Rub the herbs together, crush them, and inhale the aroma. Try recognizing spices without using labels or blindfold yourself and guess with your friends and family, using only your senses of smell and touch.

• Collect unusual containers or jars to store your spices. Make personalized labels for whole spices and your favorite mixes. Making labels is an art form in and of itself.

• Play around. The ability to play is 9/10 of magic. Although a pestle and mortar are traditional, an electric spice grinder is a top choice.

1. Consider toasting some spices before grinding.

2. Smell a herb or spice after crushing it.

3. When tasting, sprinkle some salt on some popcorn. It may take several minutes for your flavors to meld.

• Follow the rules. Here are a few good rules from the world of magic.

Begin with whole spices. The oils in herbs and spices give us a taste, and those oils go rancid after a while. Throw away any spices that have previously been ground. They are not magical at all! Sumac powder, cinnamon powder, garlic powder, and turmeric powder are the only exceptions. You should buy everything else whole and grind them yourself.

When you first start, concentrate on learning traditional recipes. Make excellent recipes and then experiment with them later. It's critical to understand how others combine spices and in what proportions. Use your imagination after you've played with recipes for a while. It'll come naturally in no time.

Keep your spice mixtures near at hand and visible so you remember to use them. You'll want to use them all within a few months.

Herbs with Magical Properties in the Kitchen:

Herbal magic has been performed for centuries in numerous civilizations around the world. Many tribes and faiths utilize these plants to protect themselves from negativity and to bring wealth and success into their lives. As witchcraft has become more commonly accepted, herbal magic has experienced tremendous rebirth. Here are five culinary herbs with magical properties that you can easily obtain at your local market. These herbs can be used for more than just seasoning your food!

• **SALT: Protection & Purification**

Salt has been used for magical purposes for millennia. It is most commonly used for cleansing, protection, and healing. Because salt is associated with riches, many people combine it with green vegetables to draw fortune into their lives. Some individuals put salt around their windows or doors as a protective measure or to ward off negativity. Salt can also be used in sigil work, which means it can be used to create a sigil for a certain magical action.

- **STAR ANISE: Increased Psychic Awareness**

Star anise is best burned as incense with charcoal and a fire-safe burner to increase psychic awareness and vigor. Star anise is an excellent offering to a god/goddess, individual deity, or entity you work with. While casting spells, star anise can also be used to deflect anything that is not from light.

- **ROSEMARY: "All Use Herb"**

Rosemary is described as the "pure quartz of herbs" due to its numerous applications. Most people use this plant to replace herbs that are in short supply for spells. Others grow rosemary outside their front door for safety. Similarly, rosemary bundles (like white sage) are used to purify their homes, while some people may wear rosemary immediately before an exam or test to help them recall things and materialize accomplishment. Rosemary can also be used in dream pillows to aid sleep and prevent nightmares.

- **BAY LEAVES: Manifestation, Wishes, and Spell Work**

Bay leaves have a wide range of magical applications. By burning one Bay Leaf, you can purify the vibe of your room and any negative or sluggish energy. Similarly, many people use the herb to communicate their desires to a higher power for them to be fulfilled. To send your desires to the "universe," write them on Bay leaves and then burn them. The ash from burned Bay leaves can also be used in magic bottle workings. Use a cauldron to burn the leaves and then collect the ash securely.

- **BASIL: Purification, Money, Love, Protection**

People who are looking for love often wear Basil on their bodies. Many ladies offer Basil to men they plan to marry to show their commitment. Basil is frequently used for purification and money magic. When Basil is strewn outside any business, it brings financial success and good fortune. Mix some Basil with any brilliant green crystal chips in a spell bottle to manifest abundance, then carry it with you or wear it as a necklace.

Rose Plant

Rosa (genus Rosa) is a genus of almost 100 perennial shrubs in the Rosaceae family. Roses grow throughout the temperate zones of the Northern Hemisphere. Many roses are planted for their beautiful blossoms, which range in color from white to different hues of pink and yellow to dark red and maroon; most have a nice perfume that varies depending on the kind and climate.

Most rose species are native to Asia, with a handful unique to North America, Europe, and northwest Africa. Roses from all over the world frequently hybridize, resulting in variations that overlap their parental shapes and make it difficult to distinguish between fundamental species.

Fewer than 10 species, most of which were native to Asia, interbred to produce today's varied range of garden roses.

Roses are susceptible to many illnesses, most of which are caused by fungus. Powdery mildew appears as a gray-white mold-like development on the surface of juvenile leaves and stems. Because of the visible black patches caused by the black spot fungus, leaves break off. Roses are also prone to rust. Aphids, a common insect pest on young stems and leaves, are a common bug problem.

Physical characteristics

Roses are bushes that grow erect, trailing, or climbing and have many prickles of varied shapes and sizes on their stems, which are commonly referred to as thorns. The leaves are pinnately compound (feather-shaped) and alternate, with oval, coarsely serrated leaflets. Wild rose blossoms normally have five petals, although cultivated rose flowers frequently have two (i.e., with varied sets of petals).

Rose blossoms range in size from tiny miniatures with a 1.25 cm diameter to hybrid flowers with a diameter of more than 17.5 cm. The rose plant's fleshy, occasionally delectable, berry-like "fruit" (actually the floral cup) is known as a hip, and it is typically red to orange in color.

Pick your roses with care.

Roses are classified into various classes, ranging from micro-miniatures to grandifloras, groundcovers to climbers, and some classes contain hundreds of different varieties. While it may be tempting to plant a wide range of roses in your rose garden, you will most likely end up with a disorganized jumble and far too many plants for the available space. A few well-chosen types will provide more enjoyment than dozens of mismatched plants that need fixing. Shrub and other landscape roses, such as the Oso Easy collection, are low-maintenance choices for a carefree rose garden.

Find the appropriate location.

For the best flower display and healthiest plants, rose bushes should be exposed to six to eight hours of sunlight daily. They must also be grown in soil that is well-drained and organically rich. Roses grow better in hotter climates when they are shaded from the sun in the afternoon. Planting your rose bush near a west or south-facing fence or wall may help reduce winter freeze damage in colder climates.

Check that the timing is right.

Roses should be planted in the spring or fall. Planting in the fall allows the roots to develop before the plants become dormant for the winter.

Because bare-root roses tend to be available only in the early spring, they should be planted as soon as possible after purchase. Roses purchased in pots allow you to plant them at a later date.

Plant correctly

If you plant your bare-root/container roses correctly, they will get off to a great start.
• The planting hole must be deep and wide enough to accommodate the plant's roots. Because roses dislike wet feet, the site must have good drainage.
• Combine the soil from the planting hole with peat moss, garden compost, or other organic ingredients. Before inserting the rose shrub, place a small amount of this mixture in the bottom of the planting hole.
• In temperate climates, the plant's crown should be at ground level; in cold climates, it should be 2 - 3 inches below ground level.
• Add some slow-release fertilizer and fill the hole partially with a soil mixture.
• After properly soaking the hole, finish filling it with the remaining soil.
• Water again, then mound loose soil over the canes to protect the rose as it adjusts to its new home.
• If you're planting several rose bushes together, space them at least three feet apart to allow for growth as they mature.

Fertilize your plants regularly.

To create a beautiful display of blossoms, a rose shrub must be fertilized regularly. Organic methods provide continuous delivery of nutrients over time. Compost, composted manure, and other natural and organic fertilizers, such as organic fish emulsion, can be used monthly. Organic amendments also help promote healthy soil bacteria and maintain pH balance in the soil. Slow-release fertilizers, like Jobe's Natural Fertilizer Spikes, provide a balanced supply of nitrogen, potassium, phosphorus, and other minor nutrients. They provide the nutrition that rose bushes need to thrive.

Bare-root plants that have been freshly rooted: Treat the soil with organic amendments when it's time to plant. Wait until the plant has developed its first blossoms before applying full-strength fertilizers to avoid burning the young roots.

Displaying them

Rose cut flowers have long been valued for their beauty and fragrance. However, no roses are more beautiful than those gathered from your own garden. Here are some tips to keep your cut roses fresh:

• Roses last the longest when cut just after the bud stage, when the petals begin to open.

• Use hand pruners or garden scissors with sharp blades to clip the stems without damaging their water intake pathways.

• Clip roses when they are dewy and hydrated (in the morning and evening), rather than when the heat stresses the plant.

• Recut the rose stems before arranging them in a vase.

• Remove any air bubbles that may be blocking the stems from absorbing water. Also, trim the stems at a 45-degree angle to prevent them from sitting flat on the bottom of the vase.

• Remove any lower leaves that fall below the waterline to prevent decay or bacterial growth. Leave as much foliage as possible above the waterline to help draw up water.

• If possible, change the water frequently to eliminate bacteria. Recut the flower stems every few days to enhance water absorption.

Use water wisely.

The soil must be kept evenly moist during the growing season. The amount and frequency of watering will depend on your soil type and climate. Roses thrive with one inch of rain every week during the growing season. Roses grown in sandy soil require more water than those in clay soil. Roses will quickly wilt in dry, hot, and windy conditions. How you water is just as important as how often you water. To keep rose leaves healthy, avoid wetting them. Use a soaker hose, a watering can with a long spout, or a watering wand aimed directly at the soil.

Rosebush maintenance

Rose maintenance is simpler than you would think — anyone can cultivate them. Plant them in a sunny, dry location. To ensure lovely blooms, fertilize them regularly. Water them evenly to keep the soil moist. Prune established rose plants in the spring. Keep an eye out for symptoms such as powdery mildew and black spots.

Don't panic if you've been putting off beginning a rose garden. Roses require the same basic maintenance as other flowering bushes. Follow these ten basic tips to learn how to cultivate roses:

Prune like a pro

Over-pruning a rose shrub is nearly impossible. However, following a few simple recommendations will achieve more professional results and a healthier plant. Many of the newest rose varieties require little, if any, pruning, and using rose-to-prune gloves and a good set of bypass pruners can make the job much easier.

Pruning is usually best done in early spring. Begin by removing any dead or damaged canes from your roses. For varieties that require severe pruning, cut back one-third to half of the previous year's growth until you see new, white centers within the cane.

Simply trimming your roses can keep them looking good all season.

Certain reblooming rose varieties will require deadheading throughout the season to encourage reblooming. Cut spent flowers back to the first 5-leaf stem to promote regeneration. If the rose bushes are "self-cleaning," no deadheading is required (that is, they do not produce rose hips). The blooms will naturally fall off, and the plants will continue to produce flowers.

Container-grown roses

Because they are easy to cultivate and establish, container roses are great for inexperienced gardeners. They can also be acquired from local nurseries during the growing season, allowing you to plant them when the weather is cool and gloomy.

Roses from the ground: One advantage of bare-root roses is the greater diversity of varieties available. They are also inexpensive and can be purchased online. Unlike container roses, bare-root plants must have their roots soaked in water overnight before planting. Also, the roots should be kept moist during the first few months following transplantation.

Keep them healthy.

Choosing disease-resistant rose varieties is the most effective way to prevent rose diseases. These roses have been bred and selected to resist the most common rose diseases, such as powdery mildew and black spot.

Powdery mildew is most prevalent in the summer when the days are hot and dry and the nights are cool and wet. Warning signs include curling and twisting leaves and the development of a white powdery coating on the leaves. To reduce powdery mildew, water plants near ground level in the morning, as damp leaves (especially overnight) create an ideal environment for growth. Allowing air to circulate through the foliage of a rose bush can also help prevent the buildup of powdery mildew. A simple mixture of baking soda and horticultural oil can help prevent the spread of black spot. Another option is a three-in-one organic fungicide.

Common insect pests that feed on rose plants include Japanese beetles, aphids, sawflies, and spider mites. Most of these pests can be controlled with neem oil or insecticidal soap.

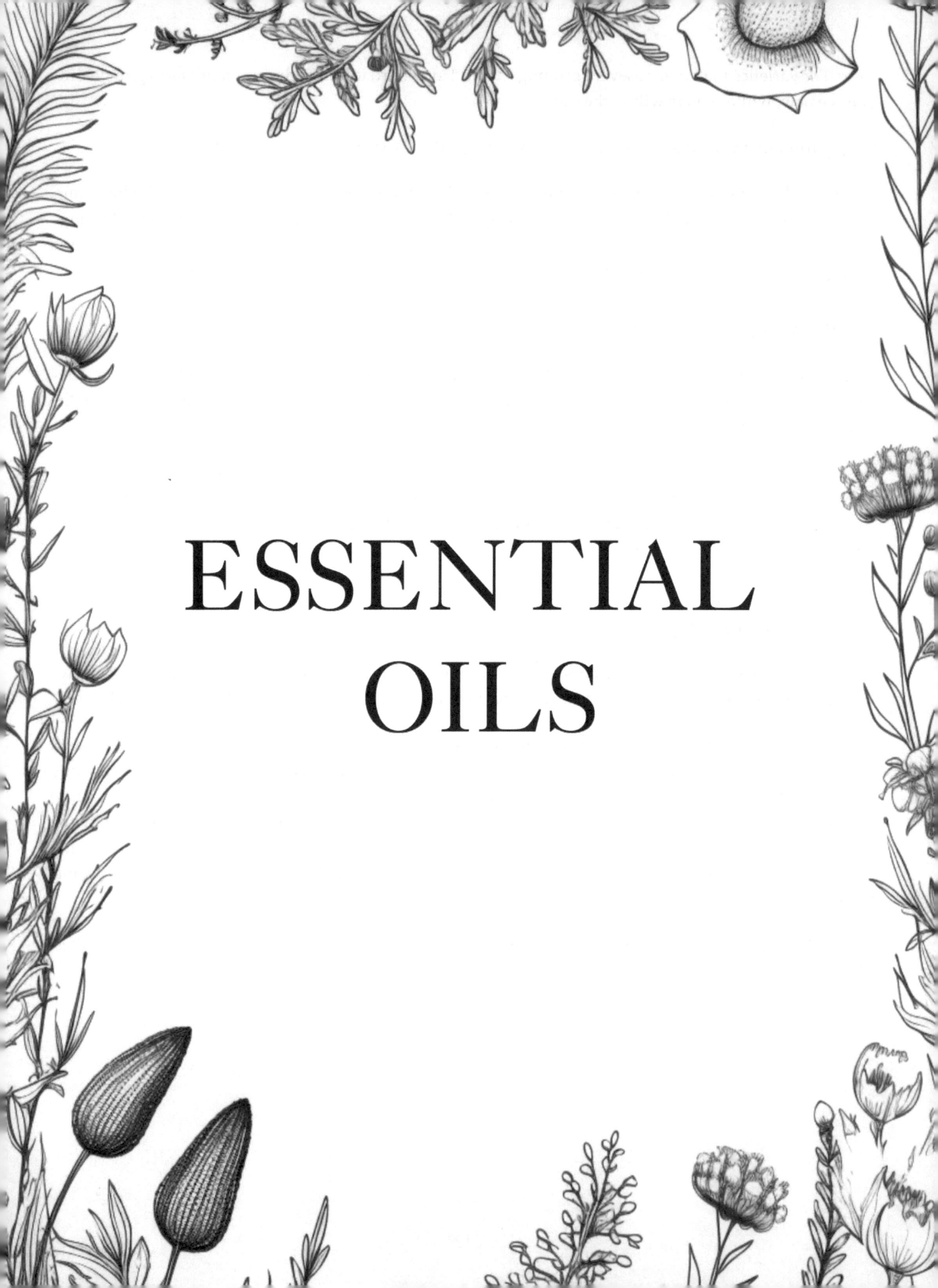

ESSENTIAL
OILS

HISTORY OF ESSENTIAL OILS

The world is filled with various fragrances, and we rely on our sense of smell to help us find food, recognize new individuals, and even appreciate the air we breathe. But how did we come to value this?

Humans have used essential oils since ancient times, but it was in the 1800s that scientists began systematically extracting chemicals from plants. Essential oils have been used since time immemorial when people extracted oils from plants by soaking them in water.

The Ancient World

The ancient Egyptians were the first to apply scented flowers and plants to improve their mental state. They practiced what was known as "perfumery," derived from the Latin term "perfumare," meaning "to smoke through" or "to perfume." Perfumers at the time combined flower essences with animal fat to create solid perfume.

The ancient Greeks followed suit, using fragrances to heal both physical and mental ailments. The Romans employed perfumery to entertain guests and worship the gods, but the practice declined during Europe's Dark Ages.

Life in the Middle Ages

Essential oils made a comeback in the late Middle Ages. In fact, contemporary researchers believe that apothecary monks preserved and continued their knowledge of aromatherapy even after it disappeared from Western civilization. One notable figure was Baldassare Pisanelli, a young monk considered Europe's first perfumer and an influential figure in the Roman Catholic Church. Another was Hildegard von Bingen, a renowned 12th-century Benedictine abbess and writer from Germany. She incorporated flowers into her medicinal concoctions and wrote about the "immense power which the Almighty gave to herbs" in her book called "Physica."

People accepted their fate when these remedies didn't work. In the early 1900s, researchers discovered that the US Patent Office had documented over 5000 patents for various inventions and remedies. According to Dr. Bill Olcott of Carnegie Mellon University in Pittsburgh, the number of pharmaceutical patents issued between 1980 and 2000 exceeded those issued between 1790 and 1980 by 207%.

The Chinese also used essential oils for healing. Cassia and camphor, both derived from the bark of Southeast Asian trees, were among the most popular.

The Modern Period

A significant moment in the history of aromatherapy occurred in 1937 when French chemist René-Maurice Gattefossé burned his hand while working in his laboratory. Although the injury was not severe enough to require hospitalization, it caused him excruciating pain. During this incident, Gattefossé happened to notice a plant known for its soothing properties on his window ledge. He crushed the leaves and applied them directly to his wound, resulting in a decrease in pain within minutes.

Gattefossé conducted further research on the essential oils in his laboratory and discovered that several of them had similar analgesic qualities. He outlined how to use essential oils for both physical and mental

111

disorders in his book "Aromathérapie: l'Art d'utiliser les Huiles Essentielles" (Aromatherapy: The Art of Using Essential Oils).

Health Advantages

The Top 10 Health Benefits of Essential Oils!

1. They can alleviate nausea and vomiting - Lavender has long been used to relieve nausea and vomiting in pregnant women, and goldenseal has the same effect.

2. They can help you relax - Some essential oils, such as lavender, lemon balm, bergamot, and peppermint, are believed to relax the body.

3. They can aid in weight gain - Lemon essential oil is recognized for its fat-burning properties, while peppermint essential oil is claimed to aid in weight gain by increasing the release of various hormones that stimulate appetite.

4. Essential oils aid in weight loss - Sage is used in aromatherapy to promote sweating, which can accelerate weight loss effects.

5. They can help your skin - Some essential oils have been shown to help reduce skin inflammations and infections. Tea tree oil is an anti-fungal and anti-bacterial agent, and bergamot and lavender can help remove acne, pimples, and other facial disorders.

6. They can increase alertness - Some individuals find it easier to focus without disrupting their day by adding peppermint essential oil to their drink or inhaling peppermint oil before engaging in activities.

7. They can help you sleep better - Certain essential oils have been shown to enhance peaceful sleep by relaxing muscles and soothing nerves. Camphor is believed to reduce tension and promote relaxation, and bergamot is said to do the same by easing digestion.

8. They can improve your immune system - Fennel essential oil is beneficial for enhancing the body's resilience to illness and reducing inflammation. Lavender is also known for its anti-inflammatory effects.

9. They can aid with depression - Certain essential oils, such as lavender, are believed to be useful in treating symptoms of depression.

10. For example, bergamot has been used both internally and externally to treat sinusitis and other related disorders like upper respiratory infections.

Aromatherapy and Native Americans

Aromatherapy is a natural complement to conventional medicine. It is used to cure many ailments and is especially useful in times of crisis, such as natural catastrophes, injuries, and serious illnesses.

Native American Indians have incorporated essential oils into their daily lives for millennia. Native

Americans in the Pacific Northwest engaged in considerable trade with Asia following contact with Europeans in the late 1600s. As a result, they would frequently come into contact with Asian aromatics such as cedarwood, clove, frankincense, juniper berry oil, or Madagascar Vanilla. Not only were essential oils used to treat illnesses, but also in skincare. When the indigenous people were sick or exhausted, they would utilize the oils in their baths.

Native Americans were reputed to have acute senses, so much so that they could discriminate between different oils based solely on the aroma. This ability was put to use when they were hunting for specific oils for various uses. When it comes to healing, American Indian tribes would always rely on holistic treatments such as herbalism and aromatherapy, among other things. Native Americans in America employed several strategies to care for themselves, including essential oil mixes to improve their quality of life.

Many tribes used essential oils to treat a variety of diseases. For example, the Abenaki tribe would use clove oil to ease migraines and vapor rub to reduce aches. The Navajo utilized frankincense oil to treat wrinkles on the face, clay to treat kidney stones, and jalapeño pepper oil combined with honey to treat rashes. The Ojibwa tribe utilized cedarwood oil to treat sunburns, crushed coral to treat dandruff, and birch bark tea as an anti-inflammatory agent.

Other nations have decided to incorporate Native American techniques into everyday life, making them more successful than ever before. Aromatherapy is now widely used as an important component of alternative medicine worldwide, and the use of essential oils for medical purposes is still prevalent today.

HOW TO PREPARE ESSENTIAL OILS BY YOUR OWN

Essential oils, such as lavender and rosemary, are concentrated oils derived from fragrant plants. They can be extracted using various methods, with distillation being the most common. While essential oils can be expensive, home distillation is a cost-effective option.

Putting Together an Essential Oil Still:

• Purchase an essential oil still: These stills can be easily obtained online, although they can be expensive. If you plan to produce large quantities of essential oil, it is advisable to hire a professional.

• If you prefer not to buy one, you can make your own still: There are numerous designs to choose from, and many stills are hand-built. A still should include the following components:

  - A heat source, typically a direct fire.

  - A pressure cooker.

  - A 10 mm diameter glass pipe.

  - A tub filled with cold water to chill and condense the steam.

- An essencier to separate essential oils from unwanted substances in the final product.

- Use stainless steel and glass components whenever possible. Avoid using plastic tubing as it can affect the oil quality. Some plants are sensitive to copper, but extensively tinned copper is safe in all conditions. Aluminum elements can be used with certain herbs containing phenols in their oils, such as cloves or wintergreen.

Bend the pipe to fit into the cooling tub. The plant matter will be heated in the pressure cooker, and the resulting steam will pass through the pipe. Transform the steam into liquid by immersing it in cold water or an ice bath. The pipe may need to be bent in different ways depending on the cooling tank used, such as coiling it in a basin or bending it at a 90-degree angle to pass through a bucket of ice.

• Plug the pipe into a pressure cooker valve: If using a single 10 mm pipe, use a short, flexible hose that fits tightly over both apertures. Secure the connection with a jubilee clip from a hardware store. Ensure the hose is long enough to allow for little bending. If necessary, make a 90-degree bend in the pipe to enter the cooling tub.

• Insert the pipe into the cooling tub and pass it through: If using an open basin, ensure the coil is fully contained within the tub. When the basin is filled with cold water or ice, bury the coil. Drill a small hole in the bottom of the bucket to allow the pipe to exit the ice bath, and seal it with silicone sealer or epoxy.

• Keep all your instruments in a safe location: Depending on the equipment and pipe configuration, you may need to experiment to establish a stable setup. Place the pipe-attached cover on the pressure cooker, thread the pipe through the cooling tube, and onto your essential.

Preparation of Plant Materials:

• Determine the ideal time to harvest: Each plant species has a specific time in its life cycle when the oil content is optimal. Research when and how to harvest each plant you want to distill. For example, lavender should be picked after half of the flowers on the stalk have faded, while rosemary should be harvested when fully flowered.

• Harvest your plants correctly: Proper handling and harvesting techniques are essential for maximizing oil output. Only use the blooming tops of rosemary bushes for essential oil production. Avoid damaging or breaking the plants, as this can reduce the oil yield. Handle them with care and minimize touching.

• Be selective when purchasing plants: If buying harvested plants, look for healthy and undamaged ones. Ask the vendor about the harvest date. Organic plants are preferable to avoid pesticide or herbicide contamination.

• Ensure the plant material is well-dried: Although drying reduces the oil yield per plant, it increases the overall essential oil produced in each batch. Dry the plants slowly, away

from direct sunlight. Lavender and peppermint can be left to dry with an infield for a day or two after cutting. Different plants have different drying requirements, but avoid overheating. Drying in shade or a dark environment helps retain the oil.

Distillation of Essential Oils:

• Fill the still's tank with water: If using a homemade still, the pressure cooker serves as the tank. Use fresh, pure water that is filtered or distilled. Follow the manufacturer's instructions for a commercial still. Ensure you have enough water to complete the distillation process, which can take varying times depending on the plant and quantity.

• Add the plant materials to the water: Fill the tank as much as possible with the plant materials. Ensure they don't obstruct the steam vent in the pressure cooker lid. No need to cut or prepare the plants, as this may result in oil loss.

• Bring the water to a boil: Close the lid, allowing only outgoing steam to pass through the pipe attached to the steam valve. Most plants release their essential oils at the boiling point of water, around 100 degrees Celsius.

• Monitor the still closely: The distillate should start flowing through the condenser and into the separator after a while. Ensure there is enough water in the cooling tub, replacing it if necessary to maintain the cooling process.

• Optional: Filter the collected oil: After distillation, you can filter the oil using cheesecloth or dry cotton fabric. Ensure the fabric is clean and dry to prevent contamination.

• Transfer the oil to a storage container promptly: Essential oils have a shelf life of one to two years, or even shorter for some. Store them in dark glass bottles or stainless containers. Use a clean funnel when pouring the oil, and keep it in a cool, dark place.

• Decide what to do with the hydrosol: Hydrosol is the distilled water infused with plant fragrance. Some hydrosols, like rose or lavender water, can be used independently. If not storing the hydrosol, add it to the still for the next batch or dispose of it.

Safety and Side Effects

Many people like to utilize essential oils because they promote healing and wellness. Essential oils can be applied topically or inhaled. When applied topically, they are frequently combined with a carrier oil before being applied to the skin. However, there is considerable concern about essential oil side effects and safety considerations. Continue reading to find out more!

In small amounts, essential oils are typically considered safe to use. They contain very few chemicals that can cause adverse reactions in those with sensitive skin or respiratory disorders. However, certain essential oils may include potentially irritating compounds. This implies they have the potential to irritate the skin, eyes, nose, throat, and lungs. These consequences are usually minor and transient, but if not managed properly, they can become life-threatening.

Here are some essential oils that may cause discomfort:

When using essential oils, precautions should be taken to avoid causing additional stress to the body. Stress can hinder healing by inducing the fight-or-flight response. When this happens, the body produces hormones such as cortisol and adrenaline, which cause blood glucose levels to drop and lead to additional inflammation.

Follow these steps to reduce the detrimental effects of stress on your body:

- Do not use essential oils on injured or irritated skin.

- If you are on any medications or drugs, consult your doctor before using essential oils. Some essential oil preparations may enhance the effects of certain drugs.

- Keep all essential oils in a cool, dry place away from heat sources such as heaters and sunlight. Light, heat, and air can degrade some of the more fragile components in essential oil molecules. This degradation process changes the structure of the molecule, which can have negative consequences.

- Always use the recommended doses and administration methods for essential oils. Some essential oils are safe to ingest internally, while others should not be ingested. Consult a medical practitioner if you are unsure.

- Avoid using essential oils close to electrical equipment or appliances, as some may cause interference with electronic devices.

- If you have any concerns about using essential oils, consult your doctor before using them. If you have a specific health problem or are sensitive to certain chemicals, it is recommended to avoid certain essential oils entirely. If you have allergies, do not put lavender oil under your nose.

Preparation techniques

Essential oils are not the same as flowers, herbs, incense, or incense burners, but they can be blended with other essential oils for excellent results.

All you need is a diffuser pot, an essential oil diffuser, and some water. The diffuser should be 6-8 inches tall to accommodate the water. Fill the diffuser halfway with water before adding your essential oil blends. The next step is simple: pour your oil mixture into the diffuser and place it near a heat source to release the scents into the room.

Have you ever wanted to learn how to extract essential oils from plants you grew yourself? Knowing how to distill essential oils can provide another natural remedy in your home apothecary, especially considering recent research on the therapeutic and medicinal effects of aromatherapy. Many of our favorite culinary herbs can also be used to produce essential oils. For example, peppermint plants can be used to flavor meals year-round and produce essential oils through the steam distillation method.

Here are three of the most common methods for producing essential oils:

Steam Distillation

The most common method for making essential oils at home is steam distillation, which can be done in a crockpot or with a still. You can purchase a good still made of non-reactive metals and glass for a few hundred dollars or build your own.

Steam distillation involves boiling the plants and herbs until the essential oils separate and float on the water. The oil can be collected from the water's surface and stored in an amber or blue glass container. However, it's important to note that this method may not produce a completely pure essential oil, which could diminish its medicinal benefits.

Expression

Expression involves squeezing flowers, plant material, or fruits to extract the oils. This method is commonly used for citrus oils. Citrus peels are placed in a commercial press and squeezed to extract the volatile oils. These oils are readily available in most natural food stores as they are a byproduct of the citrus agricultural business and are relatively affordable.

Solvent Extraction

Solvent extraction is primarily used for commercial purposes and involves the use of highly harmful chemical solvents. If you're new to essential oils, there are better options to consider. This method requires careful handling and application of commercial-grade solvents, which can be dangerous if not used correctly. It should only be used in well-ventilated environments.

How Does it Work?

The most common application of essential oils is aromatherapy, where essential oils are inhaled through various methods. It is important to note that essential oils should never be taken orally.

Essential oils consist of chemicals that interact with the body in different ways. When applied to the skin, several plant chemicals can be absorbed. Certain application methods, such as applying heat to specific body areas, are believed to enhance absorption. However, more studies are needed on this topic.

The aromas of essential oils can stimulate the limbic system, a region of the brain responsible for scent, emotions, long-term memory, and behavior. Interestingly, the limbic system plays a vital role in memory formation, which may explain why certain fragrances evoke memories and emotions. Additionally, the limbic system is thought to regulate various unconscious physiological functions like heart rate, breathing, and blood pressure. As a result, some people believe that essential oils have physical effects on the human body. Nevertheless, further research is required to confirm this.

Essential oils are naturally occurring chemicals known as "volatile compounds," meaning they easily evaporate into the air or water vapor. Think about the fresh-cut roses and how their molecules quickly dissipate into the air. Terpenes, found in plants such as citrus blossoms, lemongrass, and ginger, as well as phenols, found in plants like thyme and oregano, are the main chemical components present in essential oils. They also contain other aromatic molecules that, when inhaled, affect the brain.

When inhaled, essential oils disperse into the bloodstream and get absorbed by the capillaries throughout the body. These essential oils have the ability to cross the blood-brain barrier, a semi-permeable membrane that protects the brain from external chemicals. Since the brain and nervous system are primarily composed of water, essential oil molecules are transported throughout the body via fluid exchange. In other words, as blood circulates through the brain, it exchanges water for chemicals from other body parts. This allows the essential oils to rapidly spread throughout the body and reach different areas of the brain. Once there, they can influence specific hormones and neurotransmitters that regulate mood, sleep, cell growth, and energy production.

How Should It Be Used?

Essential oils are concentrated plant oils with powerful medicinal and therapeutic properties. They have been used for generations, not only in aromatherapy but also for cleaning, cooking, and many other purposes. So, if you want to learn more about this ancient wellness practice, keep reading!

People have been using essential oils to heal their minds and bodies for thousands of years. With our beginner's guide to essential oils, you can make the most of these natural remedies!

Relax your muscles with lavender or peppermint oil. Use rosemary or tea tree oil to clean around the house. Diffuse orange oil in your bedroom before bedtime for an aromatherapy session. The applications for essential oils are practically limitless!

There are various ways to work with essential oils. You can add them to your bath, incorporate them into your meals, inhale them through a diffuser, or apply a few drops to your hands and rub them together. We are here to guide you through the essentials of using essential oils, from the calming effects of lavender to stress reduction.

Follow along as we explore different oils, how to use them for specific conditions, and even some enjoyable DIY projects you can try!

What are you waiting for? Start your essential oil journey today!

Lavender oil is a popular choice for many diffusers due to its ability to reduce stress and anxiety. Similarly, peppermint oil is an excellent option for any diffuser because it has similar effects on both the mind and body.

How to Keep Them

The way essential oils are stored can affect their shelf life, beneficial properties, quality, and safe use. When stored in the proper containers and at the appropriate temperature, essential oils can have a maximum shelf life of at least one year. Well-cared-for essential oils can last 10 years or longer, depending on the type of oil and the storage conditions.

Is there an expiration date for essential oils?

All essential oils will eventually expire and become unsafe to use. Careful storage and handling are essential for maintaining the quality of oils. Over time, oil quality deteriorates due to oxidation, resulting in the loss of fragrance and nutritional benefits.

While citrus essential oils are known to oxidize faster than others, losing their scent and benefits as soon as 6 months after being opened, essential oils with woody or earthy aromas, such as Patchouli and Sandalwood, tend to improve with age and may take longer before weakening in potency and aroma. The lifespan of an oil can vary greatly depending on the quality of the source plant, harvest, extraction technique, distillation conditions, storage, batch/lot, and treatment of the oil.

It is influenced by the methods used by the provider, the client, and the supplier for bottling, storing, and controlling the oil.

How can you tell if your essential oils have become contaminated? What are the odor and appearance of expired oil?

There are four primary indicators that an essential oil may have degraded:

- The aroma may have become stronger and unpleasant or faded.

- The color may have darkened, lightened, or become colorless.

- The oil may appear murky or muddy.

- The texture may have thickened.

These are general guidelines as not all oxidized essential oils exhibit the classic signs of degradation. Therefore, all oils should be properly stored, handled, and used before they expire.

Are there any places where essential oils should not be kept?

Essential oils should not be stored in bright, hot, or humid environments such as the bathroom, near a stove, on a windowsill, or in any sunny spot. Constantly changing room temperatures can also accelerate the degradation of oil quality.

What factors influence the shelf life of essential oils?

Oxygen: Exposure to oxygen/air can cause oils to oxidize, resulting in the depletion of volatile constituents and the loss of fragrance and other qualities. To prevent oxidation and evaporation, essential oil bottles should be tightly closed when not in use.

Heat: Essential oils should not be placed near open flames, candles, sunlight, or stoves, as they are combustible. High temperatures can cause oils to reach their individual flashpoints, leading to potential ignition and accelerated degradation.

Moisture: Leaving essential oil bottles uncapped for extended periods can allow moisture to seep in, causing oils to become cloudy. Water beads may also form inside the bottles.

Light: Direct sunlight can substantially affect the attributes of essential oils, including fragrance, appearance, and effectiveness. Oils are typically sold and stored in dark-colored bottles to prevent UV radiation from entering. Despite the dark bottles, oils should still be kept out of direct sunlight to slow down the oxidation process caused by continuous heating and cooling.

Key Considerations for Oil Storage While Traveling:

Travelers' carrying cases designed to accommodate multiple oils are available for safely transporting essential oils on vacation. These cases can hold up to forty oils, ensuring proper and secure storage of essential oils on the go.

How to Extend the Shelf Life of Essential Oils and Track Their Freshness:

Follow the handling and storage instructions provided in the oil company's SDS documentation or on the product's website.

- Store essential oils in cool, dark settings, away from direct sunlight.

- Replace any oxygen in the bottle's "headspace" with nitrogen gas, which does not react with essential oil components, to avoid oxidation.

- Keep track of the purchase date of each essential oil, typically found on the product's label or cap.

- Avoid storing undiluted essential oils in dropper bottles as the rubber can become sticky and compromise the oil's purity.

- Fill essential oil bottles as close to the brim as possible to minimize the oxygen-filled headspace. If necessary, transfer the oil to smaller containers with less empty space.

- Instead of pouring directly into the bottle, pour the required amount onto sterile equipment, dilute as needed, and then apply.

What are the potential risks of using expired essential oils?

Using expired essential oils that have been contaminated can be harmful to one's health. Reported side effects include skin sensitivity, peeling, irritation, rashes, burning, and inflammation.

Can essential oils be stored in the fridge?

Yes, essential oils can be stored in the refrigerator, which is particularly useful for those who use their oils infrequently.

Can you keep essential oils in the freezer?

Yes, essential oils can be stored in the freezer. If they freeze or form crystals, allow them to gradually return to room temperature. The time it takes for the oil to thaw depends on the type of oil and can range from several minutes to many hours. Some crystalline oils will liquefy when handled, while others may benefit from a warm water "bath" by placing the bottle in a bowl of warm water. In any case, keep the bottle cap loosely closed to prevent the escape of volatile ingredients. Tightening the cap while heating can cause pressure to build up inside the bottle, resulting in spraying when the cap is removed. To avoid this, leave the bottle cap unfastened.

How to Mix

To begin, combine your essential oils to create a nice and therapeutic aroma. Essential oils must be diluted before being applied to the skin using a carrier oil, dispersion agent, or alcohol. After combining these ingredients, store your oil properly, especially if you intend to age the mixture.

Making a Blend:

- Determine the type of aroma you want: Scents of all kinds are regularly used to treat a wide range of ailments. Consider the type of fragrance you want.

- Essential oils are classified into groups depending on their scent. Each category complements the others effectively. However, you can mix perfumes from different categories. Experiment with various scents to see what you can create.

1. For floral notes: Lavender, jasmine, neroli, rose, ylang-ylang.

2. For herbal ones: Marjoram, basil, rosemary, thyme.

- Choose top, middle, and base notes: The note refers to the amount of time it takes for the oil to evaporate. High notes fade rapidly, while base notes last longer. If you want your oils to last long, choose a nice foundation note that complements the middle and top notes.

1. Top notes (gone after 1-2 hours): Anise, citronella, basil, eucalyptus, orange, lavender, lemongrass, and spearmint.

2. Middle notes (gone after 2-4 hours): Fennel, tea tree, nutmeg, chamomile, and jasmine.

3. Base notes (may linger for several days): Balsam, ginger, cedarwood, oakmoss, and patchouli.

- Put your blend to the test: Take a cotton swab dipped in each oil bottle. Each vial should have one swab. Swirl them around in the air, holding them about a foot away from your nose. This will give you an idea of how the scent combination will smell. If you don't like it, remove one of the cotton swabs and try again. You can also use cotton balls or fragrance testing strips to analyze your fragrances.

- Combine the oils: Once you've agreed on a mixture, start blending the essential oils. Fill a clean mixing bowl with the calculated amounts of the top, middle, and base notes, and use a glass vial with a pipette/dropper to drop the required amount of droplets according to the recipe. If you're unsure about the quantities, consider the following principles:

1. The 30-50-20 rule: Your blend should include 30% top note, 50% middle note, and 20% base note.

2. The 1-2-3 rule: Use 2 drops of the middle note and 3 drops of the top note for every drop of the base note.

3. Combine the essential oils before adding any carriers or diluting agents.

Diluting Your Essential Oils:

You'll need a carrier oil if you want to apply it to your skin: To utilize essential oils on your skin, you must dilute them with a carrier oil. Essential oils are very concentrated, and using them on the skin without a carrier oil risks causing irreversible damage. Some of the best carrier oils are:

- Almond oil
- Avocado oil
- Olive oil
- Hemp seed oil
- Rosehip oil
- Sesame oil
- Jojoba oil

If you intend to use it in the bath, include a dispersion agent: If you don't want to apply the essential oil directly to your skin but prefer to use it in the bath, you should use a dispersion agent to help the oil spread evenly

While some vegetable oils like coconut oil can be used as a dispersant, others are too thick for this purpose. Use a lighter and more liquid viscosity. Some outstanding agents are:

- Milk
- Honey
- Sweet almond oil
- Jojoba oil

Combine it with alcohol to make perfume: If you want to make perfume, you can combine essential oils with alcohol. Perfumes are only used sparingly. While jojoba oil can be used to produce perfume, the most common diluting agent is alcohol. Use ten to fifteen drops of the essential oil blend for every half-ounce of alcohol/jojoba oil.

Finishing Your Blend:

- Determine the proportions of your ingredients: After blending the essential oils, add them to a carrier oil or a dispersion agent, depending on how you intend to use them. The amount of each ingredient depends on your intended use.

- For massages, use fifteen to twenty drops of the essential oil combination per ounce of carrier oil.

- In lotions/skin oils, use three to fifteen drops per ounce of carrier oil.

- For children, use three to six drops per ounce of carrier oil.

- In baths, use two to twelve drops of essential oil for every ounce of the dispersing agent.

- If you only use essential oils for inhaling/smelling, you won't need a carrier oil.

- In a mixing dish, combine your essential oil blend and diluting agent: You can combine the ingredients in a dish or container. If you're mixing oils in a bowl, stir them together with a spoon or wooden stir stick. If you combine the oils in a bottle, gently swirl them in your palm to mix them.

- Store it in a bottle: Essential oil blends can be kept in bottles, glass vials, or sprayers. Essential oils are often stored in amber vials with capacities ranging from two to four millimeters. Carefully pour the blended oil into the container, using a funnel if required. Place the mixture somewhere cool and dark.

- Essential oils have a longer shelf life than carrier oils. Blends with sesame, rosehip, and sweet almond oil can be stored for 6-12 months. Jojoba and coconut oils are incredibly stable and can be stored indefinitely. The combined oil can also be stored in the fridge, except for combinations that include avocado oil. Allow three to four days for the essential oil to settle before smelling it again. Note any significant changes in the scent to track how the blend evolves over time. Aging the blend can improve its aroma.

How to Make an Equally Balanced Essential Oil

Blend Aromatherapy, healing, and well-being are all benefits of essential oils. When it comes to balancing an essential oil blend, keep the following in mind:

1. When necessary, dilute oils with a carrier oil.

2. Choose the appropriate carrier oil for your needs.

3. Avoid imbalances or using too much of one oil in the essential oil blend.

4. Know when to leave an essential oil blend alone because it is fine the way it is.

5. Create only the amount of essential oil blend required for each use.

6. Use a greater or lesser quantity of an essential oil blend to achieve specific results.

7. Use carrier oils such as sweet almond, rice bran, grapeseed, avocado, sunflower seed, hemp seed, and others that are highly beneficial to the skin without causing any negative reactions.

8. Avoid carrier oils that have been exposed to sunlight or other forms of light.

9. Use a few drops of skin-friendly essential oil in the blend as a face toner or finishing booster.

10. To provide optimum therapeutic impact, ensure your essential oils are pure and undiluted.

11. Use only therapeutic-grade oils from reputable companies that have been tested for quality, purity, and potency.

12. Avoid using oils from other sources that may harm your skin or introduce undesirable attributes to the blend.

13. Develop an essential oil blend that perfectly matches your individual needs.

14. Balance the attributes of the oils you use so that the blend only has positive properties.

15. Learn how to use essential oils correctly to enjoy the benefits without experiencing negative side effects or reactions.

16. Avoid blending different essential oils in one mixture because they can negate each other's effects and may result in unwanted negative effects.

Carrier Oils

Carrier oils dilute essential oils, making them easier to apply and less potent. They contain a high concentration of plant sterols, which are emollient, anti-inflammatory, and beneficial for dry skin. Transportable carrier oils are available in both small and large bottles. Examples include almond oil, coconut oil, and grapeseed oil. The highest quality carrier oils are cold-pressed from natural materials without any additional ingredients such as alcohol or preservatives.

Carrier oils have numerous applications. They can be used in aromatherapy sprays and for in-home massages to enhance their benefits. Carrier oils are also utilized in lotions, soaps, shampoos, body treatments, massage creams, and other products to aid in the absorption of essential oils.

How to Select the Best Essential Oils

Tip #1:

We can assist you in determining the best essential oils for your needs! All you have to do is choose an oil and then read about all the fantastic benefits of each one. Check out lavender and frankincense for stress relief - they both assist your body in releasing relaxing hormones. Do you need a pick-me-up? Breathe in peppermint and lemon, and your senses will be awakened in no time! No matter your mood or purpose, there is one or more oils for it. "The beauty of nature lies in its diversity," as the saying goes. "Just as no two people are alike, no two essential oils are alike."

The procedure for selecting an essential oil is straightforward. Choose your favorite aroma or the aroma that best suits your situation. These fragrant chemicals have a wide range of impacts on both the mind and the body and are used for everything from home decoration to therapeutic support. If you need help with what you're searching for, take a look at the most popular oils:

- Lavender essential oil is one of the world's most well-known essential oils. Its relaxing scent can be used as a general mood booster to lift one's spirits and relieve stress. It has also been found to have powerful antiseptic qualities that aid in treating stress-related illnesses and other disorders.

- Peppermint essential oil immediately relieves stomach pain and nausea. When inhaled or applied topically to the skin, it provides rapid relief. It's also an effective stress reliever, helping with migraines and muscle tightness. Peppermint can also be used topically or aromatically to relieve tight muscles and minor skin irritations.

- Rose essential oil is one of the most versatile essential oils available today, and its deep, pleasant aroma is a great addition to any space. Although it is most recognized for its skin-calming properties, it can also be used as a general stress reliever. It relaxes and moisturizes the body, making it ideal for the start of a yoga session or a relaxing bath.

"Nature's beauty lies in its diversity." Essential oils, like humans, are unique. With so many alternatives, you can choose the appropriate one for you.

Tip #2:

Are you getting the real thing or a cheap knockoff?

When it comes to essential oils, there are numerous options, especially when shopping online. But how do you know if you're receiving a genuine article or a cheap knockoff? Here are some guidelines to help you select high-quality essential oil.

- Find the Latin Name: High-quality essential oils state the Latin name of the plant species from which the oil is derived. For example, a bottle of lavender essential oil could be labeled as Lavandula Angustifolia/English Lavender. If the oil has a Latin name, you can know what you are buying.

- Knowing the Difference Between Essential and Fragrance Oils: Essential oils are distilled plant oils that have been condensed. They have a pleasant aroma as well as the helpful chemical components found in the plant from which they were harvested. Fragrance oils, on the other hand, are mostly synthetic and do not contain any beneficial natural ingredients. They are less expensive to produce because they are diluted with artificial ingredients. Check to see if the oil you're buying is an essential oil or a fragrance oil.

- Consider the Cost: Essential oils are expensive substances per ounce. Creating one small bottle requires a significant amount of plant resources - think hundreds to thousands of flowers. Everyone enjoys a good deal, but the price of the oil should make sense considering the plant's rarity and the effort required to distill it. If the price seems too low, it almost always is.

- Smell it out: Essential oils have a powerful aroma due to their high concentration. Some, like rose or chamomile, have milder but still distinct scents. When shopping for oils, make sure they smell pleasant and natural. Trust your intuition. If you detect a whiff of alcohol or an odor that resembles household cleaning rather than aromatherapy, avoid it. If you're purchasing online and need help with the scent, read the reviews to see if anyone has had a negative experience.

- Don't be deceived by the "Grade": The term "Therapeutic Grade" is used for a wide range of oils. However, it is important to remember that the FDA and other regulatory authorities do not control this phrase. While many reputable companies label their oils as "therapeutic grade" to signify purity, any company can do so without meeting any quality standards. A "Therapeutic Grade" label isn't always a bad thing, but don't place too much faith in it.

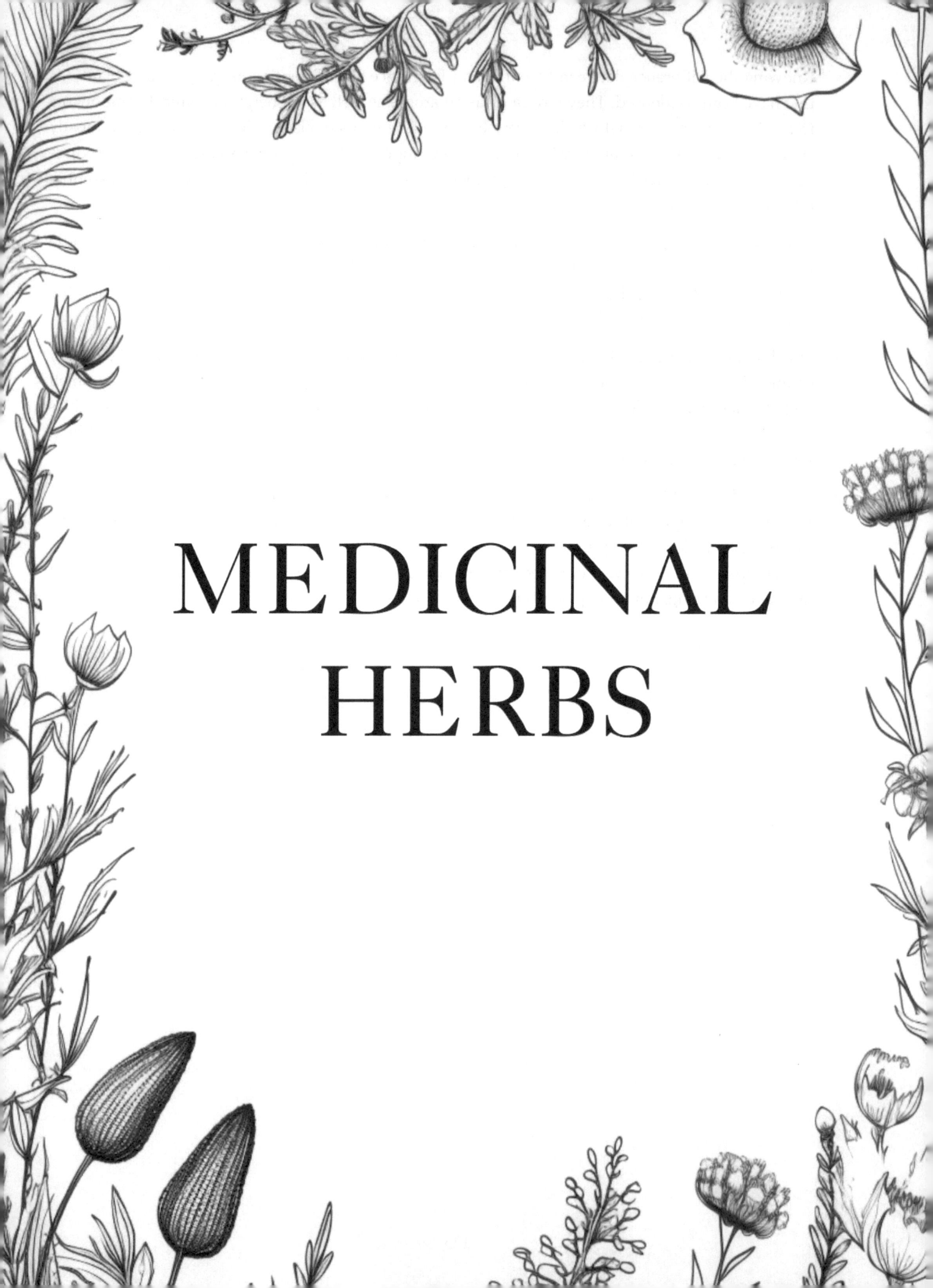

MEDICINAL HERBS

INTRODUCTION

Herbal medicine (H.M.) is the heart of alternative and complementary medicine, which has grown in popularity recently and is gradually making its way into conventional healthcare systems worldwide. H.M. is used across gender, social, and ethnic lines in both developed and developing countries. Due to the growing popularity of herbal medicine, stakes in global markets (both local and foreign) are rapidly increasing, and annual sales are quickly approaching $62 billion USD. Minimal cost, wide acceptability due to its reputation as a natural substance with limited efficacy, toxicity in specific problematic conditions, and flexibility in its availability, preparation, and administration are all important elements in this surge in patronage and use.

H.M. refers to a class of biologically active natural substances primarily composed of herbs/herbal materials but may also contain fungal and bee products, minerals (kaolin, bentonite), shells, ash, insects, and animal parts. They are used to maintain health and treat a variety of illnesses. H.M.s can provide numerous benefits, but they can also have negative repercussions. Secondary metabolite activities have been linked to H.M.'s pharmacologic and potentially dangerous effects. In various settings, H.M.S has been used rightly, abused, and misconstrued.

With so many people resorting to herbal remedies, safety is becoming a serious concern. Indeed, certain H.M. has been associated with various serious adverse effects, including cardiotoxicity, neurotoxicity, nephrotoxicity, and cancer. H.M.s can produce toxicity, and the severity of the toxicity varies depending on the herb/herbal material, user, and preparation: minor to severe and occasionally deadly. Other areas of concern include adulteration and the concurrent use of herbal and conventional drugs, which necessitate strict regulation, education, and oversight.

What's exactly is a Herb

Herbs are the leaves of plants used in cooking; they can be fresh or dried.

Spice is simply any other dried component of the plant. These include barks (cinnamon), berries (peppercorns), seeds (cumin), roots (turmeric), flowers (chamomile), buds (cloves), and flower stigmas (saffron).

Herbs are a fantastic way to add color and flavor to savory and sweet foods and drinks without adding oil, salt, or sugar. They each have their own set of health-promoting properties, flavors, and colors.

Fresh herbs have a delicate flavor, so use them in the final few minutes of cooking to get the most out of them. Taste your dish as you go to see if you've added enough seasoning. When not enough herbs are used, the flavor of your food suffers; nevertheless, if too many herbs are utilized, their flavor overpowers the other components.

Herbal health benefits

Herbs may aid in the prevention and control of heart disease, cancer, and diabetes. They also possess anti-inflammatory and anti-tumor properties, which may help avoid blood clots.

Although research is ongoing, studies have revealed that:

• Garlic, fenugreek, linseed, and lemongrass all have cholesterol-lowering qualities.

• Garlic is useful for people with moderately high blood pressure.

• Fenugreek can help regulate blood sugar and insulin activity.

• Many herbs, including onions, garlic, leeks, chives, basil, sage, mint, oregano, and other herbs, can help prevent cancer.

• Herbs, especially cinnamon, cloves, oregano, sage, and thyme, are high in antioxidants and can help decrease low-density lipoprotein cholesterol.

Fresh herbs usually contain higher antioxidant levels than processed or dried herbs. If you're using herbs for their health advantages, use them near the end of the cooking process or right before serving to preserve their characteristics.

Herb-based cuisine

Herbs are only limited by your imagination when it comes to using them in the kitchen; they can be used in practically every meal. Herbs can be mixed into:

• Desserts
• Custards
• Drinks
• Stews and casseroles
• Marinades
• Salad dressings
• Sauces
• Bread
• Soups
• Mustards
• Butters
• Vinegar
• Stocks
• Yogurts
• Vinaigrettes

Adding herbs after a dish has been served is another fantastic way to improve your dish's flavor, fragrance, and visual aspect. For example, a Bolognese sauce with fresh basil leaves on top or a pumpkin and chicken dish with sage leaves on top.

Suggestions for herb-based cuisine

Herbs can be used in a variety of ways, including:

• Fresh herbs have a more intense flavor than dried herbs. A teaspoon of fresh herb is equivalent to four teaspoons of dried herb.

• If you frequently use herbs, make a 'bouquet garni' by tying chopped and blended herbs into small muslin bags that may be mixed into your dish for flavor but must be removed before eating. Some herbs (such as rosemary and parsley) are tougher than others and will retain their flavor during cooking; these should be added at the start.

• Other herbs, such as bay leaves, are only used to flavor food and should not be consumed.

• Because herbs lose flavor over time, discard them after 12 months.

• The flavor of dried whole herbs is superior to loose leaves sold in packets or jars because the leaves are still attached to the stem.

Utilize herbs in creative ways

• Herbs are versatile and can be used in a variety of ways.

The more you use herbs, the more adventurous you will become.

• Not sure where to begin?

• Make a recipe using one or two herbs you've never used before.

• To see how a dish turns out, consider replacing different herbs with the ones listed in the recipe.

• Make your own bouquet garni.

• Grow some herbs in pots on the windowsill or in the yard for cooking.

• Experiment with different flavors at the market.

Aside from boosting your meal's flavor, smell, appearance, and texture, the more you experiment with herbs, the more health benefits you're likely to gain.

Storing Herbs

Dried herbs should be stored in unopened jars in a cool, dark, and dry spice rack. Fresh herbs will last the longest if cleaned, dried correctly, wrapped in a paper towel, placed in a zip-top bag, and refrigerated.

Where can I get advice?

• Market

• Supermarket

• Greengrocer

• Nursery

Digestive System

The digestive tract is now seen as vital to our overall health in several traditional medicine systems. Our digestive system has an impact on our neurological, hormonal, and immune systems.

Auto-immune diseases such as rheumatoid arthritis and multiple sclerosis; behavioral and mental disorders such as ADHD, depression, and autism; degenerative disorders such as Alzheimer's and arthritis; and allergy afflictions such as asthma and eczema, are all instances of problems where foods play a role. Inflammation is at the foundation of these and most chronic diseases, including obesity, heart disease, and cancer.

We can change the foods we eat or how we eat them to reduce these damaging inflammatory reactions. Understanding how to use foods, herbs, and supplements to cure common ailments - such as heartburn, constipation, and indigestion - could be beneficial.

Other factors such as our diet, stress load, alcohol, weight, sleep, circulation, smoking, exercise, liver function, chemicals, food quality, mood and so on, all impact our digestive health. Still, you can begin to support your digestive health by understanding the basic digestive functions and being aware of your body.

Here are some common digestive herbs to include in your diet, as well as the health benefits they provide:

Fennel

Fennel is also a liver stimulant and can help with bloating. It increases milk production, improves appetite and soothes colic. It reduces upper respiratory catarrh and helps as an eyewash for conjunctivitis while also balancing estrogen levels.

Ginger

Ginger is digestively relaxing and warming, as well as anti-nausea and anti-microbial against a range of stomach diseases. When your hands and feet are cold, warm them up.

Garlic

Garlic's antimicrobial and probiotic qualities, as well as its inulin and other components, aid in heart and circulation health. For example, onions, shallots, and leeks are Allium genus members with similar roles.

Turmeric

Turmeric has carminative properties, which means it can help with bloating. It's also antibacterial, anti-inflammatory and liver-friendly.

Caraway

Caraway is a digestive plant that reduces stomach cramps and nausea, aids in gas ejection from the intestine, and prevents stomach fermentation.

Allspice

Allspice soothes and warms the stomach. Eugenol has anti-bacterial properties and stimulates digestive enzymes. It's better to drink it as tea after a meal.

Cinnamon

Cinnamon is a warming appetite stimulant and circulatory stimulant. There are antiviral, antifungal, and antibacterial activities present. Reduces blood sugar and the bacterium that causes ulcers, Helicobacter pylori.

Peppermint

Peppermint is an antispasmodic, cooling, anti-microbial, and refreshing herb. When used topically, it cures coughs and colds, stimulates liver function, and decreases itching.

Dill

Dill is a sedative with a calming effect. It can help you get a good night's sleep while relieving colic and cramping pain. It is an essential component of gripe water.

Circulatory System

In terms of volume, the blood that runs through your veins accounts for 7% of your body weight. The normal adult human body has 4.5 to 5.5 liters of blood. This fluctuates depending on factors such as a person's gender, height, weight, and overall health. This red fluid is quite remarkable in many respects, providing a variety of critical purposes, including carrying oxygen to different body parts, regulating body temperature, and fighting infection and disease.

The importance of healthy blood circulation cannot be emphasized enough. Loss of appetite, prolonged numbness in limbs, unexplained digestive troubles, frequent exhaustion, skin discoloration, varicose veins/brittle nails, and hair — these appear to be symptoms of poor circulation.

What is blood circulation, and how does it help your body function properly?

The thumping heart is in charge of pumping blood around the body. The heart and blood vessels collaborate to maintain blood flow throughout the body. Arteries transport oxygen-rich blood from the heart to every part of the body, whereas veins return carbon dioxide-rich blood to the heart.

What factors contribute to impaired blood circulation?

Several factors influence blood circulation inside the body, including:
- Smoking is one of the primary causes of impaired blood circulation because carbon monoxide damages the cell layer, allowing lipids and plaque to stick to vessel walls, impeding normal blood flow.
- Due to our sedentary lifestyle, we lack time to exercise, and a lack of exercise or movement in daily life can also contribute to poor blood circulation.

- Regular fast food consumption leads to obesity, which obstructs blood flow.

- High/low blood pressure and cholesterol are two of the most common reasons for decreased blood circulation.

What steps can you take to improve your blood circulation?

- **Avoid alcoholic beverages.**

While it is acceptable to drink on occasion, excessive alcohol consumption can contribute to a variety of health problems, including cardiac problems. When you drink alcohol regularly, it's time to cut back on how much you drink each month. Choose healthy alternatives, such as red wine, which is rich in antioxidants and has been shown to improve cholesterol levels and blood flow when consumed in moderation.

- **Keep your hydration up.**

Our organs require water to function properly. Water cleanses our systems of pollutants and improves blood circulation, assisting the body in avoiding health problems.

- **Green tea warning.**

If you drink milk tea all the time, switch to green tea, which is healthier and more stimulating to your body. Green tea helps dilate blood vessels in the body, resulting in enhanced blood flow. Matcha tea is another alternative.

- **Avoid stimulants.**

Limit your intake of stimulants such as coffee to allow your blood to circulate freely. Reduce your intake of sweets and coffee, which dehydrate your body, because improving your blood circulation requires an adequate amount of fluids.

Consider taking circulation-boosting vitamins or increasing your dietary intake of these herbs and other supplements:

- **Honeybee pollen**: Many people take bee pollen pills to help with allergies and colds, but few realize they can also help with circulation. Bee pollen contains rutin, an antioxidant that may help strengthen blood vessels and prevent blood clots, which can cause serious health problems and even death. It may help avoid arterial hardening.

- **Parsley**: Consider eating fresh parsley the next time you sprinkle something on your food. The herb is utilized in many products designed to improve circulation because it can help open up blood arteries, allowing blood to circulate more freely throughout the body. Parsley is particularly high in vitamin C, which is essential for blood vessel health.

- **Hawthorn**: When shopping for supplements, you may discover that many contain Hawthorn. This is because it has been demonstrated to increase circulation and make the heart healthier. By boosting the health of your heart muscle, hawthorn may improve the rhythm of your heart.

- **Ginkgo Biloba**: Gingko Biloba is legitimately used by German doctors to improve their patients' circulation and a range of other health issues. It is intended to help those with asthma and improve cognition due to increased brain circulation. It also increases blood flow to the heart and heals blood vessels.

- **Cacao**: Although you don't need another reason to love chocolate, studies have shown that the beans used to manufacture everyone's favorite sweet treat can help your circulatory system operate better. It contains an antioxidant that encourages your body's production of new blood vessels, resulting in improved blood flow. It's also thought to keep your veins and arteries healthy.

- **Cayenne Pepper**: Cayenne pepper has been used for years to cure anything from toothaches to headaches, but it can also increase circulation due to a component called capsicum. In fact, when you consume cayenne pepper or take a tablet, your blood flow improves almost immediately. Some paramedics are believed to keep it on hand and administer it to stroke or heart attack victims. To gain health benefits, take cayenne pepper as a supplement or incorporate it into your diet.

Before taking any herb or supplement, talk to your doctor about how it might affect you or if there are any potential side effects. Some supplements may conflict with medications you are already taking or exacerbate pre-existing health concerns.

Integumentary System

Sage: Sage appears to be an antioxidant powerhouse, which means it is a rock star in anti-aging, combating free radicals, and acting as a natural astringent for oily, acne-prone skin.

It's also high in vitamin A and calcium, both necessary for cell regeneration. To control sebum production, make a nice-smelling toner out of it. Boil the leaves for your hair, then rinse with cool water.

Hot Peppers: Chili, cayenne pepper, paprika, and jalapeño do more than thrill your taste buds; they also help protect your skin. "Vitamins A and C in peppers help resist free radicals, reducing collagen degradation and maintaining the integrity of your skin. Capsaicin, contained in colorful peppers, acts as a sunscreen, protecting the skin from UV radiation damage. Peppers must be consumed to reap the benefits of their healing characteristics, as capsaicin, which improves the skin from within, may burn if applied topically. "Hot peppers are just so easy to incorporate into any dish," says Wolfson. Use jalapeno, cayenne, and chili peppers in guacamole.

Mint: Because of the salicylic acid (which also helps with excess oil), mint is an effective natural acne treatment. Mint juice is also anti-pruritic, meaning it soothes itchy, irritated skin.

To remove cracked feet, boil mint leaves and soak them in water. You can also prepare a paste from a few leaves to treat pimples on the spot, or you can construct a DIY mask using oatmeal and honey. Mint can be used to make a cooling and relaxing astringent.

Lavender: Lavender is an antibacterial and anti-inflammatory powerhouse that will soothe your mind as well as treat itchy, inflamed skin.

Infuse dried or fresh flowers into creams, toners, and facial steams. Your mixture will not only smell wonderful, but it will also help improve circulation and calm your skin.

Calendula: Calendula contains a high concentration of flavonoids and carotenoids (both powerful antioxidants), so it's no surprise that it can help with everything from chapped lips to wrinkles. It has been shown to improve wound healing, plump skin through circulation and hydration, and reduce inflammation.

One of the most lovely ways to use calendula is to drop the flower heads into a bath and soak up the benefits.

Chamomile: Several of the most potent ingredients found in your favorite natural skincare products began their lives on Earth. So, why not grow your own naturally attractive foods for a change? Here are some skin-friendly herbs you can grow in your backyard or window herb garden.

Chamomile relieves acne, rashes, and eczema by reducing inflammation. Due to its lightening properties, the chemical has been shown to aid in discoloration caused by sunburns/acne.

Make yourself a cup of chamomile tea. Allow it to cool. It should be used to thoroughly cleanse the entire body. Additionally, a homemade facial treatment can help decrease wrinkles and fine lines, and using chamomile as a hair rinse can help retain and nourish color-treated hair. Alternatively, a tried-and-true method for puffiness and dark circles is to place tea bags over your eyes.

Thyme: According to research, thyme is more effective than typical store-bought acne treatments because of its antibacterial protection over problematic areas.

Combine witch hazel, brewed green tea, and thyme for a less-drying acne-fighting toner. This combination can also be used to construct a mask with cosmetic clay (such as bentonite).

Aloe Vera: Aloe Vera is rich in minerals, vitamins, and other skin-beneficial substances. It's hydrating, anti-inflammatory, moisturizing, and anti-aging, and it can help with skin cell turnover.

No DIY is required here. Cut the leaves apart with a sharp knife, scoop out the gel, and use it as a skin soother, moisturizer, leave-in conditioner, scalp mask, or aftershave treatment. If you want to get creative, add it to a skin-quenching smoothie for inside-out benefits.

Rosemary: The potent small leaves of the rosemary plant can aid with anything from skin moisturizing to collagen synthesis to fighting free radicals. It's also high in minerals, which protect the skin from environmental damage like sun exposure. It also helps with skin suppleness as you age.

To fight acne, dilute rosemary oil with water and use it as a natural astringent. Massage the oil into your scalp to promote hair growth and eliminate dandruff. Use rosemary oil with a cleanser to enhance circulation and refresh skin.

Cinnamon: Cinnamon adds a spicy flavor to pastries and hot drinks but is also abundant in antioxidants, which fight skin damage. According to Keri Glassman, author of The O2 Diet, "cinnamon contains more antioxidant power than 1/2 cup of blueberries." For an easy antioxidant boost, sprinkle 1/2 teaspoon of cinnamon on the coffee grounds shortly before brewing.

Glassman suggests throwing out spices that are more than two years old and storing them in a dark closet because heat from the stove and sunlight will impair their efficacy.

Nervous System Treatments

One of the remarkable aspects of herbalism is that it acknowledges healing as a holistic process that promotes the balance of the mind, spirit, and body. According to herbalists and traditional healers, stress and life perspectives greatly impact our health, and every fiber of our being is intertwined. While stress is mostly an emotional state that many people in the twenty-first century encounter, it also has physical implications. As a result, every healing process must incorporate an understanding of and support for our nervous system.

Nervous System Supporting Herbs

You may be wondering where herbs fit into all of this. We use two herbs to help the nervous system in Western herbalism: nervines and adaptogens.

Nerve relaxants include herbs such as chamomile, valerian, and passionflower. We use these herbs in blends such as Nighty Night tea to help with occasional insomnia and Chamomile with Lavender tea for a worried stomach because they provide rapid relief from nervous tension. These herbs can help with stress that affects your sympathetic nervous system, sometimes called "fight-or-flight."

If your nervous system is frequently overworked and requires full-body support, adaptogens are another excellent family of herbal companions. Adaptogens like reishi, astragalus, and ashwagandha can help you boost your stamina and rebalance your body, allowing you to better defend yourself against the negative effects of stress.

Adaptogens are named after the Latin word 'adaptare,' which means "to adjust" or "to change." We like to think that these powerful botanicals help us deal with the stress and exhaustion of life's trials. These healing plants can be safely incorporated into everyday rituals and foods.

In fact, herbs are only one component of a full nerve-soothing regimen. Taking a warm bath, eating healthy meals, meditating, and spending time outside are good practices that can help reduce stress and improve your quality of life. Stress-relieving herbs may be useful functional nutrients for the human body, assisting in physiological process balance, healing, and normalization.

Herbs that Help You Manage Stress Healthily

Chamomile: Chamomile is commonly called the "mother's hug" herb. Chamomile leaves can be soaked in water to make a relaxing tea related to better sleep patterns.

Passionflower: Passionflower is another safe, fast-acting herb related to anxiety alleviation and restoration of tranquility.

Kava: The effects of kava on stress and anxiety have been carefully studied. It has a long history of alleviating tension and anxiety in Polynesia.

Lemon balm: Lemon balm leaves can be used to make an herbal tea that is appropriate for people of all ages and stages of life. Lemon balm can provide immediate relief by calming your nervous system without being sedative.

Ashwagandha: Ashwagandha is an adrenal adaptogen, which means it regulates cortisol levels. Ashwagandha is known to have a calming effect on the nervous system, especially during tiredness, and is connected to increased immunity.

Herbs for Stress, Anxiety, and Exhaustion

When your adrenal glands produce too much cortisol, it activates your sympathetic nervous system, activating the "fight or flight" reaction. Adrena-adaptogenic herbs, such as ashwagandha, help the body healthily respond to stress by reducing cortisol production. Due to a shortage of nutrition, your body cannot produce neurotransmitters inside the nervous system when stressed.

The following nutrients are required:
• B vitamins

• Magnesium

• Calcium

Other Plants and Herbs for Stress Reduction
• Oats

• Nettle leaf

• St. John's Wort

Adrenal tonics are the adrenal cortex and adrenal medulla tissues that need to be restored. Licorice and Rehmannia are two adrenal tonics. Adrenal adaptogens help people adjust to adrenal hormone production that is "in line with what life requires." Angela describes their effect as "like a dimmer switch," resetting the body's cortisol levels to normal, baseline levels.

Herbs for a Good Night's Sleep
Many people have difficulty falling or staying asleep. Herbs can help with both of these problems. Angela recommends steeping chamomile for around 20 minutes to make it therapeutic. Eat a protein-rich meal before retiring to bed.

Children's Herbal Safety and Calming Herbs

Herbal stress treatment can benefit children since it is a gentle, discreet, and safe approach. The liquid herbs are easy to dose; start with a few drops and gradually increase the amount as needed. Stress can have an impact on children. Angela recommends lemon balm, chamomile, ashwagandha, and passionflower for this.

Compliance and Adherence of Children to Medicinal Herbs

Angela recommends administering herbs to children as a sort of medication as early as possible in their lives to help them become accustomed to the effects and taste of herbs. She also suggests that families consume herbs together in the mornings and nights, gradually introducing the herb flavor.

Roots of Healing: An Encounter with Native American Herbal Wisdom

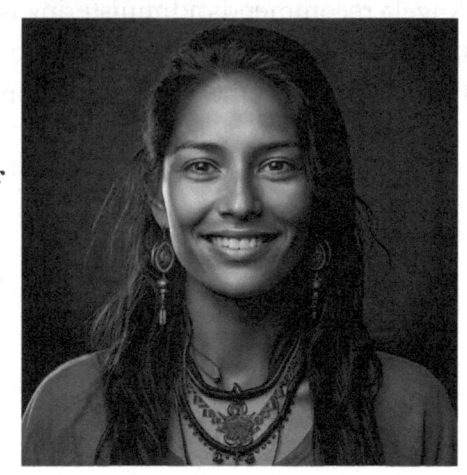

During a recent visit to a remote Native American community, deeply nestled within the untouched expanses of the natural world, I experienced an encounter that profoundly encapsulated the essence of this book's teachings. This visit was not only a journey through the majestic landscapes but also a profound exploration into the heart of traditional Native American herbalism. One afternoon, as the golden hues of the sun kissed the earth, a community elder invited me to join in a sacred gathering. The purpose was to prepare a young individual for an upcoming ceremonial rite of passage. The elder, well-versed in the ancient practices of herbal medicine, shared with us the significance of each herb we were to use, echoing the wisdom passed down through generations. As we sat in a circle, surrounded by the vibrant tapestry of the natural world, the elder began to blend an assortment of herbs, each carefully chosen for its spiritual and healing properties. Among them were sage for purification, cedar for protection, and sweetgrass to invite good spirits and positive energy. The meticulous preparation of these herbs was a living testament to the teachings enshrined in the early chapters of "Native American Herbalists Bible: 13 Books in 1." The elder explained how these herbs, when combined, create a powerful synergy that not only supports physical healing but also promotes spiritual well-being, facilitating a deeper connection with the natural world and the guiding spirits of their tradition. This practice, deeply rooted in respect for the Earth and its bounty, was a profound demonstration of the holistic approach to health and healing that is a cornerstone of Native American herbalism. This encounter was a vivid reminder of the timeless relevance of the knowledge preserved within "Native American Herbalists Bible: 13 Books in 1." It underscored the importance of not only understanding the healing properties of herbs but also appreciating the cultural and spiritual dimensions that imbue these practices with deeper meaning. As I left the gathering, the elder's parting words resonated deeply within me: "The plants are our oldest teachers. Listen to them, and they will guide you." This profound experience reaffirmed my commitment to

sharing the rich heritage of Native American herbalism, hoping to inspire others to embark on their own journey of discovery, healing, and connection with the natural world. As we explore the *"Native American Herbalists Bible: 13 Books in 1"* together, I hope that you, too, can sense the profound connection to the Earth and its healing gifts that Native American herbalism fosters. This book is not merely a collection of remedies; it is an invitation to partake in a living tradition that nurtures holistic well-being.

If you find resonance and insight within these pages, I encourage you to share your journey with others. Your reflections can illuminate the path for more individuals to rediscover and embrace this ancient path of wellness. When crafting your review, consider reflecting on aspect such as:

- **Depth of Information:** Did the book comprehensively cover the topics, making you feel informed and prepared to use herbal remedies?
- **Practical Application:** How did you find the real-world application of the remedies and techniques? Did the book instill confidence in using herbs for health and healing?
- **Educational Value:** Which sections or teachings have been most beneficial in your herbal journey?

To share your thoughts, simply visit the ORDERS section of your Amazon account and click on the "Write a product review" button, or scan this QR Code

Additionally, if you have any suggestions for enhancing the book or wish to share your experiences with Native American herbal remedies, your insights are warmly welcomed at *info@herbfulharmony.com*.

Together, let us honor and propagate the legacy of Native American herbalism, paving the way for a future enriched by its wisdom and healing power.

With gratitude and solidarity,
__Aiyana Tessay__

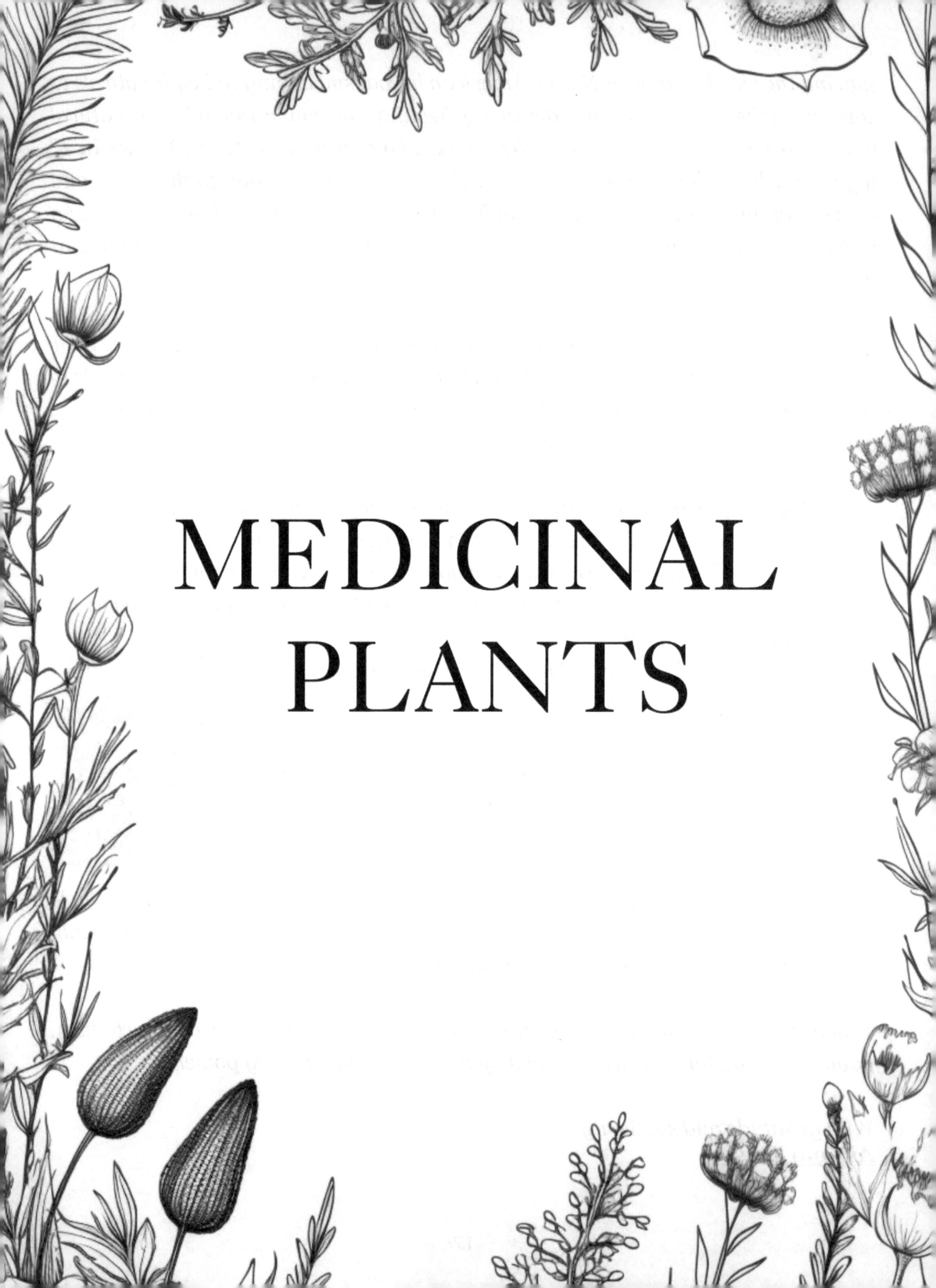

MEDICINAL PLANTS

1. ACAI

Acai is a fruit that can help reduce inflammation and enhance blood circulation. It may be useful when there are other causes of implantation problems, such as endometriosis, fibroids, or scar tissue from past surgical treatments. Acai Berries. Acai (Euterpe oleracea Mart.) is a South American palm tree that grows widely in Brazil, Colombia, Surinam, and the Amazonian floodplains.

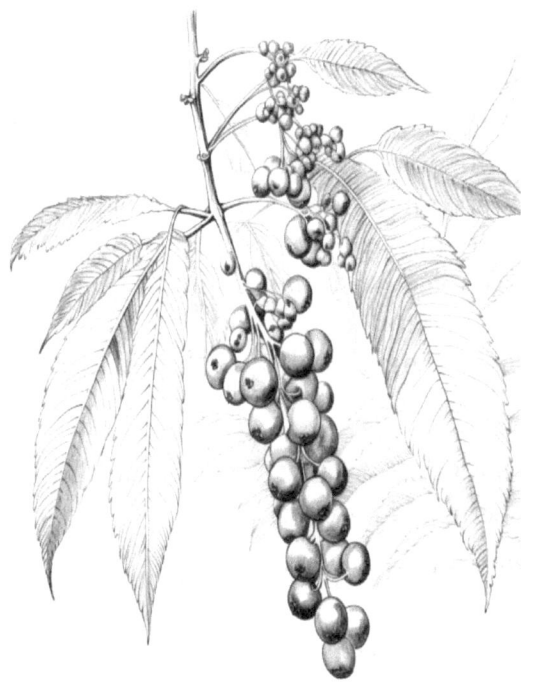

NATIVE AREA: Brazil, Colombia, and Suriname

MEDICINAL PART: Berries.

MEDICINAL USES: Arthritis, erectile dysfunction, skin appearance, weight loss, high cholesterol detoxification and general health.

SCIENTIFIC NAME: Euterpe oleracea.

2. ALFALFA

Alfalfa (Medicago sativa) is a plant that has been used for millennia as animal feed. It has long been valued because it contains more minerals, vitamins, and protein than other feed sources.

Alfalfa is a member of the legume family, but it is also categorized as a herb. It appears to have come from South and Central Asia. It has continued to grow for millennia all throughout the world.

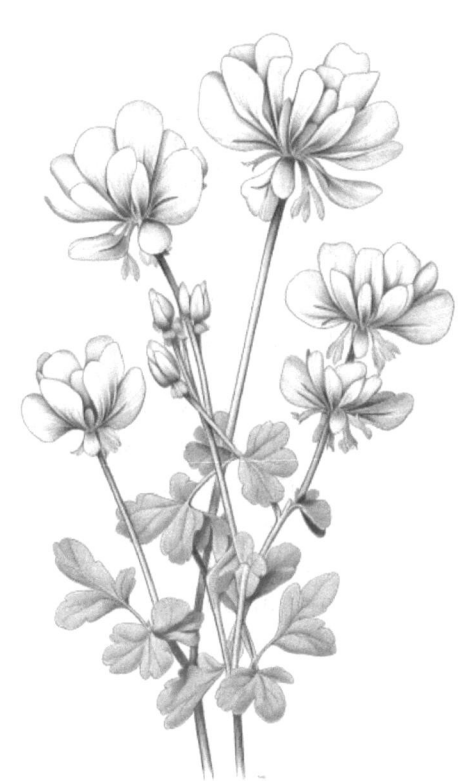

Alfalfa has been used for centuries to help with fertility concerns since it can enhance uterine blood flow and promote healthy menstrual cycles. This makes alfalfa a suitable choice if you have irregular periods, no periods, or have lately been unable to conceive despite ovulating frequently.

NATIVE AREA: Southwest Asia.

MEDICINAL PART: Leaves, sprouts, and seeds.

MEDICINAL USES: Increase blood flow.

SCIENTIFIC NAME: Medicago sativa.

3. ALLSPICE

This spice is utilized in spells and rituals because it can attract all things financial. The aroma of allspice can be utilized to attract customers or enhance sales. Allspice is a spice manufactured from the dried berries of the plant Pimenta dioica, which belongs to the Myrtle family. Allspice has a flavor similar to cinnamon, cloves, nutmeg, and pepper. Allspice is utilized in various cuisines, including Caribbean, Middle Eastern, and Latin American dishes.

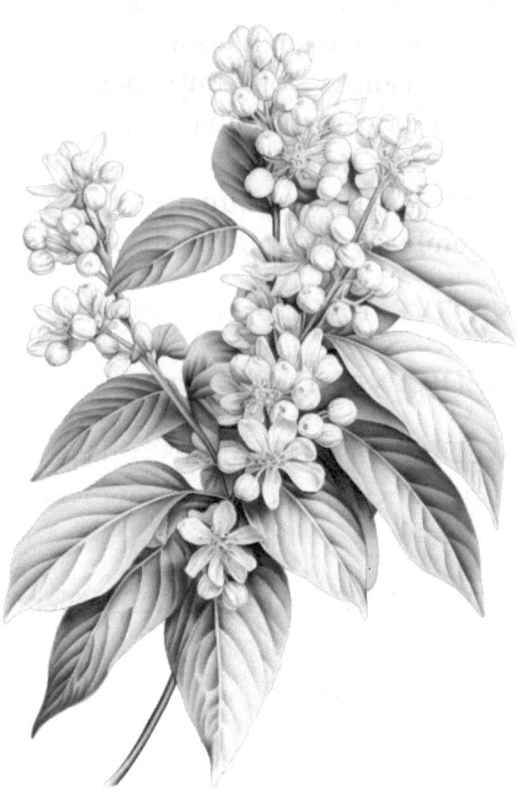

NATIVE AREA: Greater Antilles, southern Mexico, and Central America.

MEDICINAL PART: The unripe berries and leaves.

MEDICINAL USES: Vomiting, diarrhea, fever, cold, indigestion, intestinal gas, abdominal pain, heavy menstrual cycles, high blood pressure, diabetes, and obesity

SCIENTIFIC NAME: Pimenta dioica.

4. ALOE VERA

Although it is commonly used to cure sunburns, aloe vera can also be used to heal small burns from various sources, as well as bug bites. Aloe vera's anti-inflammatory qualities aid with gout pain but can also help with dry skin or dermatitis. This plant is frequently used to heal scrapes, diabetes, skin problems such as acne and psoriasis.

It contains toxins that can gradually act within the body to aid complete healing. Aloe vera has received much attention for its capacity to promote healthy skin and weight loss by increasing metabolism and burning fat while aiding in cell regeneration. It was utilized as a conventional cure for many various ailments in ancient times, and it still holds true now.

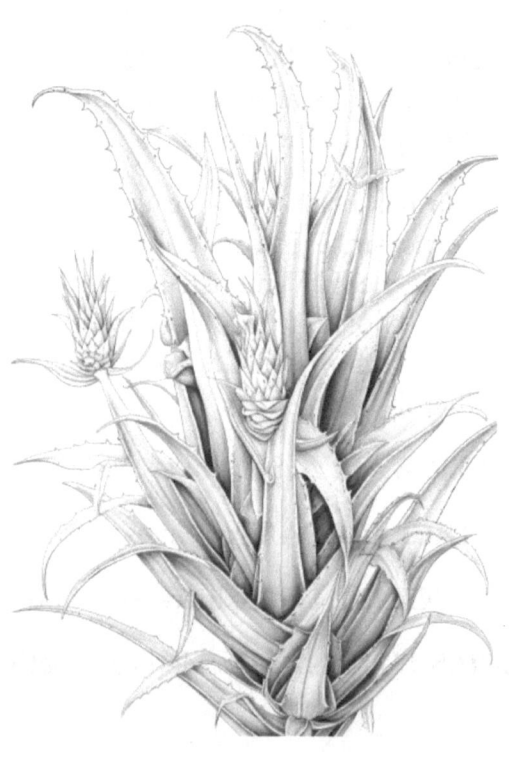

NATIVE AREA: Africa, Madagascar, Arabian Peninsula.

MEDICINAL PART: Leaf.

MEDICINAL USES: Treat sunburns, relieve heartburn, battle dental plaque, and reduce blood sugar levels.

5. AMARANTH

Amaranth stems and leaves were used as a substitute for coffee beans by the Incas, and for this reason, it's commonly known as 'The Grain of the Incas' in Spanish. Along with their tasty leaves, amaranths are also known for their brilliant colors in the fall when they die.

Chemicals found in amaranth function as antioxidants. Some animal study suggests that amaranth can lower total cholesterol and "bad" LDL cholesterol while enhancing "good" HDL cholesterol, which has sparked interest in utilizing it to treat high cholesterol. However, amaranth does not appear to provide these advantages in humans.

NATIVE AREA: Mexico and Central America.

MEDICINAL PART: Entire plant.

MEDICINAL USES: Ulcers, swelling of the mouth or throat, diarrhea and high cholesterol.

SCIENTIFIC NAME: Amaranthus caudatus, Amaranthus tricolor.

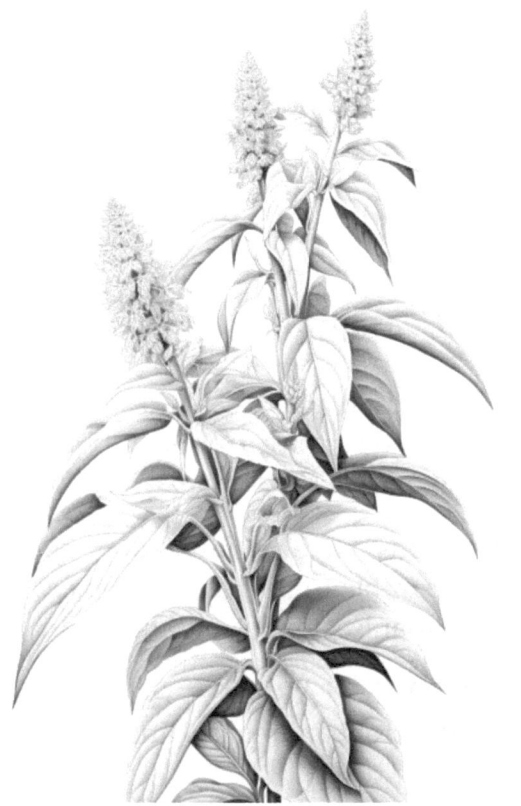

6. AMARYLLIS

Because it can bloom into gorgeous white blooms in 24 hours, the Amaryllis plant has become particularly popular throughout Christmas. This is why it is also known as the 'Instant Flower.'

It is a tiny genus with two species of flowering bulbs. Amaryllis belladonna is the most well-known of the two, a native of South Africa's Western Cape region, namely the rocky southwest area between the Olifants River Valley and Knysna.

Because it is commonly given during Christmas, most people associate the bright red Amaryllis with the holiday season. This flower comes in various colors: red, white, pink, orange, yellow, and purple.

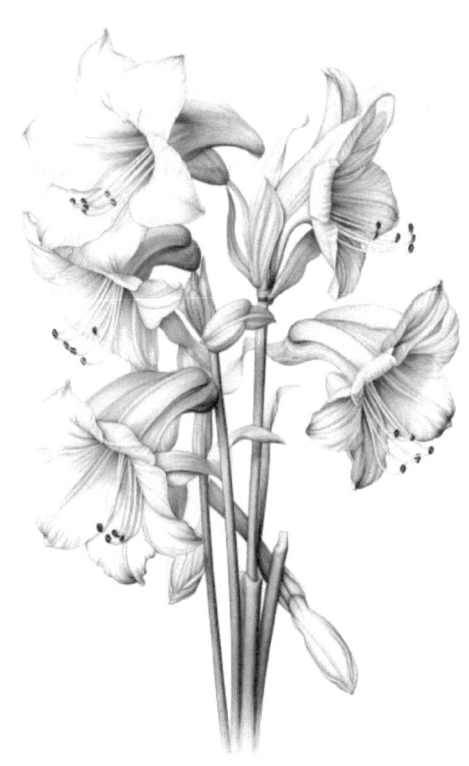

The name Amaryllis is a little puzzling. Hippeastrum is a flowering genus with the common name Amaryllis. In the early nineteenth century, this genus was split from Amaryllis. On the other hand, the genus Amaryllis is still alive and well today: the nude lady is the most common species. Hippeastrum and Amaryllis share similar forms, except for the Hippeastrum's hollow stem. Hippeastrum is a genus that has approximately 90 species and over 600 hybrids.

NATIVE AREA: South Africa.

MEDICINAL PART: Leaves and bulb.

MEDICINAL USES: Depression, seizures, and anxiety.

SCIENTIFIC NAME: Amaryllis belladonna.

7. ANISE

This plant has a sweet and spicy aroma and is sometimes used with honey as a cough suppressant. It is used to attract prosperity and abundance in protection and money spells. Anise, commonly known as aniseed or anix, is a flowering plant in the Apiaceae family.

Its seeds have a flavor and perfume comparable to that of other spices such as star anise, fennel, and licorice.

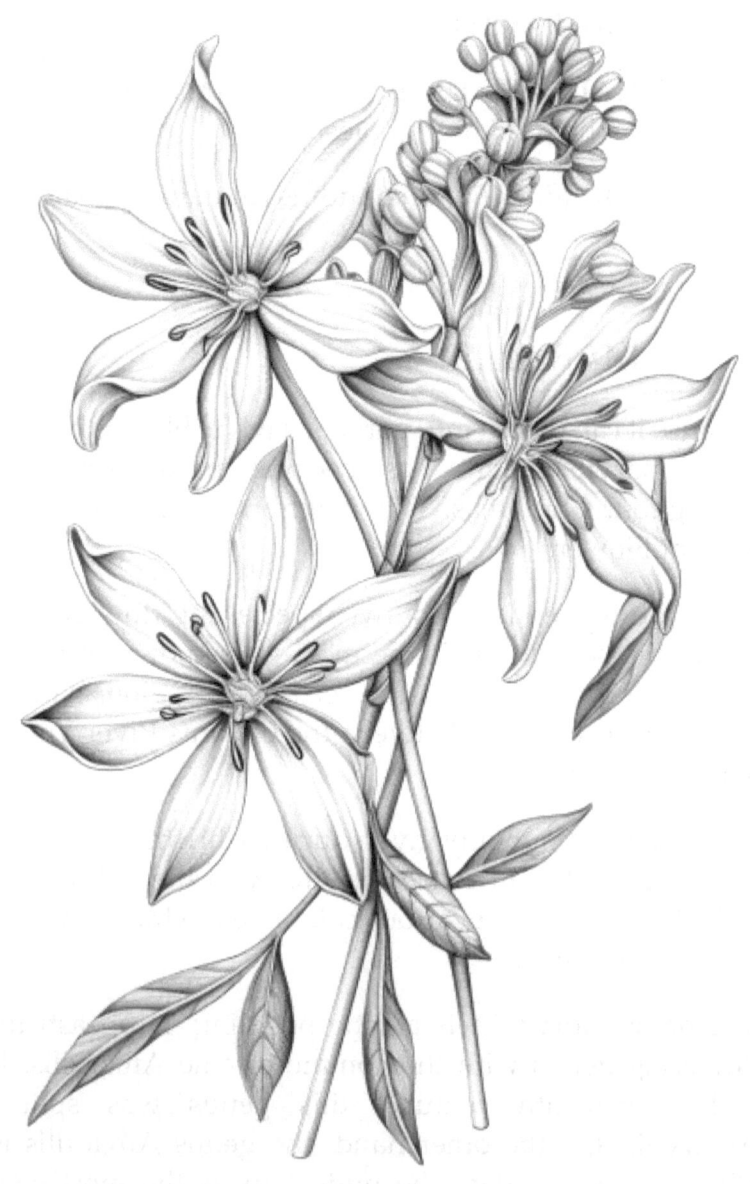

NATIVE AREA: The eastern Mediterranean region and Southwest Asia.

MEDICINAL PART: The seed (fruit), oil, the root and leaf.

MEDICINAL USES: As a diuretic and an appetite stimulant, it is used to treat stomach distress, intestinal gas and "runny nose,"

SCIENTIFIC NAME: Pimpinella anisum

8. ASTILBE

The astilbe plant is a medical herb used by persons who want to bring prosperity into their life as well as those who want to become wealthy. Many people enjoy the plant's blossoms because the petals have been used to make a healing oil that can be applied directly to the skin.

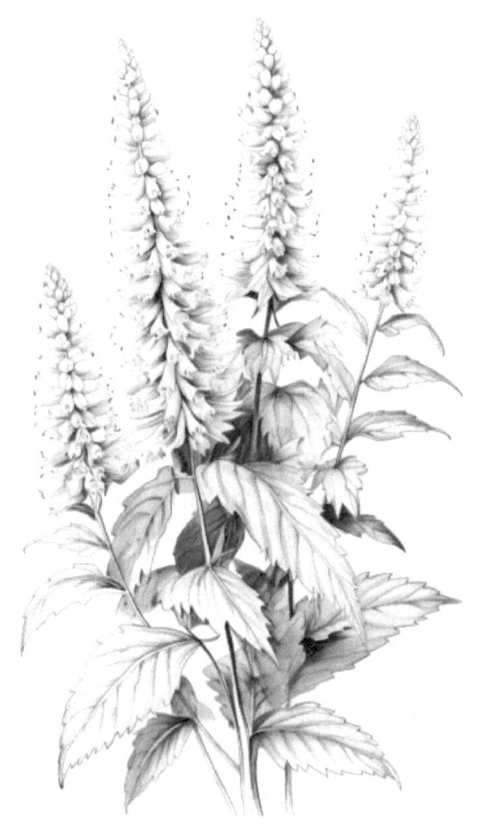

Asia and North America are home to Astilbe species. They are hardy perennials with fluffy blooms in white, pink, or crimson that add color to the landscape. They can withstand direct sunlight. They will, however, bloom more freely if they are exposed to sunlight.

NATIVE AREA: Asia and North America.

MEDICINAL PART: Leaves.

MEDICINAL USES: Diarrhea, dysentery, ulcer, inflammation and body ache.

SCIENTIFIC NAME: Astilbe Chinensis.

9. AVENA SATIVA

This plant, often known as "oat," has been utilized in Asia and Europe for almost 5,000 years for its nutritional content and because offers several health advantages for both the body and the psyche. Taoists and Buddhists have traditionally used it for its cleansing effects. Avena sativa (Poaceae), known as oat, oats, green oat, or milky oat, is a plant native to Europe, the Mediterranean, North Africa, and northern Central Asia, now grown worldwide.

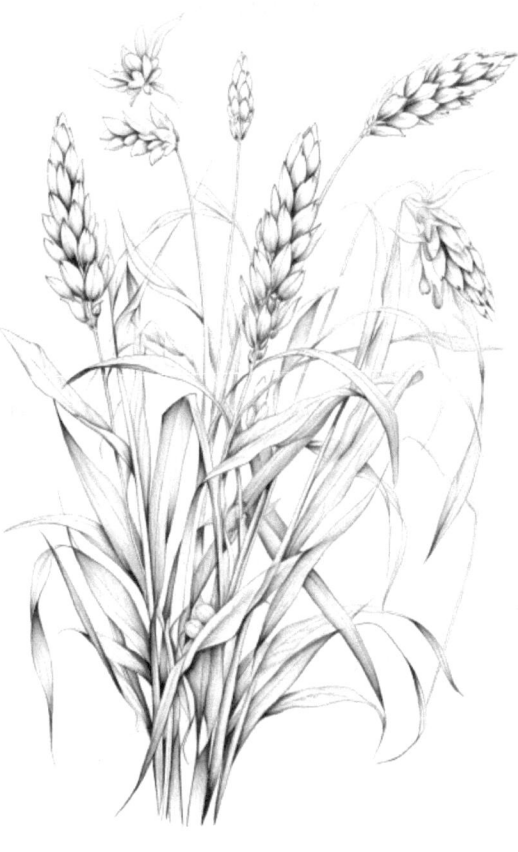

NATIVE AREA: Europe, the Mediterranean, North Africa, and northern Central Asia.

MEDICINAL PART: Plant.

MEDICINAL USES: helps in reducing weight, lowering cholesterol and improving heart health.

10.   AZALEA

This lovely flower might assist in resuming their lives after a tragedy. It can also be used in purifying spells to eliminate negative energy from a person's home. Azaleas in the yard would provide protection to any witch or wizard.

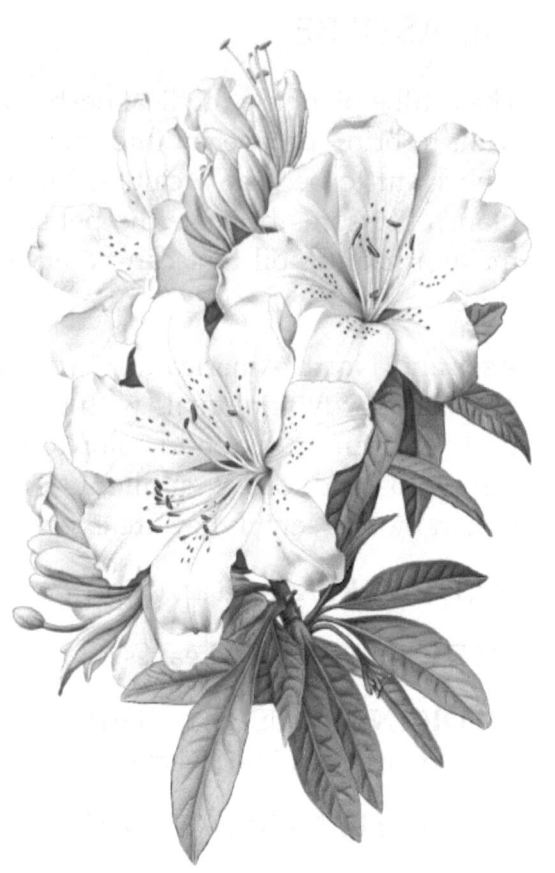

Most North American azaleas are located in the Appalachian mountains range, from Maine to Florida. All indigenous trees in North America are deciduous, with open, loosely branching patterns, and are known for their hardiness and gorgeous fall foliage. The flowers have calming, analgesic, and anesthetic properties. They treat arthritis, cavities, itching, maggots, and severe injuries. The root is used to cure arthritis, rheumatism, and severe injuries.

NATIVE AREA: North America.

MEDICINAL PART: Flowers and roots.

MEDICINAL USES: Treat arthritis, cavities, itch, maggots, and severe injuries.

SCIENTIFIC NAME: Rhododendron.

11.   BAY LEAVES

Bay leaves are sometimes used in money charms because they are supposed to bring good fortune and riches with each leaf carried or burned. Bay leaf charcoal is frequently used to drive negative energy away from an area, making it a potent cleansing plant. Preparations: The whole leaf can be used in cooking or made into tea.

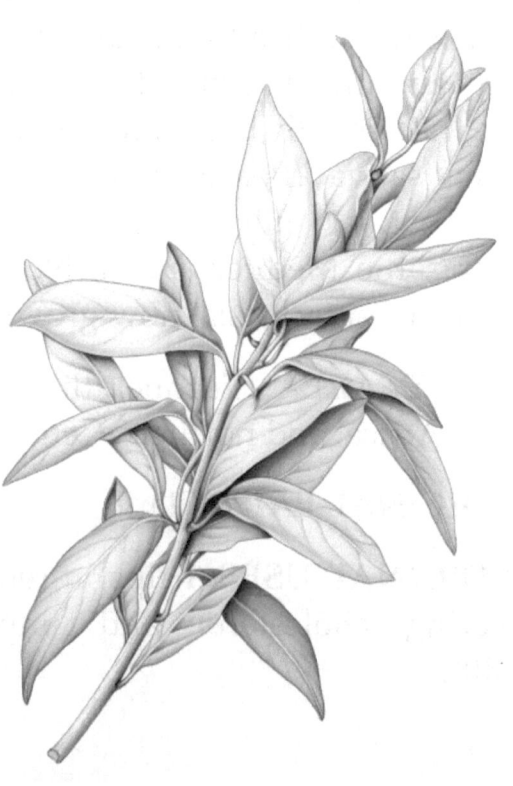

NATIVE AREA: Mediterranean and widely cultivated in North America, Central America, India, Russia, France, Italy, Turkey, Spain, and Mexico.

MEDICINAL PART: Leaves.

MEDICINAL USES: Sprains, indigestion, rheumatism, earaches.

SCIENTIFIC NAME: Laurus nobilis.

12.   BASIL

For an unexpected cash windfall; to feel bold; to be optimistic; to be satisfied; to become wealthy. Basil, sometimes known as large basil, is a culinary herb in the Lamiaceae family.

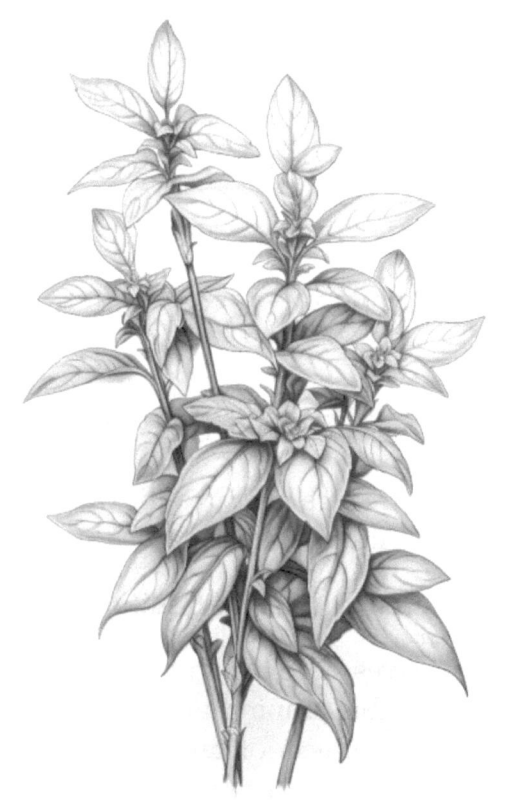

Basil is indigenous to tropical areas ranging from central Africa to Southeast Asia. It is a delicate plant that is utilized in cuisines all over the world. There are numerous basil cultivars, as well as other related species or hybrids that are also known as basil.

Basil contains anti-bacterial aromatic oils, making it effective in treating illnesses. It is useful in treating food poisoning, stomach infections, and even gum infections. Make sure you use fresh basil for this, because dried or processed basil will not work.

NATIVE AREA: India, central Africa, Southeast Asia

MEDICINAL PART: parts of the plant that grow above the ground.

MEDICINAL USES: Stomach problems

SCIENTIFIC NAME: Ocimum basilicum.

13.   BEGONIA

The begonia has been around since at least 1690 when it was cultivated by Sir Edmond Enderby of England. However, it was not until 1720 that Begonia became widely known for its beauty. The appeal of the begonia lies in its pretty leaves and bright flowers.

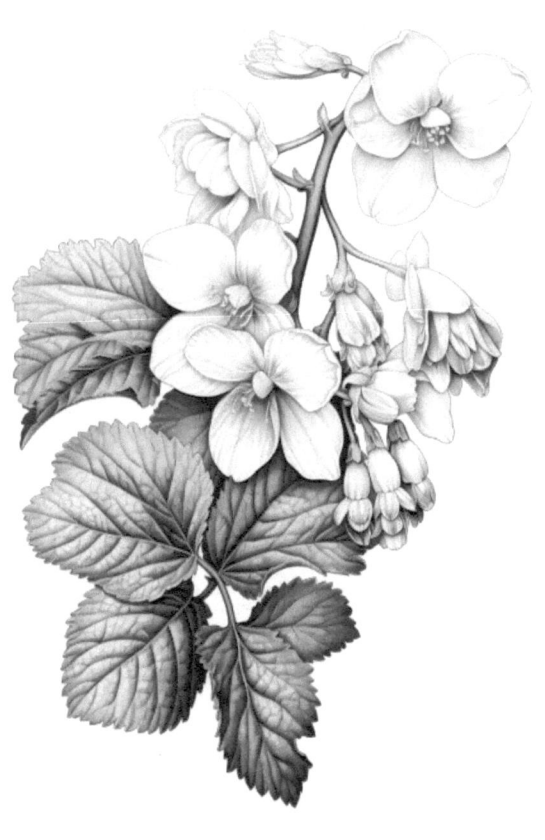

Begonias are native to the tropics and subtropics; none are native to the United States. They can be found in Central and South America, Asia, and Sub-Saharan Africa, among other places.

Many begonias prefer damp, cool woodlands and tropical rainforests as their natural habitat, but some have adapted to drier conditions. Traditionally, begonia is used as a wild herb/whole plant to soothe sore nipples. The juice of the entire plant is used to cure peptic ulcers and alleviate headaches. The paste is used to stop bleeding from cuts and wounds, as well as to treat ringworm and scabies externally.

NATIVE AREA: Central and South America, Asia and Sub-Saharan Africa.

MEDICINAL PART: Whole plant.

MEDICINAL USES: Headaches, ulcers, cuts and wounds

SCIENTIFIC NAME: Begonia semperflorens.

14.   BLACKBERRY

Blackberries are high in antioxidants, particularly anthocyanins. They are an effective treatment for skin conditions such as rashes and eczema.

Blackberry leaf tea has traditionally been used to heal sore throats, aching gums, and mouth ulcers.

The leaves are high in vitamin C, hydrolyzable tannins, and flavonoids. The astringent effects of tannins help to tone the mucosa. As a result, it is said to be beneficial for gastrointestinal discomfort and diarrhea.

NATIVE AREA: North temperate regions.

MEDICINAL PART: The leaf, root, and fruit.

MEDICINAL USES: Diarrhea, diabetes, gout, fluid retention, and pain and swelling (inflammation); and for preventing cancer and heart disease.

SCIENTIFIC NAME: Rubus.

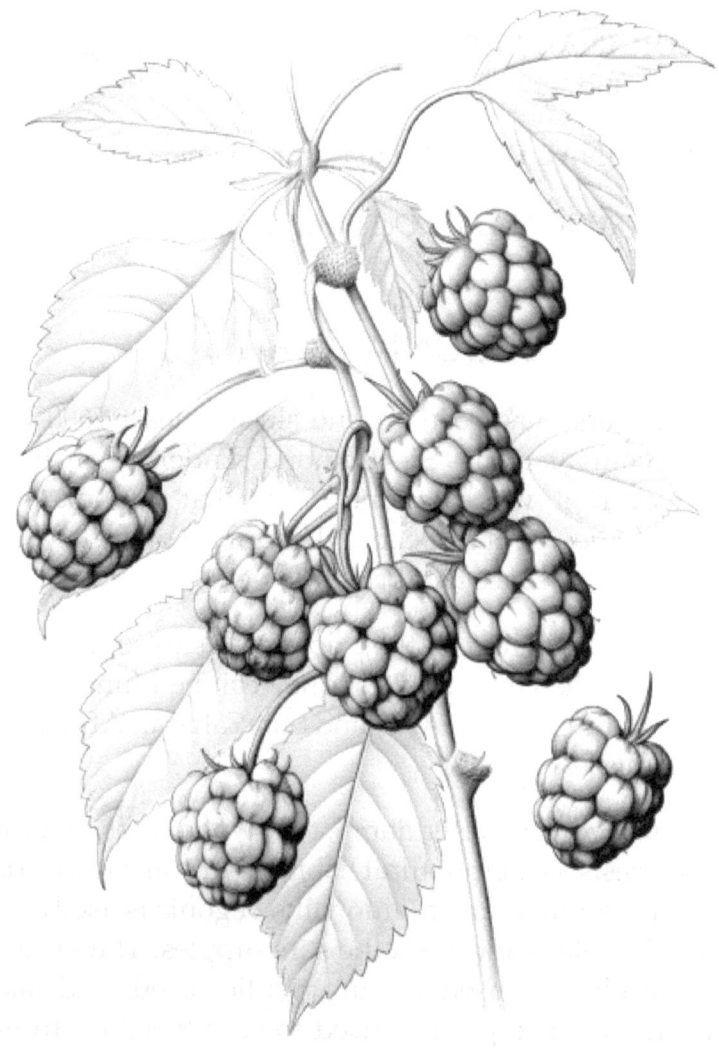

15.   BLACK COHOSH

Native Americans utilized the black cohosh root, a perennial plant native to the eastern United States and Canada, to treat colds, coughs, rheumatism, kidney issues, malaria, menstrual disorders, menopause symptoms such as hot flashes and night sweats, as well as to induce labor and lactation.

Over the last few decades, black cohosh has increased in favor of nonpharmacologic treatment for menopausal symptoms in Europe and the United States. Clinical trials, on the other hand, have yielded conflicting results thus far.

Despite the absence of conclusive evidence, black cohosh remains a popular alternative to hormone therapy, which has been linked to an increased risk of heart attacks, strokes, and breast cancer.

Black Cohosh has long been used as a natural anti-inflammatory and pain reliever, and it can aid in the reduction of menstrual cramps.

This may increase implantation rates by increasing blood flow to the uterus.

The Ranunculaceae family includes black cohosh. It is a native medicinal plant that grows in rich woodlands from Maine to Ontario, south to Georgia, and west to Missouri and Indiana.

NATIVE AREA: North America.

MEDICINAL PART: Roots and rhizome.

MEDICINAL USES: Improving weak bones.

SCIENTIFIC NAME: Actaea racemose.

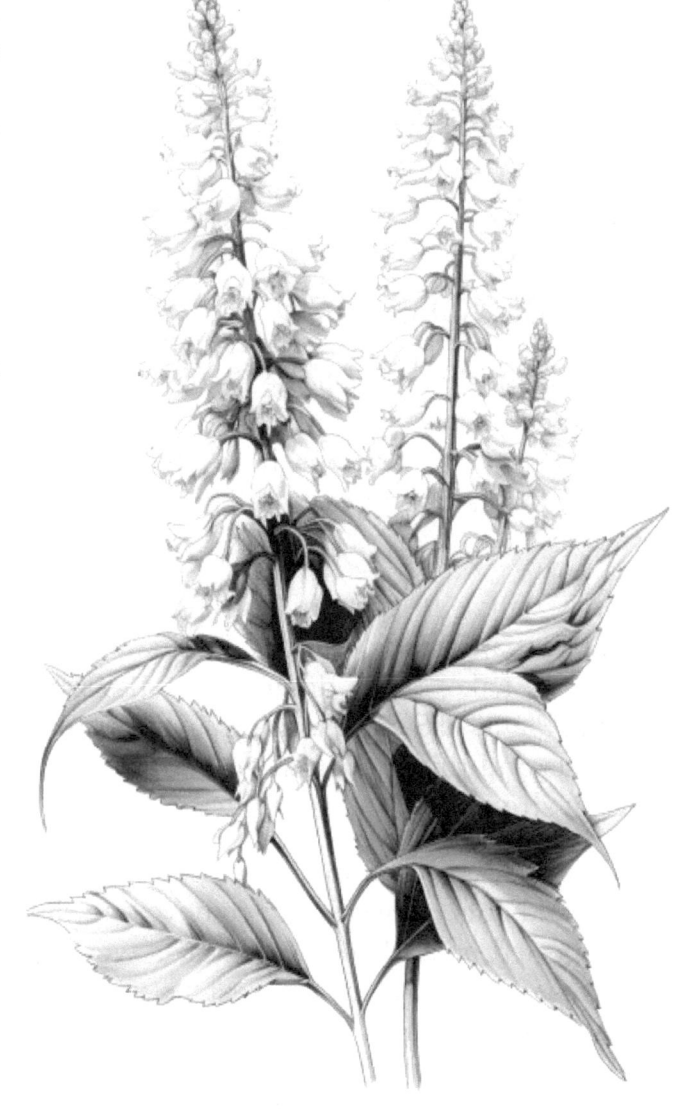

16.   BLESSED THISTLE

Blessed Thistle is a blooming plant that delivers nutrients to the body, relieves pain, inflammation and fever, promotes healing in the body and can aid with women's bleeding.

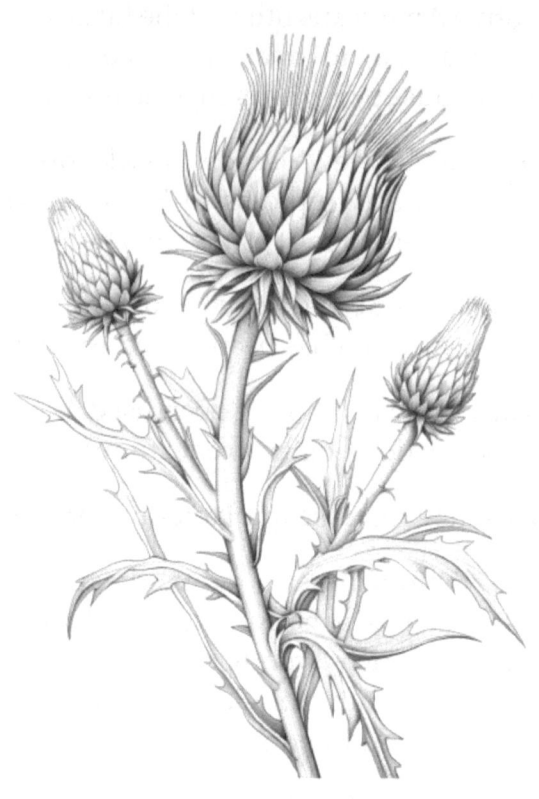

The blessed thistle (Cnicus benedictus) is a Mediterranean plant that grows from southern France to Iran. It is distinguished by its dandelion-like hairy leaves and fuzzy yellow blooms. Blessed thistle tannin components may help with diarrhea, coughing, and edema.

Blessed thistle has been used to treat indigestion, infections, wounds, and various other diseases, but no scientific evidence supports these claims.

NATIVE AREA: Mediterranean region.

MEDICINAL PART: Roots and leaves.

MEDICINAL USES: Indigestion, infections, wounds.

SCIENTIFIC NAME: Cnicus benedictus.

17.   BLOODROOT

Bloodroot is a lovely and delicate flower that grows in the eastern United States. The plant has been used for its medical powers for generations, but Native Americans also employed it for its power over evil spirits and protection against curses.

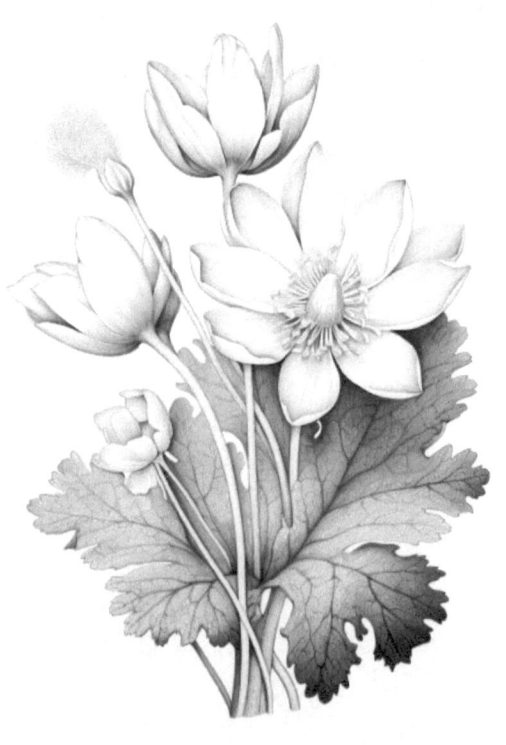

Bloodroot is native to eastern North America, stretching from Nova Scotia, Canada, south to Florida, USA, and west to the Great Lakes and down the Mississippi River embayment. Plants of Sanguinaria canadensis grow in moist to dry forests and thickets, often on flood plains and near coastlines or streams on slopes.

It is commonly used to promote the healing characteristics of wounds and cuts, as well as to remove any dead tissue from the affected area. Bloodroot extracts were applied to the chest area in the 1800s to help treat bleeding tumors and other breast-related issues.

It can also be used to reduce plaque formation on the teeth: this keeps the teeth and gums healthy and prevents tooth-related disorders.

NATIVE AREA: Native to North America.

MEDICINAL PART: The underground rhizome.

MEDICINAL USES: Fever treatment.

SCIENTIFIC NAME: Sanguinaria canadensis.

18.   BLUEBERRIES

These antioxidant-rich dark blueberries aid in the fight against malignant cells and prevent premature skin aging. Blueberries are abundant in vitamins C, E, K, A and B6, as well as manganese: all of which help to fight degenerative diseases.

They've been shown to help prevent heart disease, cancer, bone strength, mental wellness, and blood pressure control. Anthocyanin is a plant pigment in blueberries that gives them their blue color and several health benefits.

Blueberry is also used to promote circulation as a laxative and is used by some women to alleviate labor pains and as a tonic after a miscarriage. Dried fruit and leaves are used to treat diarrhea. Tea prepared from dried leaves is used to cure sore throats and swelling (inflammation) of the mouth or the skin lining the throat.

NATIVE AREA: South America, Europe and Asia.

MEDICINAL PART: Berries.

MEDICINAL USES: Prevent heart disease and cancer,

bone strength, mental health, and healthy blood pressure.

SCIENTIFIC NAME: Vaccinium sect. Cyanococcus.

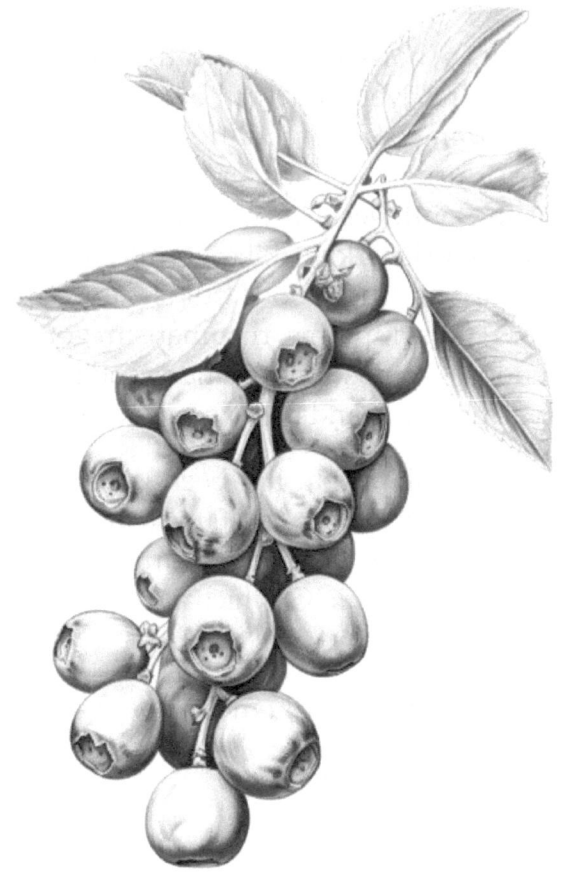

19.   BLUE VERVAIN

This plant is native to North America, with populations in both Canada and the United States. The herb was used by Native Americans to stop bleeding, heal fevers and colds, relieve stomach pains and headaches. It was also thought to guard against lightning strikes, curses and evil spirits. Blue vervain is a biennial herb in the Verbenaceae family. They have a self-sustaining development pattern and are indigenous to the United States, Canada, and North America.

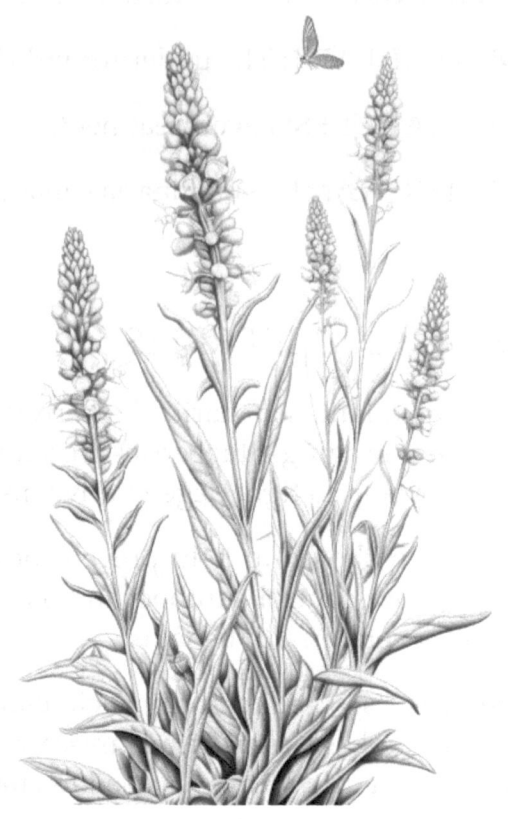

NATIVE AREA: North America

MEDICINAL PART: The root.

MEDICINAL USES: Healing wounds, abscesses and burns, arthritis, joint pain, dislocations, bone bruises and itching.

SCIENTIFIC NAME: Verbena hastata.

20.   BURDOCK

Burdock, a northern European native, is one of nature's first "velcros," with burs that attach to fur and clothing and are difficult to remove. This species is usually found as a weed than an invading plant in Southwestern wilderness areas. Burdock improves urine flow, kills germs, reduces fever, and "purifies" the blood. Colds, cancer, anorexia nervosa, GI symptoms, rheumatism, gout, bladder infections, syphilis complications and skin illnesses such as psoriasis and acne are all addressed.

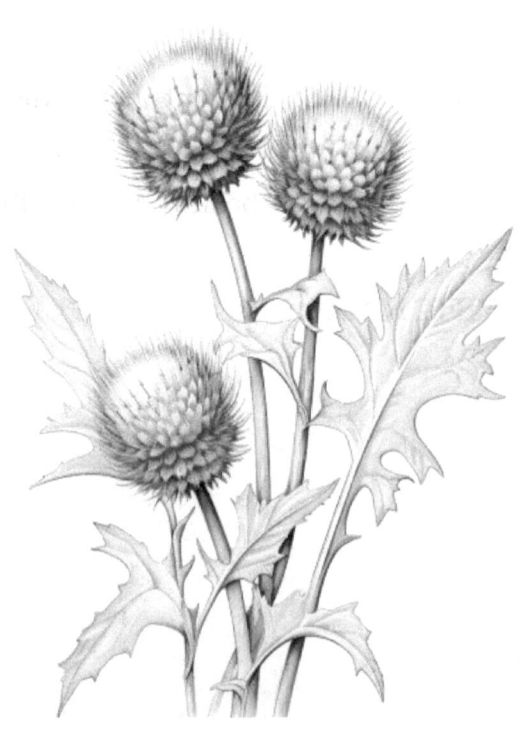

Burdock, a plant that has been used as a natural treatment for over 4,000 years, has been demonstrated to help battle heart disease; it is also abundant in vitamin C, which aids in inflammation reduction.

NATIVE AREA: Northern Europe

MEDICINAL PART: Roots.

MEDICINAL USES: Increase urine flow, kill germs, reduce fever

SCIENTIFIC NAME: Arctium.

21.   CATTAIL

Cattails are recognized for their white blooms and feathery leaves and can grow up to 15 feet tall. Native Americans used the plant as a food source and a medical herb for a variety of ailments, including bladder infections, colic discomfort, coughs, sore throats, fevers, and more. They are very little and resemble tufted nutlets. Typha latifolia grows when the soil is damp or even flooded during the growth season. Except for Hawaii, it is native to every state in the United States.

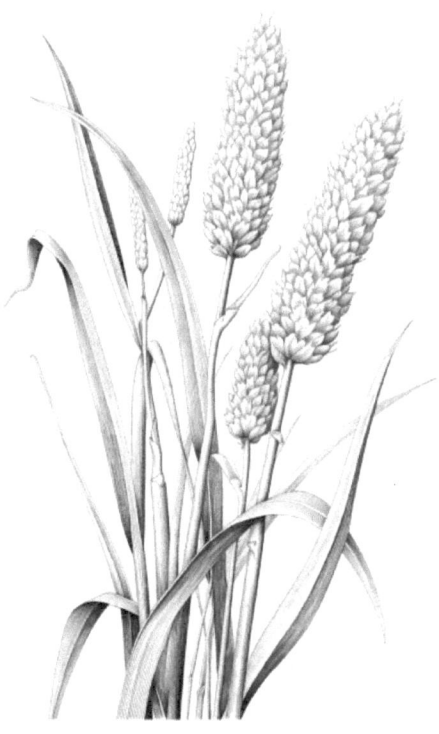

NATIVE AREA: North and South America, Europe, Eurasia, and Africa.

MEDICINAL PART: The ashes from burned cattail leaves and the droplets of sap.

MEDICINAL USES: Helps in treating bladder infections, colic pain, coughs, sore throats and fevers.

SCIENTIFIC NAME: Typha Latifolia.

22.   CARDAMOM

Cardamom is a spice derived from the cardamom plant, and the seeds and oil taken from the roots are used to make medication. In people who drink little or no alcohol, cardamom is used to treat nonalcoholic fatty liver disease (NAFLD), diabetes, and excessive cholesterol. Apart from providing taste to your foods, cardamom contains anti-inflammatory effects and is known for its antioxidant characteristics, which aid in preventing heart disease and stroke. Cardamom treats heartburn, intestinal spasms, gas, constipation, irritable bowel syndrome (IBS), liver and gallbladder problems, and loss of appetite.

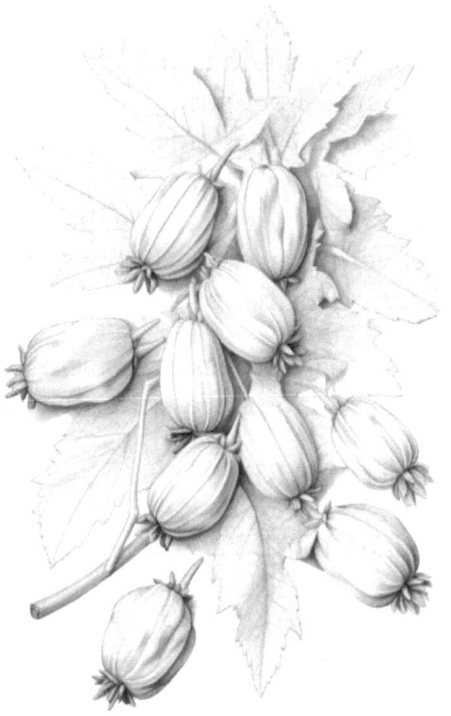

It is also used to treat the common cold, cough, bronchitis, sore mouth and throat, and susceptibility to infection.

NATIVE AREA: India.

MEDICINAL PART: Seeds.

MEDICINAL USES: Common cold, cough, bronchitis.

SCIENTIFIC NAME: Elettaria cardamomum.

23. CASTOR BEAN

Because of its form, the ancient Egyptians employed this plant as a fertility charm—and it also makes an efficient broom when ground up. Because the seeds were frequently employed as laxatives and purgatives, the plant was also supposed to be a potent aphrodisiac.

Some people use castor seed paste as a poultice on their skin to treat boils, carbuncles, pockets of infection (abscesses), inflammatory skin disorders, middle ear inflammation, and migraine headaches. Castor oil softens the skin and dissolves cysts, growths, and warts.

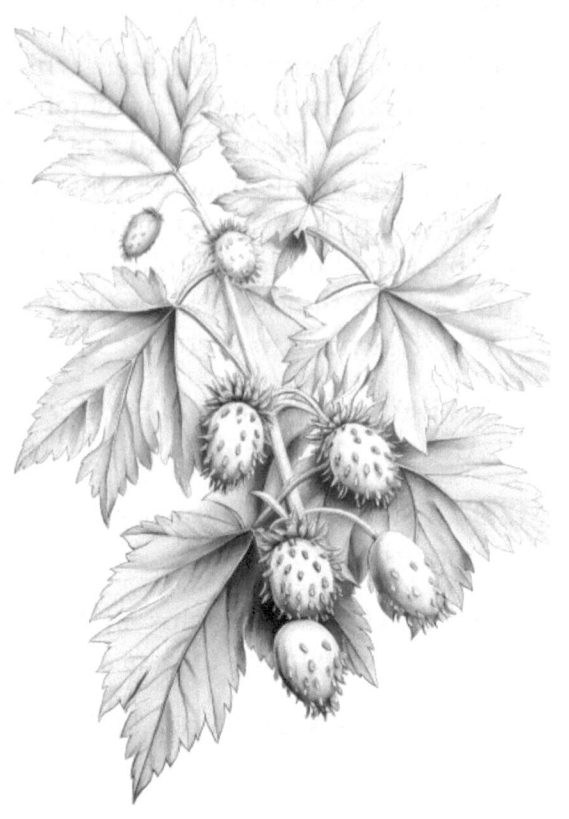

NATIVE AREA: India and China.

MEDICINAL PART: Seed.

MEDICINAL USES: Inflammatory skin disorders.

SCIENTIFIC NAME: Ricinus communis.

24. CAYENNE PEPPER

This really spicy chili pepper can significantly rev up your metabolism and aid in removing toxins from your body. Cayenne pepper includes capsaicin, a chemical component that aids in cholesterol reduction and blood circulation improvement. The pepper may improve digestion by increasing the creation of digestive fluid, delivering enzymes to the stomach to aid digestion, and offering further protection against stomach infections.

In animal studies, capsaicin has been proven to help decrease blood pressure, lowering heart disease risk.

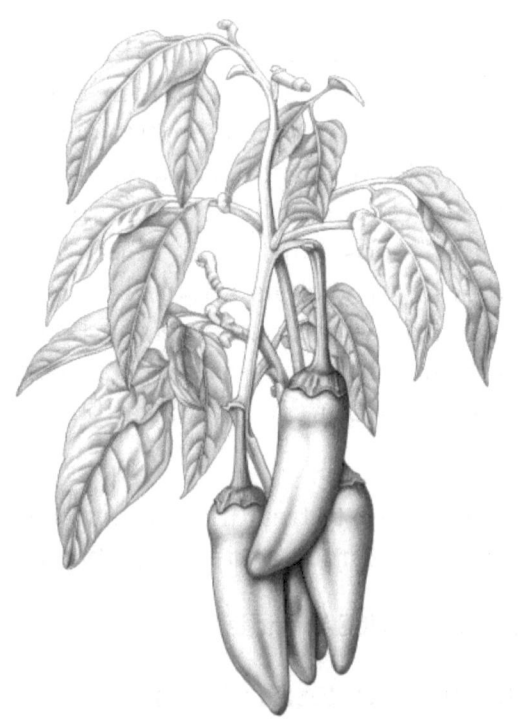

NATIVE AREA: Central and South America

MEDICINAL PART: Spice.

MEDICINAL USES: Protection to the stomach against infections.

SCIENTIFIC NAME: Capsicum frutescens.

25.   CHAMOMILE

Chamomile tea can help with a variety of problems, including insomnia and other forms of restlessness. Patients suffering from sleepiness and weariness will find that this herbal medicine can assist them in enhancing their sleep quality.

Chamomile tea has anti-inflammatory effects, making it effective in treating arthritis. Because of its antihistamine qualities, it is an effective treatment for hay fever and other allergies.

Chamomile powder can also be used in a bath to help relieve rashes and eczema after a bath.

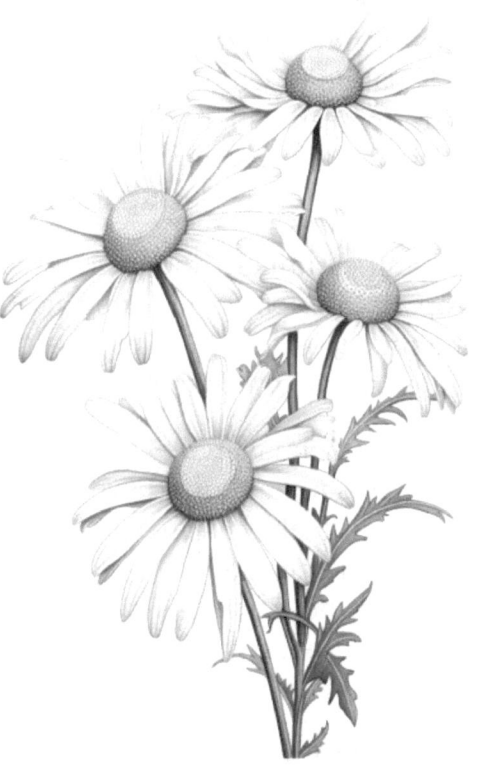

NATIVE AREA: Europe, Africa, and Asia.

MEDICINAL PART: The whole plant.

MEDICINAL USES: Digestive relaxant.

SCIENTIFIC NAME: Matricaria chamomilla.

26.   CHASTEBERRY

Chasteberry extracts were previously utilized to treat various gynecological and skin issues. Chasteberry is being marketed as a dietary supplement for PMS, menstrual cycle-related breast pain, infertility, and other diseases.

Chasteberry can aid in promoting ovulation and the thickening of cervical mucus. This enhances sperm penetration and may help prevent an early miscarriage.

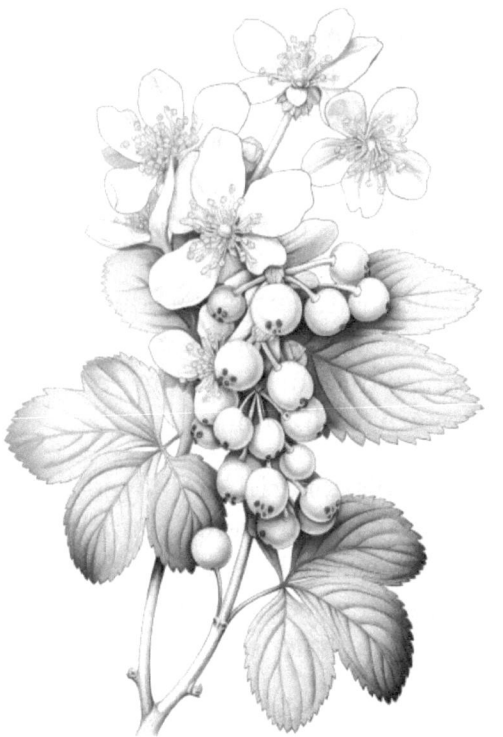

NATIVE AREA: Mediterranean regions of southern Europe, northern Africa and western Asia.

MEDICINAL PART: Dried fruits and leaves.

MEDICINAL USES: Menstrual disorders, amenorrhea, and fertility

SCIENTIFIC NAME: Vitex agnus-castus.

27. CHRYSANTHEMUM

The chrysanthemum is a gorgeous and delicate flower that is native to China and has been used in Chinese culture for generations. The plant was employed for medicinal and spiritual purposes, including ceremonies and temple offerings.

Chrysanthemums are indigenous to Asia and northern Europe. Most species are from East Asia, with China being the variety center. They may tolerate soft shade, but they thrive in full sun.

Because of their layered petals and position in the solar cycle, chrysanthemums have long been thought to make good "lucky charms" (together with other flower blossoms). Even though they don't grow well outside of Japan, the Japanese consider them lucky and frequently use them in wreaths or to embellish colorful fabrics.

NATIVE AREA: Asia.

MEDICINAL PART: Flowers.

MEDICINAL USES: Helpful for fever, cold, headache, dizziness, chest pain (angina), highblood pressure, type 2 diabetes and swelling.

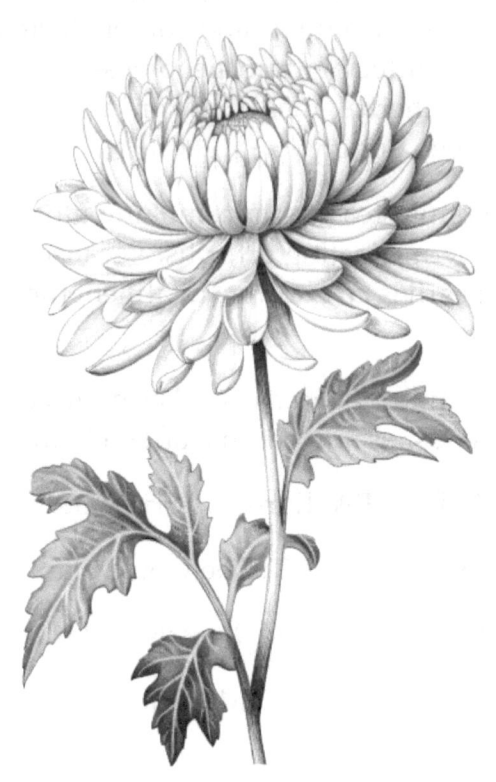

28. CINCHONA OFFICINALIS

Cinchona officinalis is a South American tropical shrub. One of its numerous names is "Jesuits' bark" since Spanish missionaries from Peru introduced the shrub to Western civilization.

These missionaries employed the plant for its medical benefits, which were found by numerous Europeans who grew to love it. Cinchona is used to stimulate hunger, the secretion of digestive enzymes, and relieve bloating, wholeness, and other stomach issues.

It is also used to treat blood vessel illnesses such as hemorrhoids, swelling modes, leg cramps, mild flu, swine flu, common deep freeze, malaria, and fever. Other applications include cancer, tongue and throat problems, an enlarged spleen, and muscle spasms. It is also used to numb the pain, destroy origins, and make

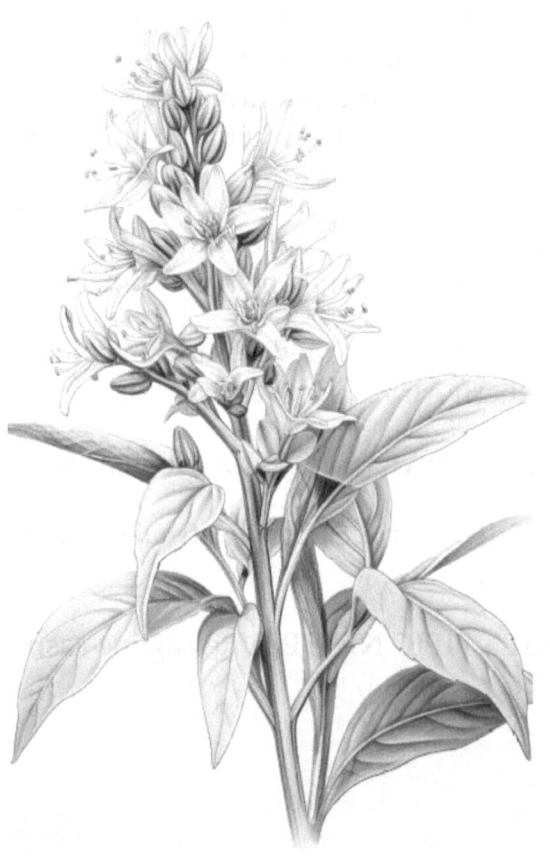

eye poultices. Cinchona extract is also administered to the skin to treat hemorrhoids, increase hair development, and manage varicose veins.

NATIVE AREA: Colombia, Ecuador, Peru and Bolivia.

MEDICINAL PART: The bark.

MEDICINAL USES: Stomach problems, blood vessel diseases and flue.

29.   CINNAMON

It increases energy levels in people who are tired or sluggish, which promotes wealth and happiness. It can also improve your stamina. This spice is obtained from a plant native to Sri Lanka. Cinnamon is commonly used in cooking, and some cultures utilize it to flavor their cuisine.

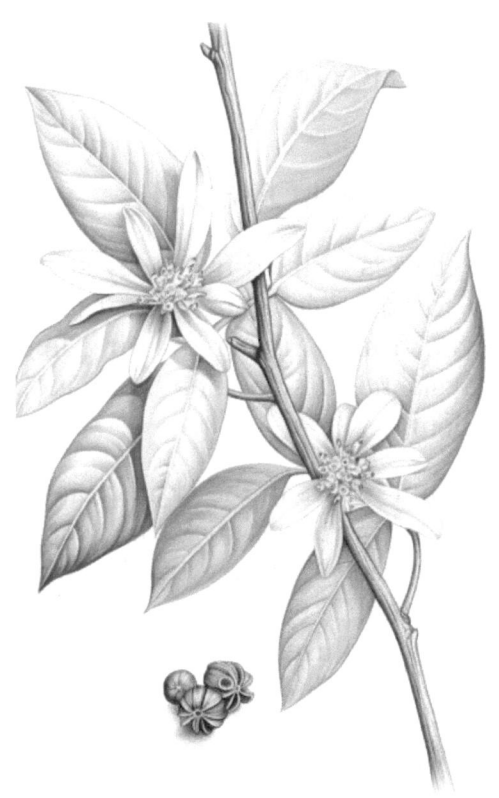

It reduces the fluid in the lungs and throat, which helps eliminate excess phlegm. This allows a person to breathe easier and cough less frequently, while also lowering cold or fever chills. The bark has been used as a spice to flavor many meals and beverages for many years. The plant's dried fruit has been utilized medicinally for various purposes.

NATIVE AREA: Pakistan, Southern Asia, Papua New Guinea, and Indonesia.

MEDICINAL PART: Fruit.

MEDICINAL USES: Antimicrobial (bactericidal, fungicidal, etc.), carminative (gas), laxative (antispasmodic), stimulant (circulatory effects).

30.   COFFEE

Coffee is high antioxidants and can be utilized naturally to keep the body and mind healthy. It helps prevent heart disease by having stimulant effects comparable to caffeine, however it does not contain caffeine. Coffee is frequently drunk to relieve mental and physical weariness and to increase mental alertness. Coffee is also used to prevent Parkinson's disease, dementia, and other diseases, but many of these claims are unsubstantiated by scientific evidence.

NATIVE AREA: Arabia.

MEDICINAL PART: Seeds.

MEDICINAL USES: Improve mental alertness.

31. CORNFLOWERS

Cornflowers can be used to relieve sore throat pain and alleviate irritable bowel syndrome. It's an effective remedy for constipation and bloating.

NATIVE AREA: Europe.

MEDICINAL PART: The dried flowers to make a tea.

MEDICINAL USES: To treat fever, constipation, water retention and chest congestion.

SCIENTIFIC NAME: Centaurea cyanus.

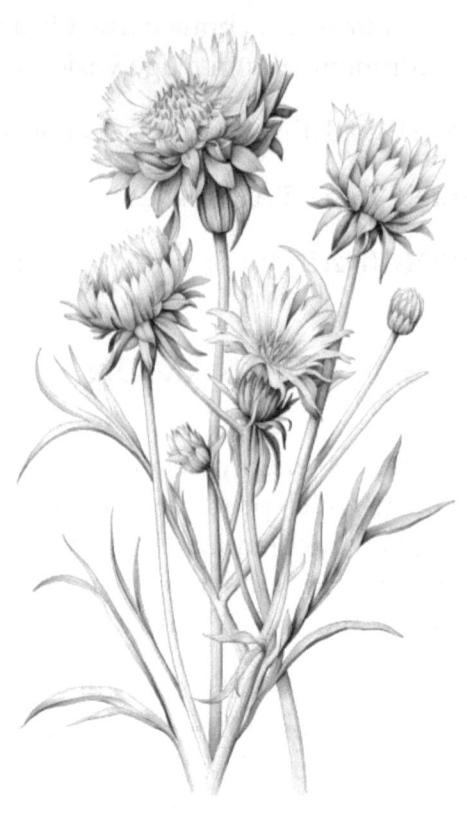

32. CLOVES

This spice is utilized in money spells and rituals. It is also used to attract love in magical love potions. This spice is derived from a flower growing in Indonesia, China, and Malaysia. It is used as a flavoring in cooking and a mosquito repellent.

This plant grows in the United States and Canada and has a variety of purposes, including cough relief. Cloves are the aromatic flower buds of the Myrtaceae tree Syzygium aromaticum. They are native to Indonesia's Maluku Islands and are often used as a spice. Cloves are accessible all year due to varying harvest seasons in various nations.

NATIVE AREA: Maluku Islands in Indonesia.

MEDICINAL PART: Leaves, oils, dried flower buds, and stems.

MEDICINAL USES: Reduce the inflammatory response in the body, lowering the likelihood of diseases like arthritis and aiding in the management of symptoms..

SCIENTIFIC NAME: Syzygium aromaticum

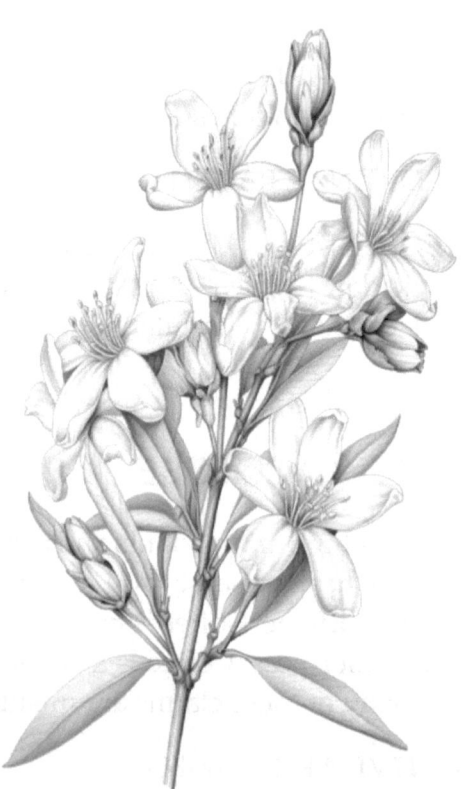

33.   CROCUS

Crocus is typically planted during the holidays in the hopes of giving a good fortune to whoever receives them as a gift. Furthermore, the ancients equated 'The Great Lover of All Things' with love, riches, and friendship.

Crocuses are native to the Alps, southern Europe, and the Mediterranean region, and they are frequently cultivated for their cuplike blooms in early spring or late fall.

NATIVE AREA: Alps, southern Europe, and the Mediterranean area

MEDICINAL PART: The seed, bulb, leaves, and flower.

MEDICINAL USES: Used for rheumatoid arthritis (RA) and gout.

SCIENTIFIC NAME: Crocus sativus.

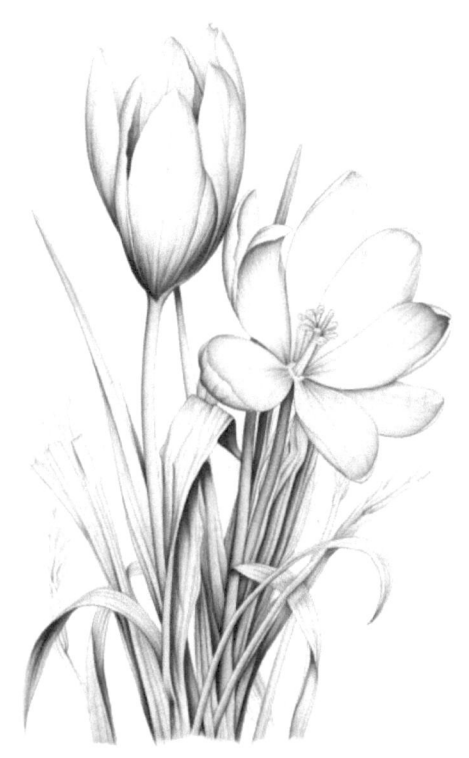

34.   DAFFODIL

The daffodil is associated with notions of spring and love because of its Latin name, 'Narcissus.'

In fact, it's been said that Narcissus fell in love with himself! This flower also belongs to the amaryllis family.

NATIVE AREA: Northern Europe.

MEDICINAL PART: Bulb, leaf, and flower.

MEDICINAL USES: Common cold, swelling (inflammation) of the main airways in the lung (bronchitis), wound healing, and joint pain.

SCIENTIFIC NAME: Narcissus.

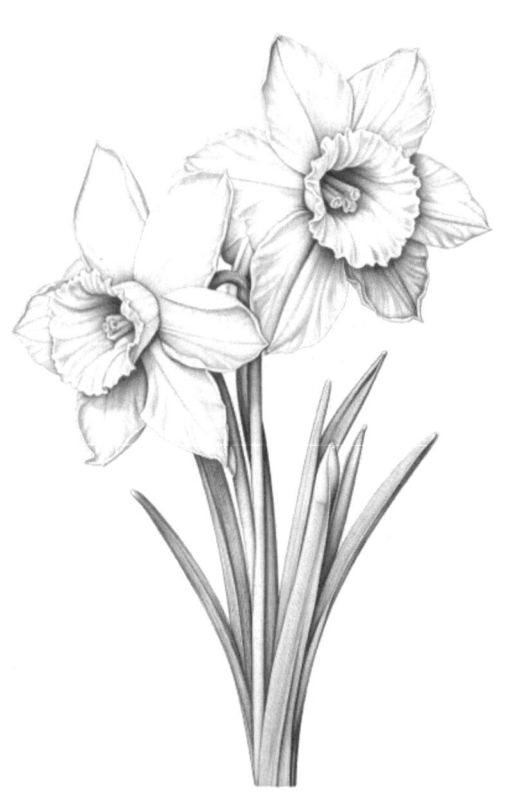

35. DAHLIAS

Depending on your preferences, these perennials can be cultivated indoors all year or outside in warm climates. They originated in South Africa and were frequently hung on entrances for good luck, particularly at the winter solstice, when the sun was at its lowest position in the sky (You can achieve a similar effect by hanging them above the entryway).

NATIVE AREA: Mesoamerica.

MEDICINAL PART: Root.

MEDICINAL USES: Food supplement.

SCIENTIFIC NAME: Dahlia.

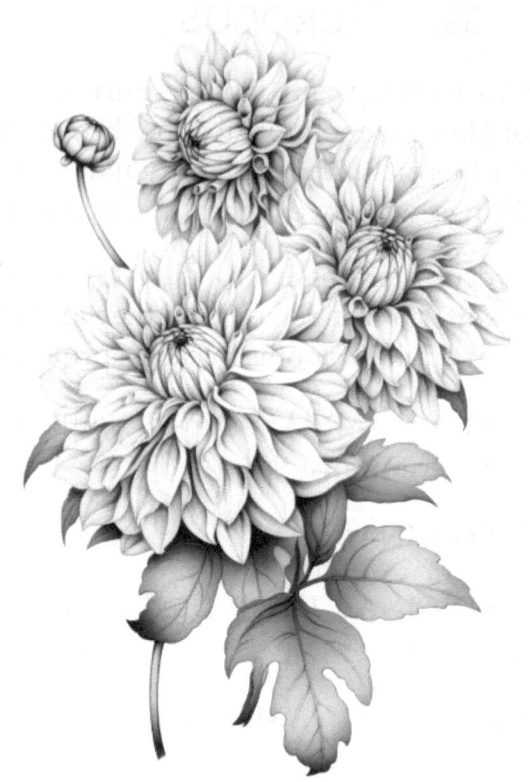

36. DANDELION

This herb is mostly utilized in money and purification ceremonies. As dried leaves, it has been traded as a sort of currency. Dried dandelion blossoms can be burned as incense to encourage wealth and prosperity.

The dandelion is a tough herb that grows practically everywhere and almost every month of the year. Because of its adaptability, this plant was frequently employed as a food source and a potent medicinal herb.

Dandelion is a yellow-flowering plant. The most widespread variety of this plant is Taraxacum officinale, which thrives in various places worldwide. The dandelion's leaves, stem, blossom, and root are all used medicinally.

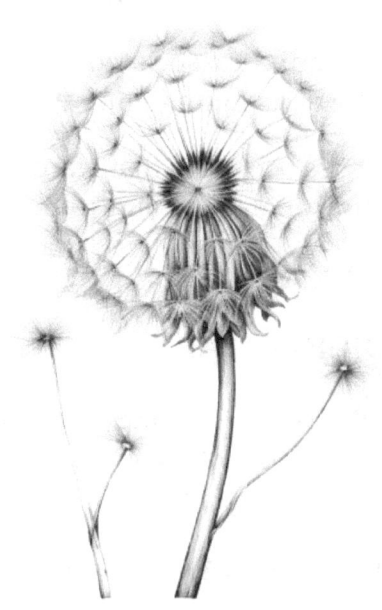

NATIVE AREA: Eurasia.

MEDICINAL PART: Flowers and leaves

MEDICINAL USES: Fever, diarrhea, boils, eye issues, and diabetes. Treat gastrointestinal issues, appendicitis

SCIENTIFIC NAME: Taraxacum officinale

37.   DEVIL'S SHOESTRING

This wildflower, native to North America, was utilized medicinally by many Native American cultures. It was mostly used to cure fevers and toothaches.

In New Mexico, a tribe employed the plant to aid a dying chief in entering the spirit realm. Devil's Shoestring is a powerful herb in the Viburnum genus that is also known as moose bush, hobblebush, cramp bark, and Goat's Rue.

This herb is native to Eastern North America, where it can be found from North Eastern Canada to Georgia. Devil's Shoestring roots are used as an antispasmodic, particularly to relieve menstrual cramps, fever, and toothaches.

Carrying the Devil's Shoestring is claimed to bring success against any attack. Use this herb in a white remedy pouch to protect against negative energy or in a green medicine pouch to bring good fortune.

It can also be bundled and placed above a doorway or fireplace to protect your home.

It was originally used as an anklet to protect against being "poisoned through the feet." North America is the native area.

NATIVE AREA: North America.

MEDICINAL PART: The roots.

MEDICINAL USES: Fevers and toothaches

SCIENTIFIC NAME: Tephrosia virginiana.

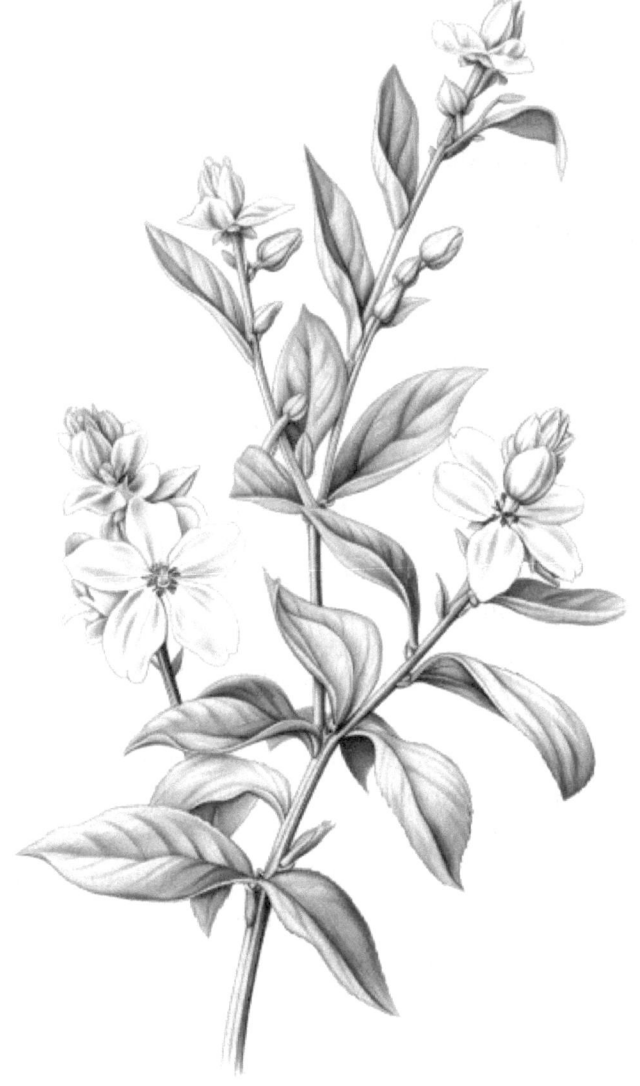

38.   DILL

Dill is considered to bring wealth and abundance in general, but it is also said that too much dill might bring devastation. That depends on how you utilize it, I suppose: if you spread it around your home or business to attract consumers, too much may imply that you must fire all of your current customers.

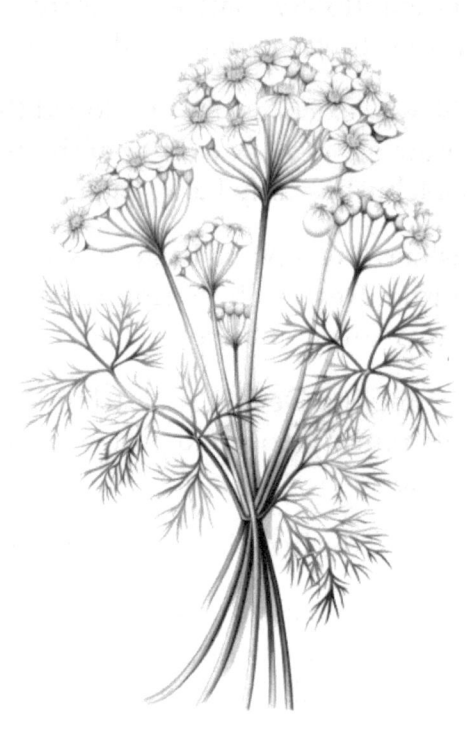

Dill seeds are also utilized in the preparation of prosperity oil. This herb is frequently used to relieve pain or inflammation in various scenarios, such as joint aches, migraines, headaches, and more. It can be boiled with other herbs to relieve stomach cramps and to encourage good bowel movements. It should be emphasized that dill should not be consumed uncooked. It is an annual plant of the Apiaceae family of celery. The genus Anethum has only one species.

NATIVE AREA: Eurasia.

MEDICINAL PART: Fruits (seeds).

MEDICINAL USES: Treat indigestion, flatulence, hemorrhoids, colic, and hiccups.

SCIENTIFIC NAME: Anethum graveolens

39.   ECHINACEA

Sunflower and ragweed relatives are Echinacea (Echinacea angustifolia, Echinacea purpurea, Echinacea pallida). The leaf, flower, and root are used to make medicine.

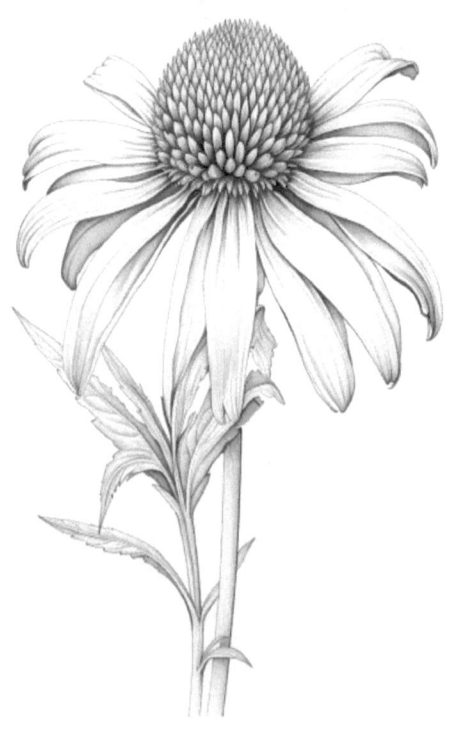

East of the Rocky Mountains, Echinacea species are native to the United States.

Echinacea appears to increase the body's production of anti-inflammatory chemicals. It may also aid in strengthening the body's immune system. Echinacea is most commonly used to treat the common cold and other illnesses and also has anti-inflammatory effects, making it effective in the treatment of arthritis, especially rheumatoid arthritis. It can aid in treating colds and flu by boosting the immune system. Because of its antimicrobial qualities, it can be used to treat eye infections and naturally lower fevers, making it useful in treating colds and other ailments. Its antibacterial characteristics may aid in the treatment of psoriasis.

NATIVE AREA: Area east of the Rocky Mountains in the United States

MEDICINAL PART: The leaf, flower, and root.

MEDICINAL USES: Decrease inflammation and increase the body's immune system.

SCIENTIFIC NAME: Echinacea purpurea

40.   FENNEL

Fennel is a plant native to southern Europe and the Mediterranean region, where it has been utilized for millennia for both culinary and medicinal uses.

It is said to have escaped cultivation in California in the mid-nineteenth century.

Fennel, a ubiquitous herb used to spice many Indian and Mediterranean dishes, is also a powerful natural cure for coughs, colds, and bronchitis.

It is also abundant in vitamin B, which aids in preventing lung cancer. Fennel is used to treat a variety of digestive disorders, including loss of appetite, heartburn, gas, bloating, and baby colic.

Coughs, bronchitis, cholera, upper respiratory infections, backaches, bedwetting, and vision problems are also treated with it.

NATIVE AREA: Southern Europe and the Mediterranean region

MEDICINAL PART: Dries seeds.

MEDICINAL USES: Digestive issues.

SCIENTIFIC NAME: Foeniculum vulgare.

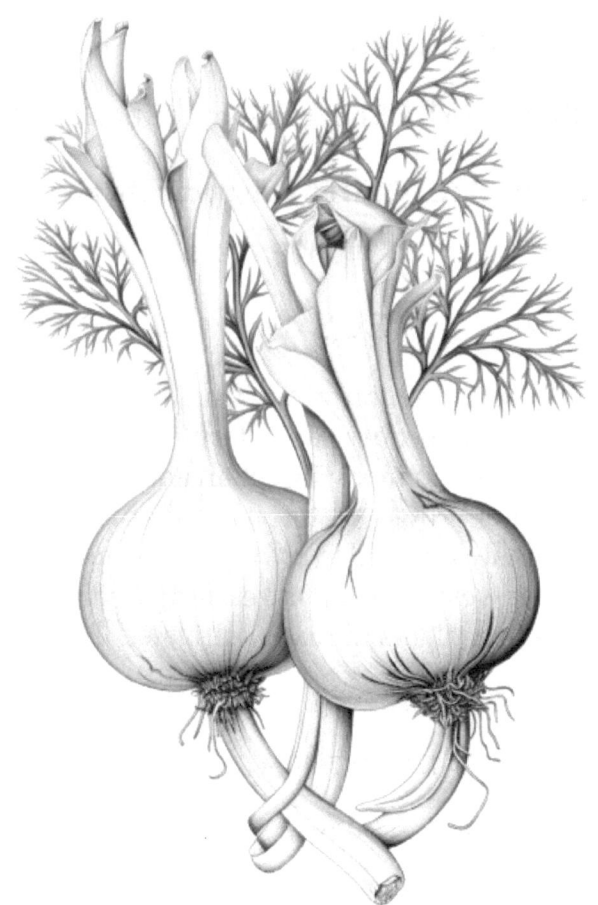

41.　FERN

Because it grows predominantly near ponds or streams, this little but powerful plant is frequently associated with the element of water in Celtic mysticism. They are also linked with Druids, which adds to their uniqueness.

This plant is a wonderful home protective charm since it repels evil spirits, and negativity, and even keeps lightning from damaging your home. The fern is extremely beneficial for dealing with divorce or betrayal—but be careful while handling this plant, as it is toxic if consumed. Royal Fern is used to treat intestinal worms, and rock cap is used to treat stomachaches and cholera. Christmas Fern is used to cure stomachaches, digestive problems, toothaches, cramps, and diarrhea. The herb bracken fern is used to cure diarrhea, nausea, vomiting, infections, weakness, stomach cramps, and headaches.

NATIVE AREA: The tropics.

MEDICINAL PART: Leaf.

MEDICINAL USES: Intestinal difficulties, toothache, cramps, and diarrhea.

SCIENTIFIC NAME: Polypodiophyta.

42.　FICUS

The most common of all fruit trees, the fig is known as a symbol of beauty and fertility. This is because of its prominence in many Egyptian and Roman sculptures, as well as Jesus's crown of thorns. It is ordinarily deciduous and commonly referred to as "fig." The common fig is a tree native to southwest Asia and the eastern Mediterranean, and it is one of the first plants humans cultivated.

NATIVE AREA: Asia.

MEDICINAL PART: Flowers.

MEDICINAL USES: Diarrhea, inflammatory conditions, diabetes, liver disorders, hemorrhoids, respiratory, and urinary diseases.

SCIENTIFIC NAME: Ficus benjamina, Ficus carica

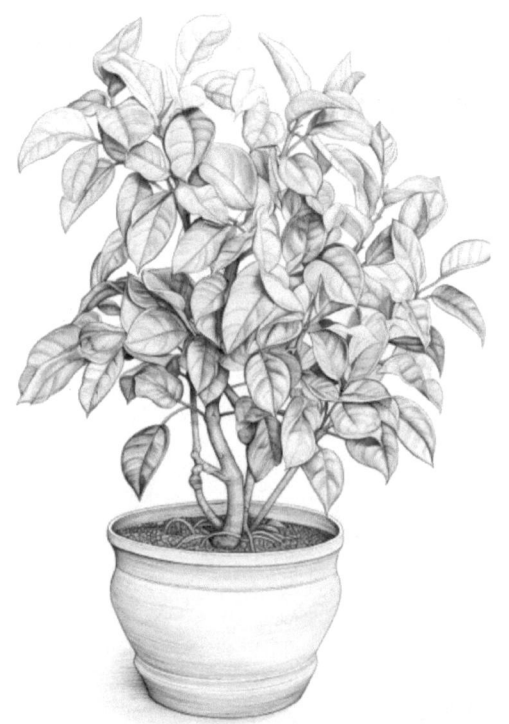

43. FOUR-LEAVED CLOVER

In some regions of the world, the four-leaf clover is considered good luck, but in others, it is considered bad luck. The Irish regard it as a divine gift, while the Chinese and Japanese utilize it to fend off evil spirits. The leaf can also be found on Celtic and Native American coins and jewelry. It is a semi-aquatic plant that grows in shallow water or loamy soils, marshes, and marshy areas. It has trailing stems and slender leaves that are simple, bright green, four-sided, and erect, like the original four-leaf clover. Leaflets obdeltoid, 2cm long, glaucous, petioles up to 15cm long; Sporocarp ellipsoid, on 2cm stalks linked to petioles.

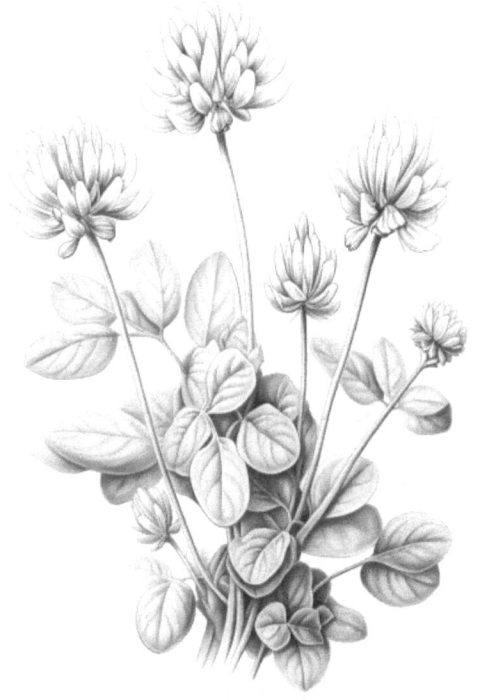

NATIVE AREA: Mexico.

MEDICINAL PART: Whole plant.

MEDICINAL USES: To treat coughing, skin problems, diabetics, eye problems and abscesses. It is used to treat snakebite.

SCIENTIFIC NAME: Trifolium repens.

44. GARLIC

Garlic is well known for its ability to lower bad cholesterol, but did you know it can also help limit the formation of malignant cells? Garlic includes allicin, a potent anti-inflammatory compound that has been demonstrated to kill carcinogenic cells in breast cancers. It is also useful for treating morning sickness. Garlic is commonly used to treat hypertension, elevated cholesterol or other lipids in the blood, and arterial hardening. It is also said to heal the common cold, osteoarthritis, and other diseases, although no scientific evidence supports these claims.

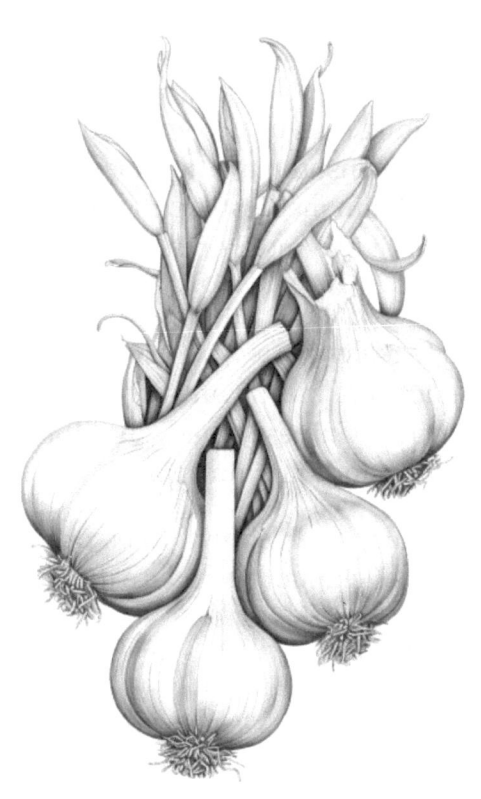

NATIVE AREA: Central Asia

MEDICINAL PART: Cloves.

MEDICINAL USES: High blood pressure, high cholesterol.

SCIENTIFIC NAME: Allium sativum.

45. GERANIUM

This lovely plant is employed in protection spells, hexes, and healing rituals. This is a wonderful option for all who are having financial difficulties or have experienced a home invasion.

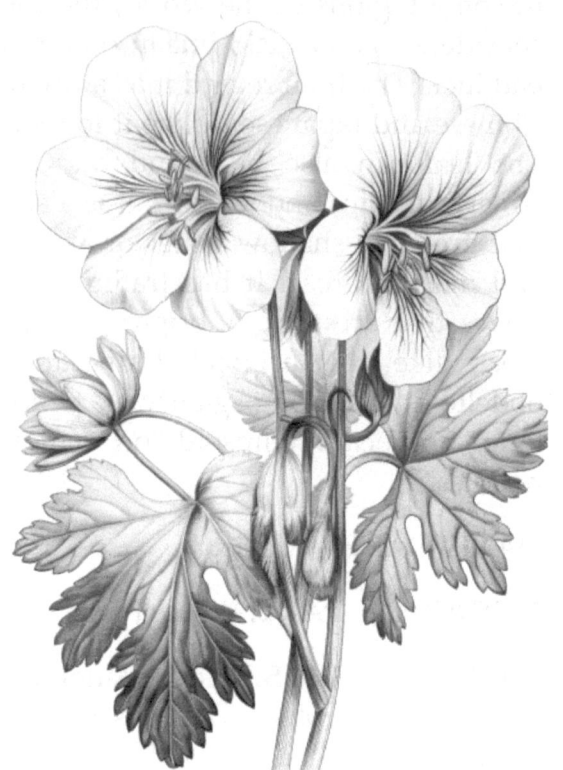

It can also be used to treat illnesses or heart disorders. Geranium (genus Geranium), sometimes called cranesbill, is any of roughly 300 species of perennial herbs or shrubs in the Geraniaceae family, native primarily to subtropical southern Africa. Geranium plants have five-petaled flowers on long stems and pinnately split leaves.

In traditional medicine, the leaves are the most essential therapeutic element. They're mostly used to brew a tasty tea with a slight rose taste.

NATIVE AREA: Africa and North America.

MEDICINAL PART: Leaves and oils.

MEDICINAL USES: Depression, infection, anxiety and pain management.

SCIENTIFIC NAME: Pelargonium.

46. GINGER

Yes, ginger can aid with anxiety relief. Many patients develop insomnia after discontinuing large dosages of opioid pain medication, therefore ginger can be used as an alternative to melatonin.

It aids in the relaxation of the body during sleep, allowing you to feel more awake in the morning when you take your medication. It is an anti-inflammatory and antiviral agent, used in Chinese medicine for generations to relieve arthritis and inflammation.

It has also been shown to be useful in alleviating the side effects of chemotherapy treatment.

The ginger is a strong charm that may protect its bearer from being possessed by a ghost and hurt or injured during a fight. Its leaves provide the power to defend their home from negative energies and can also be utilized to make protection charms. Ginger (Zingiber officinale), as an herbaceous perennial plant of the Zingiberaceae family most likely native to Southeast Asia, for its aromatic, pungent rhizome (underground stem) is so used as a spice, flavoring, food, and medicinal.

NATIVE AREA: Southeast Asia.

MEDICINAL PART: Roots.

MEDICINAL USES: Osteoarthritis, diabetes, menstrual cramps and migraine headaches

SCIENTIFIC NAME: Zingiber officinale.

47. GINSENG

Ginseng is a root produced from the roots of the American Ginseng plant, which is native to both North and South America.

The root has been utilized in Chinese culture for hundreds of years, but European traders first brought it to English-speaking countries in 1865.

It is traditionally farmed and used medicinally in Asian cultures.

NATIVE AREA: Chinese.

MEDICINAL PART: The roots and leaves.

MEDICINAL USES: Ginseng leaf-stem extract has anti-obesity, anti-cancer, anti- fatigue, anti-hyperglycemic, anti-oxidant and anti-aging properties, instead the roots are used for their antioxidant and anti-inflammatory effects.

They can strengthen the immune system, improve brain function, fight fatigue and improve symptoms of erectile dysfunction.

SCIENTIFIC NAME: Panax.

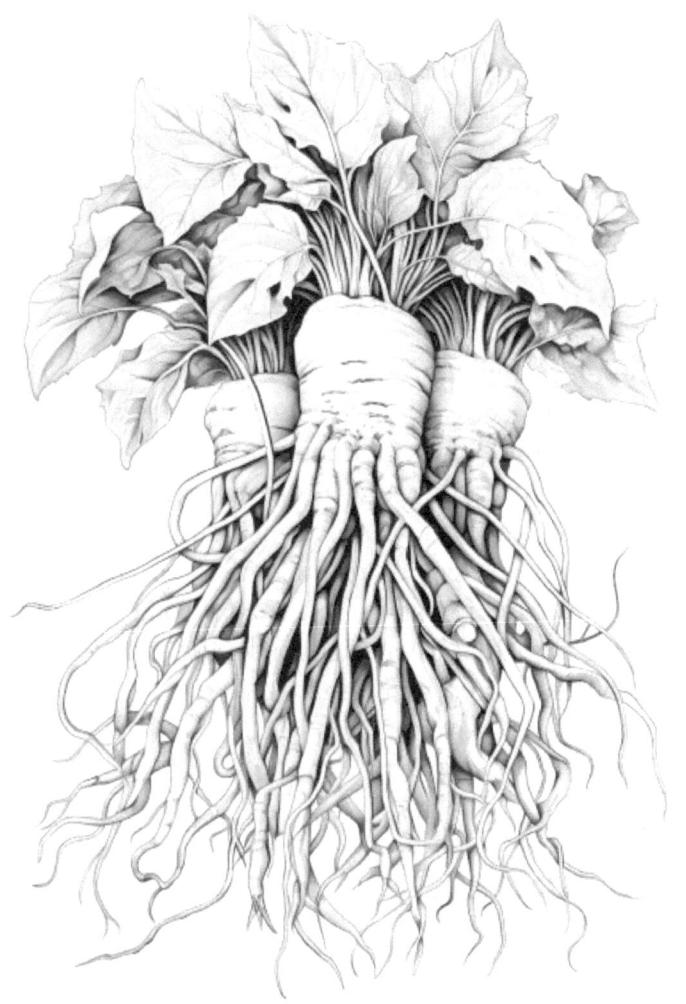

48.   GOJI BERRIES

Beta-carotene is found in goji berries. The ability of beta-carotene to support skin health is widely documented. Beta-carotene is a component in skin creams that promotes skin health. Goji berries have long been used to treat a variety of diseases, including diabetes, high blood pressure, fever, and age-related eye problems.

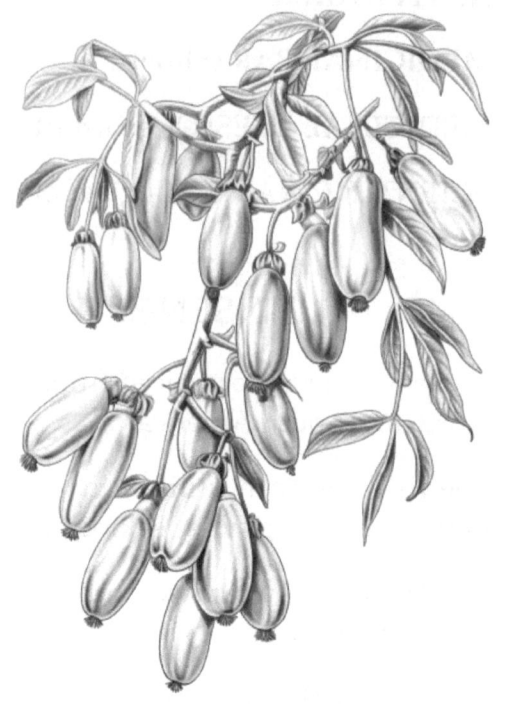

Goji berries are called a "superfood" by some and are utilized in herbal juices, teas, wines, and pharmaceuticals. They can be consumed roasted, raw, or dried (similar to raisins). These berries are not only delicious, but also high in fiber and rich in critical minerals such as beta-carotene, vitamin C, zinc, and iron, which assist in maintaining eyesight and fighting illness.

NATIVE AREA: China.

MEDICINAL PART: Berries.

MEDICINAL USES: Diabetes, fever, high blood pressure, and age-related eye problems.

SCIENTIFIC NAME: Lycium barbarum.

49.   HELLEBORES

The black hellebore tastes so bad that if eaten accidentally, it would kill a cow. In fact, cows have been known to congregate at patches of black hellebore to lick them clean of their poor taste. Eventually, they die from ingesting too much, but it's considered worth the risk.It is a native of Greece, Asia Minor, etc. The two species found wild in many parts of England, especially on limestone soil, are H. Foetidus, the Bearsfoot, and H. Viridis, the Green Hellebore; the latter has harmful effects on cattle if eaten by them.

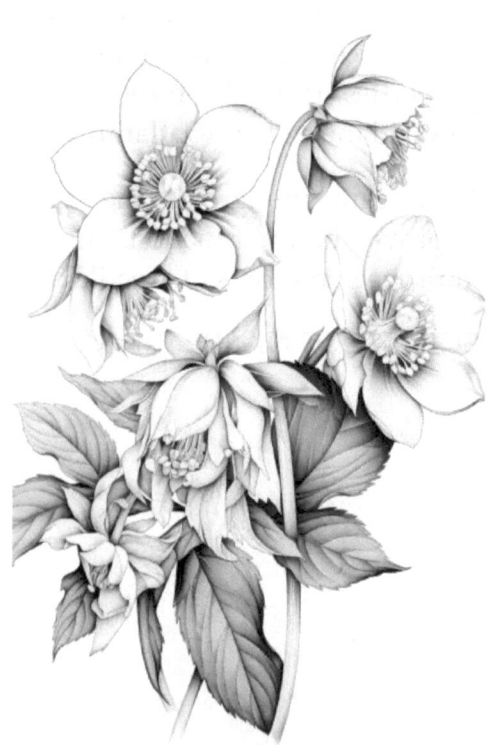

NATIVE AREA: Asia and Greece

MEDICINAL PART: Bulb and root.

MEDICINAL USES: Cholera, gout, and high blood pressure.

SCIENTIFIC NAME: Helleborus niger.

50.   GRAPE

The grape is a tranquil plant, and its juice can assist people in achieving emotional balance and overcoming emotional issues. It can also be used in healing charms. This control charm can assist in bringing serenity into the life of an angry or disturbed individual by releasing their anger and frustrations. Grapes, including the fruit, peel, leaves, and seed, are used as medicine in their totality.

Grapes contain a lot of flavonoids, which are antioxidants. They may lower the risk of heart disease and provide additional health advantages. Red grape varietals have more antioxidants than white or blush grape cultivars.

NATIVE AREA: The Middle East.

MEDICINAL PART: Fruit, skin, leaves, and seed.

MEDICINAL USES: Reduce the risk of heart disease.

SCIENTIFIC NAME: Vitis.

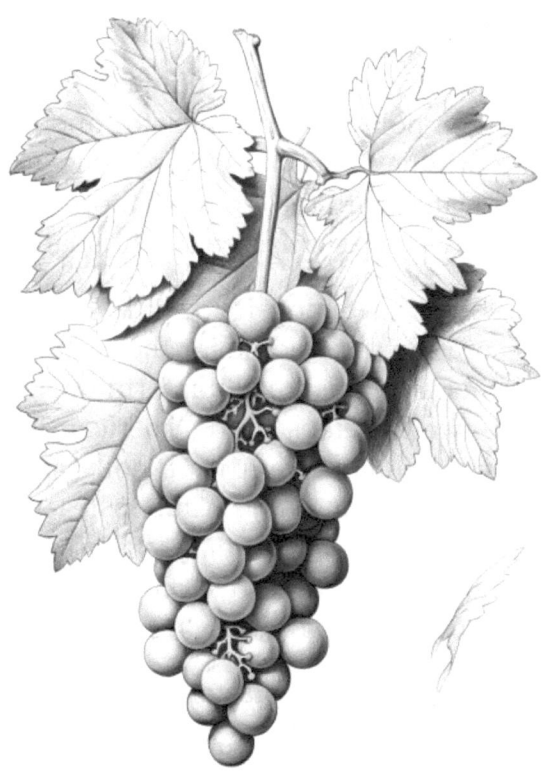

51.   HAWTHORN

This tree aids individuals in their grief process by providing comfort and recalling happy memories that might help them cope with their pain. Its berries can also be used to make protection charms. It is crucial to know that if swallowed, Hawthorn is deadly, therefore use caution when handling it. Hawthorn is used to help prevent heart disease and control excessive blood pressure and cholesterol levels. According to animal and human studies, Hawthorn increases coronary artery blood flow, improves circulation, and lowers blood pressure. It is also used to treat boils and skin ulcers.

NATIVE AREA: North America.

MEDICINAL PART: The berries, leaves, and flowers.

MEDICINAL USES: Heart disease and regulate high blood pressure and cholesterol levels

SCIENTIFIC NAME: Crataegus.

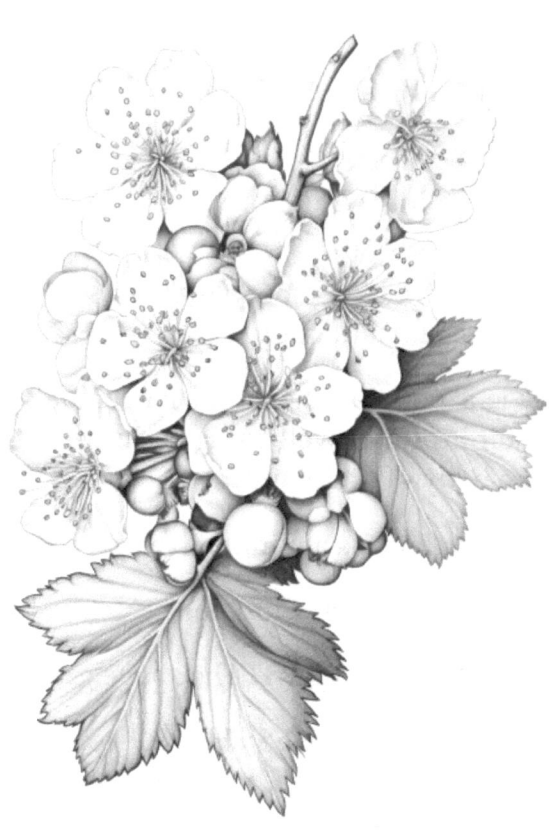

52.   HOLLY

Christmas in England would not be complete without a sprig of holly: in fact, mistletoe and holly are said to be the original Christmas evergreens. Holly is frequently associated with the crown of thorns on Christ's head on the day he was crucified in Christian legend.

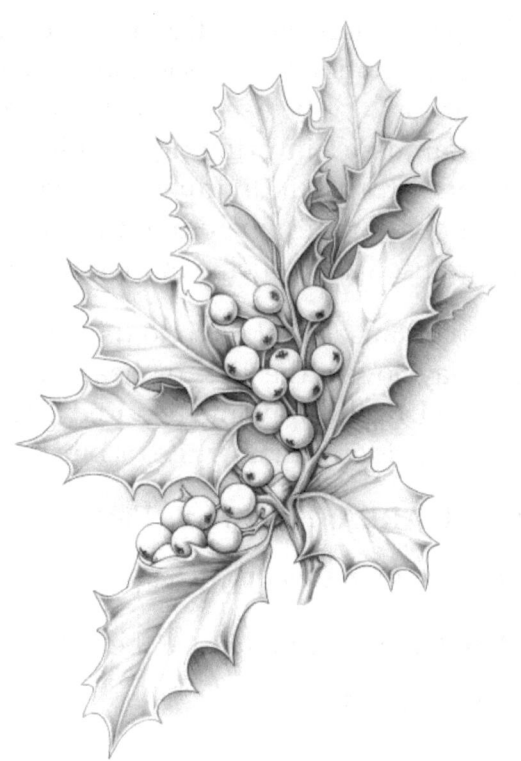

If you're searching for a little extra good luck when decorating your home for the winter holidays, look no further than this small but formidable plant. In the past, American Indians used American holly fruit tea as a heart stimulant. Yaupon, a holly species, was used to induce vomiting, and Yaupon tea was used in South America as a ceremonial "cleanser." Holly also treats coughs, fevers, digestive difficulties, heart disease, and various other disorders.

NATIVE AREA: Eastern and south-central United States.

MEDICINAL PART: Fruits.

MEDICINAL USES: Coughs, fevers, digestive problems, heart disease, and various other ailments.

SCIENTIFIC NAME: Ilex.

53.   HORSETAIL

For ages, Chinese people have used this plant both as food source and a therapy.

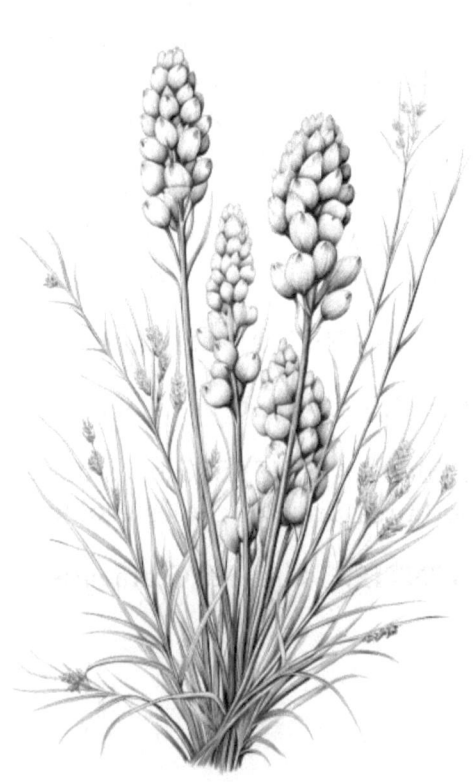

It is a popular choice for individuals looking to improve their health or well-being because of its capacity to cleanse the body of pollutants.

Horsetail tea is a popular beverage.

NATIVE AREA: Chinese.

MEDICINAL PART: The above ground parts.

MEDICINAL USES: Helpful for fluid retention, kidney and bladder stones, incontinence, urinary tract infections, and general kidney and bladder disturbances.

SCIENTIFIC NAME: Equisetum.

54.   INDIAN TOBACCO

This herb has been used for generations in North America, and many Native American cultures have employed it for its medical benefits. These people also employed the herb for spiritual and ceremonial purposes.

Indian tobacco has been used for centuries as a natural cure for respiratory disorders such as asthma, bronchitis, pneumonia, and cough. Native Americans used to smoke lobelia as an asthma cure.

The plant is recognized for its toxic and strong aroma, which comes from its blossoms and leaves and is frequently employed by Native Americans to deter their foes.

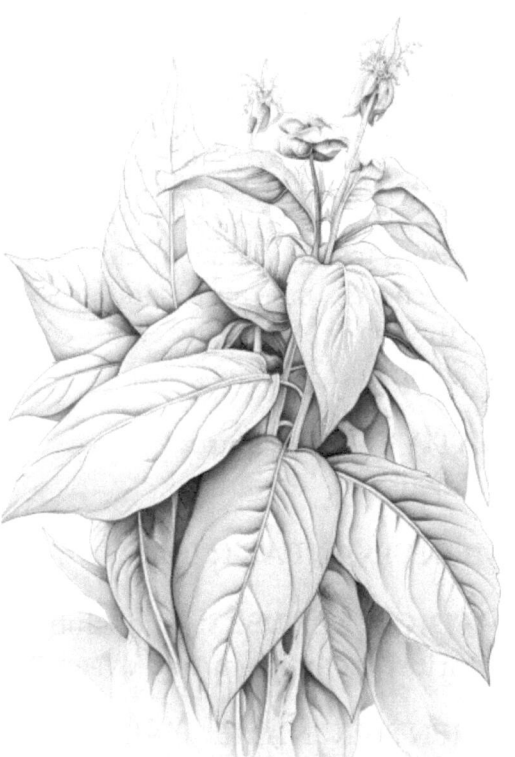

NATIVE AREA: Central Asia.

MEDICINAL PART: The leaves.

MEDICINAL USES: For respiratory conditions such as bronchitis, asthma, pneumonia andcough.

SCIENTIFIC NAME: Lobelia inflata.

55.   IRONWEED

This wildflower is found in Canada, the United States, and Central America. It has been cultivated and consumed throughout history, and it was used by Native Americans as both a medicinal herb and a food source.

Ironweed was used medicinally by American Indians, who created herbal drinks from the leaves to treat female ailments such as birth pain alleviation and blood tonic. On the other hand, I would brew herbal drinks from the roots to heal loose teeth, stomach ulcers, and bleeding.

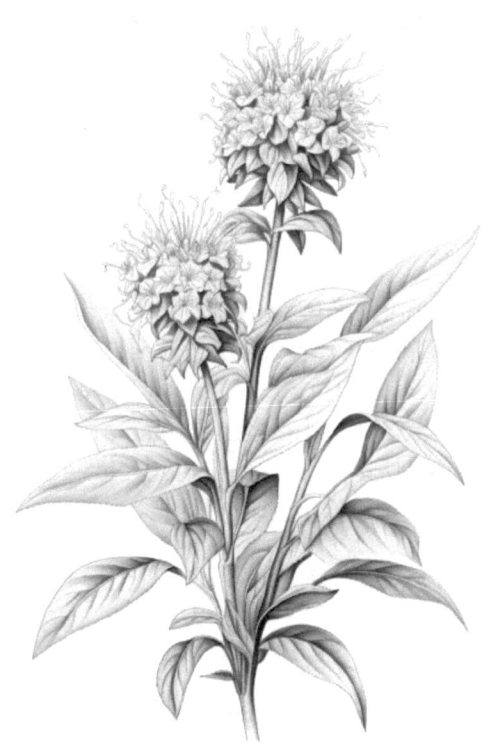

NATIVE AREA: North America.

MEDICINAL PART: The leaves and roots.

MEDICINAL USES: For female problems, stomach ulcers and bleeding.

SCIENTIFIC NAME: Vernonia fasciculata.

56. IVY

Ivy can be found in almost every garden and is known as the "Queen of the Herbs." This may be because its close cousin, Hedera, means 'Thorny Plant' in Latin. It grows so much so quickly that it has become a symbol of excess growth. Hedera, commonly called ivy (plural ivies), is a genus of 12–15 species of evergreen climbing or ground-creeping woody plants in the family Araliaceae, native to western, central and southern Europe, Macaronesia, northwestern Africa and across central-southern Asia east to Japan and Taiwan.

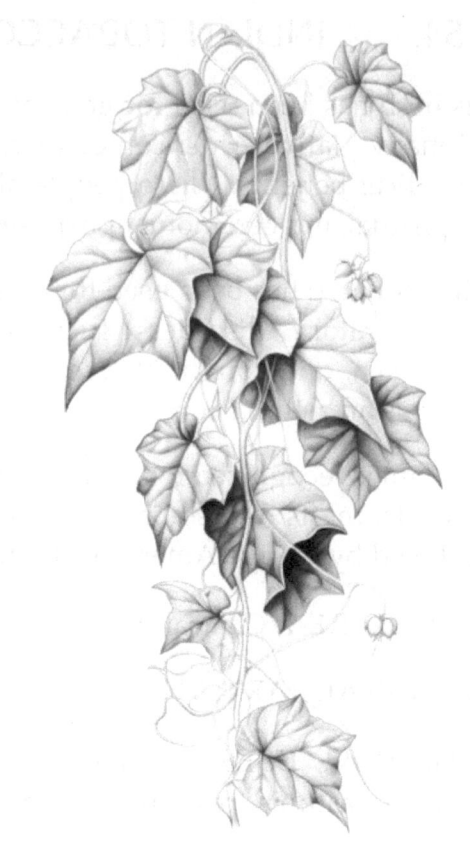

NATIVE AREA: Europe, Africa, Macaronesia, Asia east to Japan and Taiwan.

MEDICINAL PART: Leaf.

MEDICINAL USES: Bronchitis , whooping cough, arthritis, rheumatism, and dysentery.

SCIENTIFIC NAME: Hedera helix.

57. KAVA KAVA

This plant contains kavalactones, which have been demonstrated to aid in sleep. It naturally controls anxiety and tension and can be particularly beneficial whether used during the day or when attempting to conquer insomnia.

The chemicals known as kavapyrones are found in kava kava (short for "kava"). They have the same effect on your brain as alcohol: they make you feel calm, relaxed, and pleasant. The herb may also aid in pain alleviation, seizure prevention, and muscle relaxation. It's available as an herbal supplement online and in health food stores.

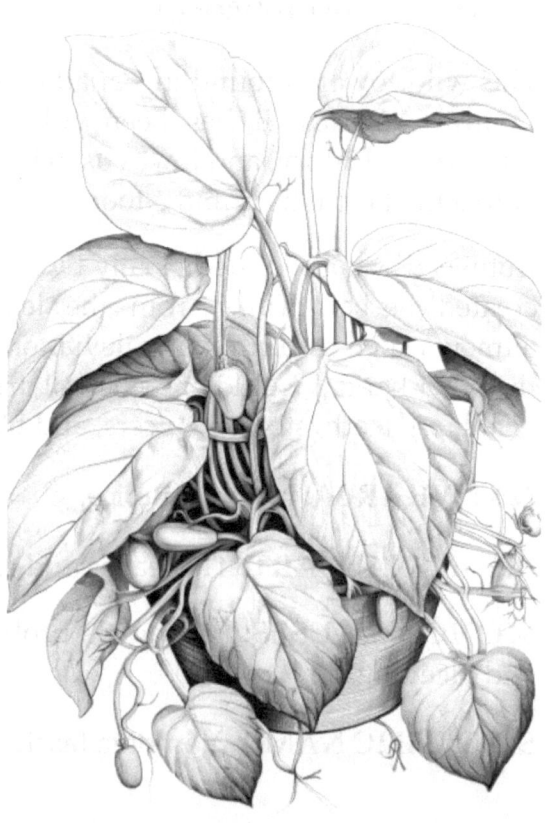

NATIVE AREA: South Pacific Islands.

MEDICINAL PART: Leaves.

MEDICINAL USES: Relieve pain, prevent seizures, and relax muscles.

SCIENTIFIC NAME: Piper methysticum.

58. LADY'S MANTLE

Lady's Mantle is a herb traditionally used in European medicine to promote menstruation and relieve the pain associated with menstrual cramps. It has also been shown to increase blood flow throughout the body, particularly to the uterus, which may aid in implantation rates. Alchemilla Mollis, often known as garden lady's-mantle or lady's-mantle, is a flowering plant in the Rosaceae family. This herbaceous perennial plant is native to southern Europe and is planted as a decorative garden plant worldwide.

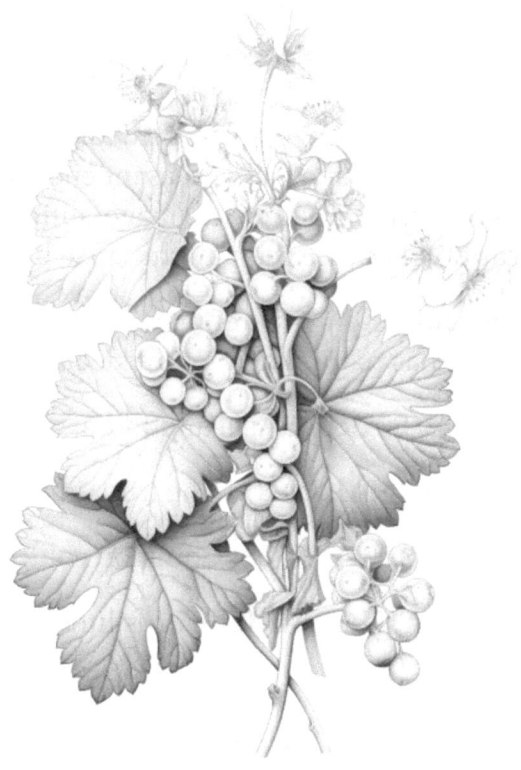

NATIVE AREA: Turkey and the Carpathian Mountains.

MEDICINAL PART: Roots and leaves.

MEDICINAL USES: For wounds and ulcers, hernias, and muscle atrophy, diuretic, anti- anemic, and anti-diabetic.

SCIENTIFIC NAME: Alchemilla.

59. LAVENDER

This herb is generally called the "herb of love," but it is also effective in attracting money. Lavender is a popular herb in love spells and is used in purifying rituals. Lavender can be used to build a relationship and promote attraction between lovers, or it can be used to end a relationship. This herb is derived from a fragrant flower native to the Mediterranean. Still, it has numerous other advantages, including aiding with confidence issues, anxiety, skin disorders such as dermatitis, and relaxation.

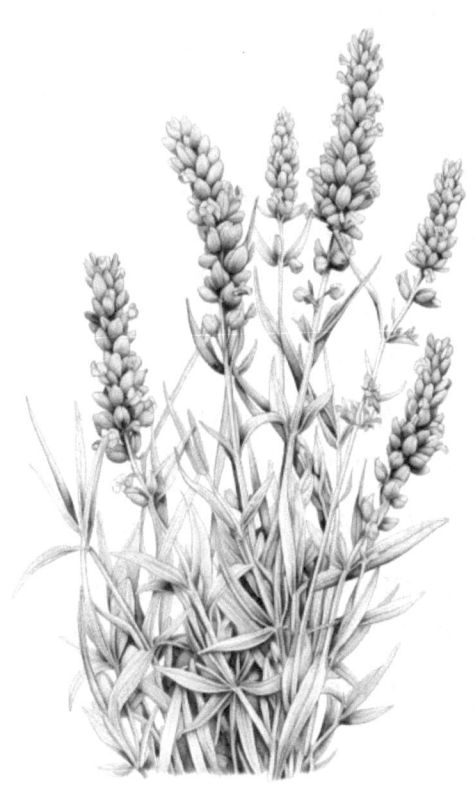

Lavandula (often known as lavender) is a genus of 47 flowering plants in the Lamiaceae mint family. The lavender plant has antibacterial characteristics that aid in healing and can be used to treat wounds and burns. It is also an effective therapy for sunburn. To treat insomnia or despair, sprinkle dried lavender petals on your pillow before going to bed.

NATIVE AREA: Europe, Africa, the Mediterranean, southwest Asia to India.

MEDICINAL PART: Oils.

MEDICINAL USES: Treat headaches, neurological disorders, tiredness, and skin conditions such fungal infections, wounds, eczema, and acne.

SCIENTIFIC NAME: Lavandula angustifolia

60.   LEMON

The lemon is a great protection charm. It attracts the excellent in your life and might assist in attracting money and pleasant energy. This can be employed in curses and hexes to ensure that the people you desire to damage suffer the brunt of their misfortune. When handling lemons, use caution because they might cause blindness if consumed.

This mint family perennial is native to mountainous areas of southern Europe and northern Africa, but it has naturalized in practically every warm or temperate region on the planet.

NATIVE AREA: Asia and India.

MEDICINAL PART: The fruit, juice, and peel.

MEDICINAL USES: Common cold, flu, ringing in the ears, kidney stones and Meniere's disease.

SCIENTIFIC NAME: Citrus limon.

61.   LEMON BALM

This herb has been used to reduce stress and anxiety for many years. It's frequently included in teas and known for its capacity to help decrease tension and induce relaxation. It relieves muscle tension, which is important while healing chronic pain.

Lemon balm is a calming herb that belongs to the mint family. Since the Middle Ages, it has been used to relieve stress and anxiety, improve appetite, promote sleep, and relieve gastrointestinal pain and discomfort (including gas, bloating, and colic).

NATIVE AREA: Mountainous areas of southern Europe and northern Africa.

MEDICINAL PART: The leaves.

MEDICINAL USES: Anxiety, increase appetite, promote sleep, and relieve gastrointestinalpain.

SCIENTIFIC NAME: Melissa officinalis.

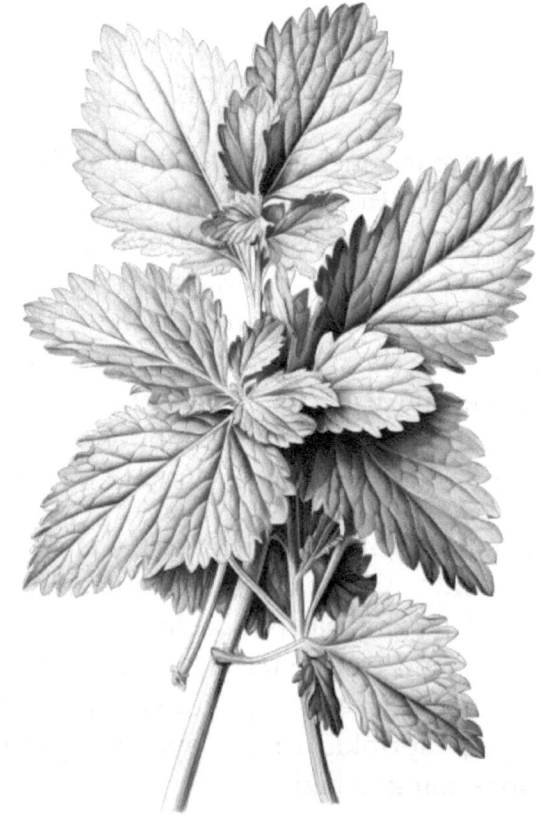

62.   LILAC

The medical properties of only the flower are still a mystery. Lilac's medicinal effects are derived from its leaves and berries. It was purportedly used as an anti-periodic tea or infusion in the past. Anti-periodic means that it prevents the recurrence of an illness, such as malaria.

According to certain research, it has a febrifuge action, which may aid in fever control. Lilac blossoms have astringent, aromatic, and possibly bitter characteristics. Astringents are chemicals that tighten, pull and dry tissues like skin.

A cool or warm infusion applied as a face toner would be excellent. An aromatic impact irritates the area with which it comes into touch (think GI tract), and irritation increases blood flow, which equals healing!

Eating raw flowers may help with gastric issues, including flatulence and constipation. Making your own fragrance oil and capturing the aromatics in herbal-infused oil could be an excellent way to capture the aromatics for medicinal purposes.

It is a plant native to Africa, Europe, and Asia that thrives in well-drained soil, particularly in temperate areas.

NATIVE AREA: Africa, Europe, and Asia

MEDICINAL PART: Flowers, leaves and fruits.

MEDICINAL USES: Anti-periodic (it stops the recurrences of diseases).

SCIENTIFIC NAME: Syringa vulgaris.

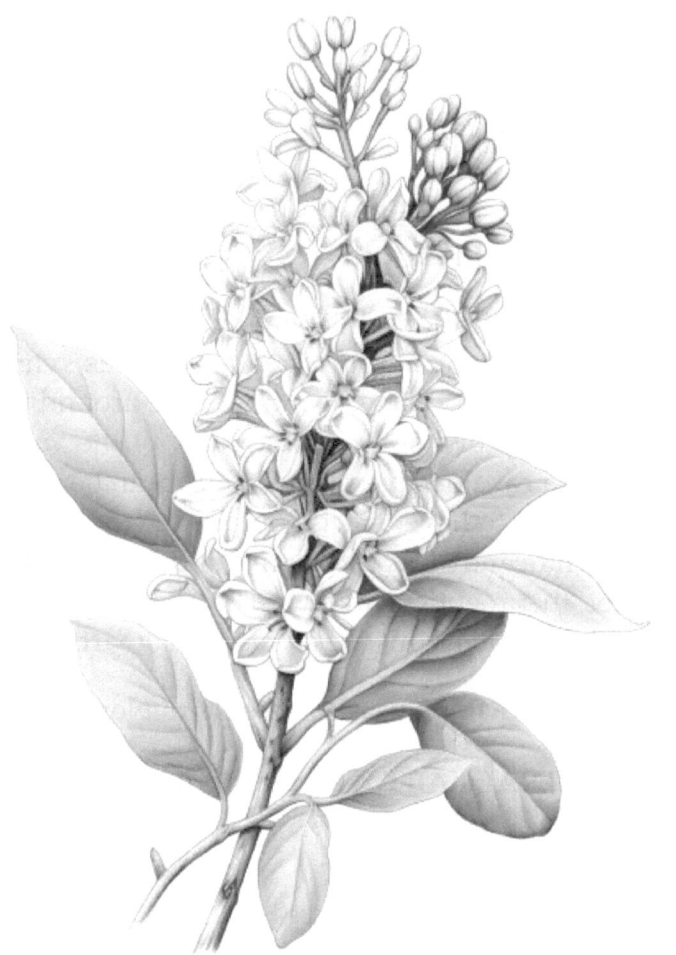

63.   LILY

Lily bulbs were thought to symbolize eternal life, and it's even said that Cleopatra would eat the bulbs by the handful.In addition, it has been said that chickens will not eat Lilium candidum because they know it will make them sick. The white lily, or Madonna Lily, is a flower that's been associated with queens, saints and Jesus' mother, Mary. It's also been thought to have magical powers by various cultures throughout history.

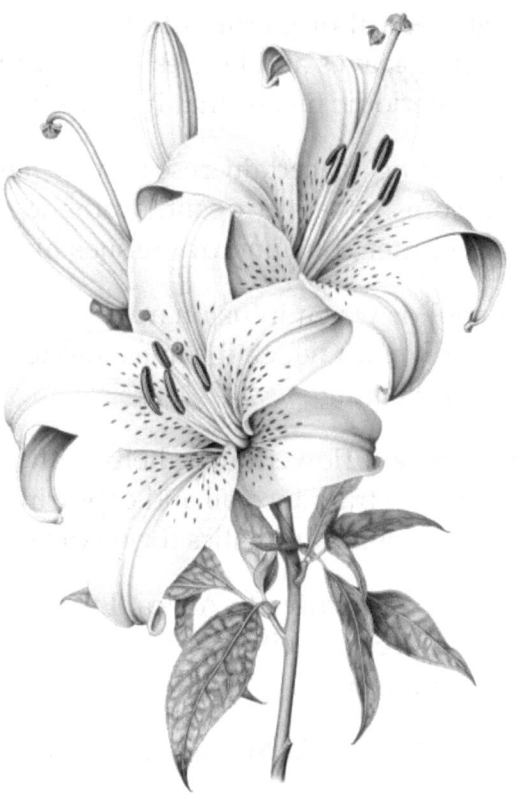

NATIVE AREA: Europe, Asia and North America.

MEDICINAL PART: The root, underground stem (rhizome), and dried flower tips.

MEDICINAL USES: Used for heart problems, urinary tract infections, weak contractions inlabor, kidney stones, epilepsy, fluid retention (edema), eye infections (conjunctivitis), leprosy, strokes and resulting paralysis.

SCIENTIFIC NAME: Lilium candidum.

64.   LILY OF THE VALLEY

In some civilizations, lilies are much more than just flowers. In some parts of Europe, they are seen as symbols of love, friendship, and purity. Planting them around your home is said to keep evil spirits at bay. Lily of the valley is mostly used as a cardioactive plant in European herbal medicine. It is expected to have effects comparable to digitalis, although it is significantly less cumulative and appears to have a much larger therapeutic window. The root, underground stem, and dried flower tips are all medicinal parts.

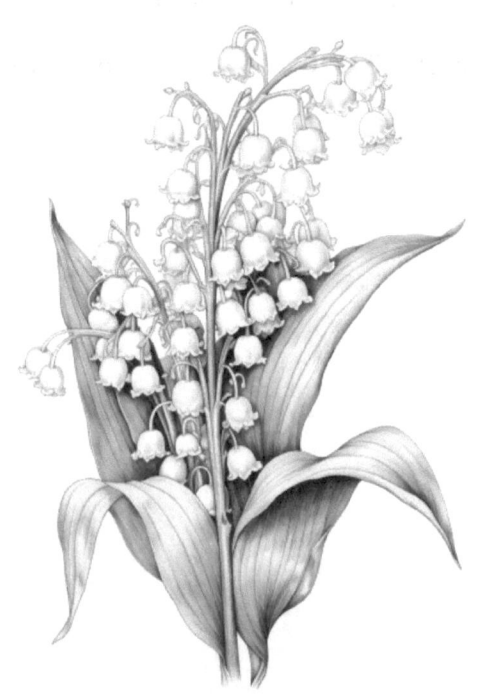

NATIVE AREA: Eurasia and eastern North America.

MEDICINAL PART: The root, underground stem and dried flower tips.

MEDICINAL USES: Heart issues such as heart failure and irregular heartbeat.

SCIENTIFIC NAME: Convallaria majalis.

65.   JASMINE

The Jasmine flower is thought to be the most popular flower for scenting lotions, creams, shampoos and perfumes. Its name is actually derived from the Persian word 'Yasmin,' meaning dew or jeweled moon, which came about because of its resemblance to the crescent moon.

It can assist in increasing libido and put people in the mood for love. As a sedative, jasmine soothes the mind, body, and spirit. It helps with tension, anger, anxiety, and sadness by bringing out pleasant and constructive feelings. It is also supposed to aid in the reduction of inflammation.

NATIVE AREA: Eurasia, Africa, Australasia and Oceania.

MEDICINAL PART: Leaf and flowers.

MEDICINAL USES: Jasmine has traditionally helped to treat liver disease (hepatitis), pain from cirrhosis (liver scarring), and abdominal pain from severe diarrhea (dysentery). It's also useful to prevent strokes, relax people (as a sedative), increase sexual desire (as an aphrodisiac), and treat cancer.

SCIENTIFIC NAME: Jasminum sambac.

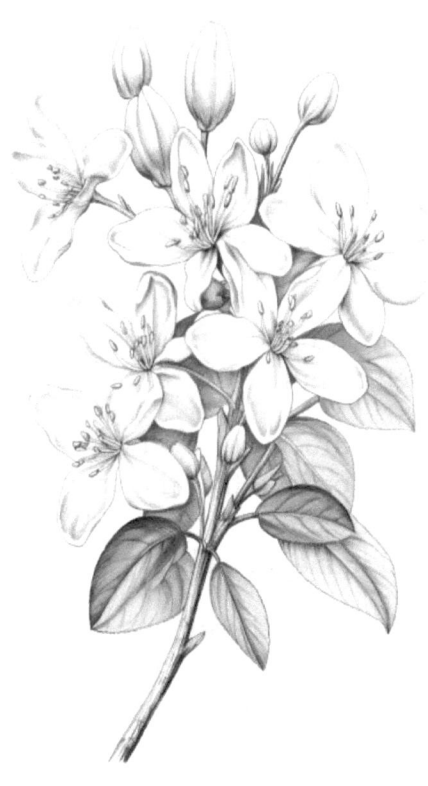

66.   JOE PYE WEED

This lovely plant is named after a Native American chief who reportedly used it as a kidney tea. There are different reports as to whether he ever existed.

NATIVE AREA: Eastern USA and Canda, and its range extends from Nova Scotia to Georgia.

MEDICINAL PART: Flowers, Leaves & Roots.

MEDICINAL USES: Diuretic and used to resolve urinary tract problems, including kidney stones. Joint stiffness, including gout and rheumatism.

SCIENTIFIC NAME: Eupatorium purpureum.

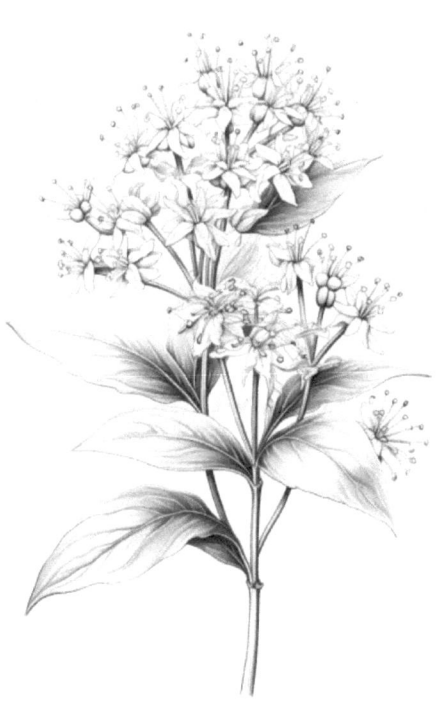

67.   MAGNOLIA

Magnolia is a type of flowering plant. The bark and flower buds are used to manufacture medication. Magnolia treats obesity, digestive issues, constipation, inflammation, anxiety, stress, depression, fever, headaches, strokes, and asthma. Stuffy nose, runny nose, common cold, sinus pain, hay fever, headache, and dark facial spots are all treated with Magnolia flower buds.

For toothaches, some people put magnolia flower buds straight into the gums. Magnolia flower bud extract is a skin whitener to lessen or counteract skin irritation produced by other chemicals in rub-on skincare products.

Magnolia bark is used in Hange-koboku-to, which comprises 5 plant extracts, and Saiboku- to, which comprises 10 plant extracts, in traditional Chinese and Japanese (Kampo) medicine.

These extracts are used to reduce anxiety and nervous tension and help people sleep better. Some experts believe that the active ingredient in these treatments is honokiol, a molecule found in magnolia bark.

Magnolia has become a popular Christmas tree since the 19th century because of its pretty white flowers and soft green leaves. In Christianity, it is thought to be a symbol of purity and childlike faith.

NATIVE AREA: Southeastern United States.

MEDICINAL PART: The bark and flower buds.

MEDICINAL USES: Weight loss, problems with constipation, inflammation, digestion, depression, anxiety, stress, fever, headache, stroke, and asthma.

SCIENTIFIC NAME: Magnolia stellata.

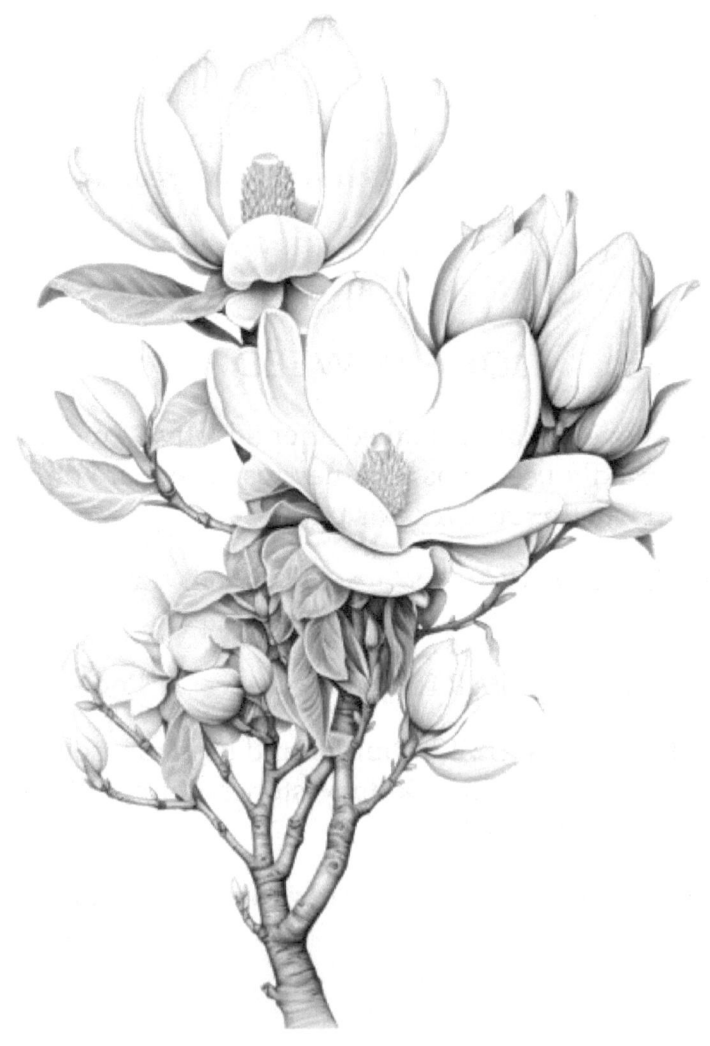

68. MANDRAKE

This root will shield from any threat, including physical harm. It will also assist in controlling negative energy and negative influences that cause unpleasant things to happen to other people. European mandrake root treats stomach ulcers, colic, constipation, asthma, hay fever, convulsions, arthritis-like discomfort (rheumatism), and whooping cough. It also induces vomiting, makes people sleepy (sedation), reduces pain, and increases sexual desire.

NATIVE AREA: Regions around the Mediterranean Sea.

MEDICINAL PART: Roots and leaves.

MEDICINAL USES: Stomach ulcers, colic, constipation, asthma, hay fever, convulsions, arthritis-like pain (rheumatism) and whooping cough.

SCIENTIFIC NAME: Mandragora officinarum.

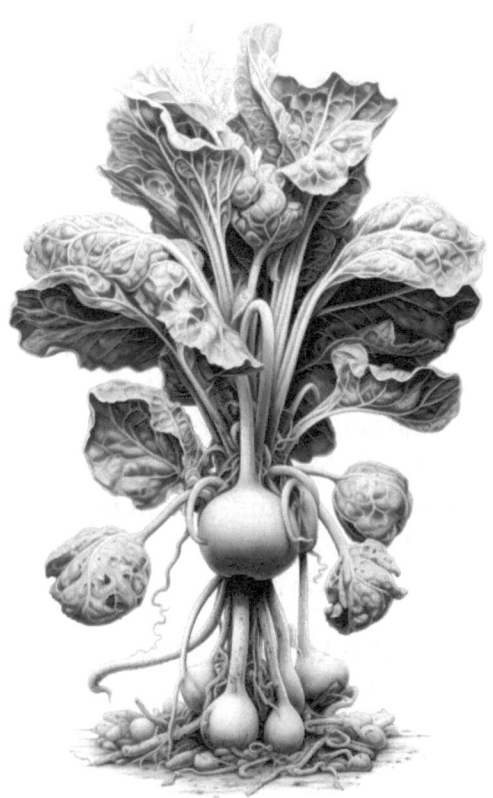

69. MARIGOLD

This gorgeous blossom serves as a wonderful protection charm, repelling negativity and evil spirits. It also protects the wearer from accidents such as vehicle accidents or falling downstairs.

Marigold (genus Tagetes) is an annual herb of the aster family (Asteraceae) native to southwestern North America, tropical America, and South America. Marigolds' most prevalent medical uses are for skin problems such as contusions, bruises, and varicose veins. Minor skin abrasions and inflammation can also be successfully addressed. Marigold ointment promotes faster healing of eczema and sunburn lesions.

NATIVE AREA: Southwestern North America, tropical America, and South America.

MEDICINAL PART: Flowers.

MEDICINAL USES: Skin disorders.

SCIENTIFIC NAME: Tagetes.

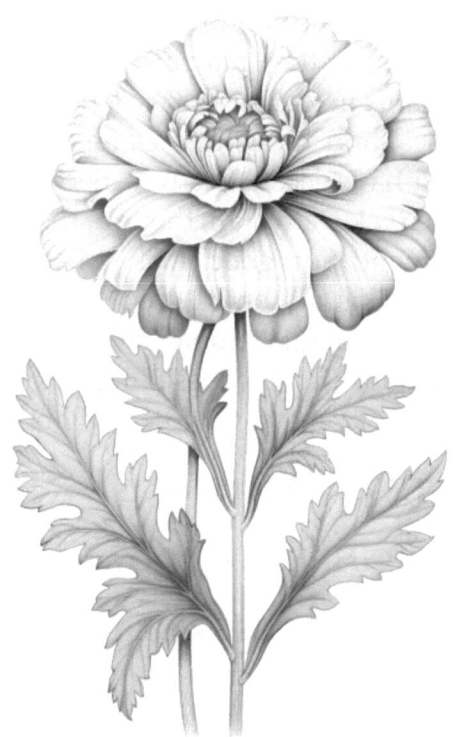

70.   MINT

Mint is frequently utilized for its cooling and relaxing properties, as well as its ability to cleanse energy. Mint tea is frequently consumed before entering a new area or ritual. It's an Herb with strong antiviral activity, useful in the fight against dangerous germs and parasites in the body. It has also increased blood flow and circulation while reducing muscle discomfort. Mentha is a plant genus in the Lamiaceae family. The precise differentiation between species is unknown; 13 to 24 species are thought to exist. Hybridization occurs spontaneously where the ranges of several species intersect, so there are numerous hybrids and varieties.

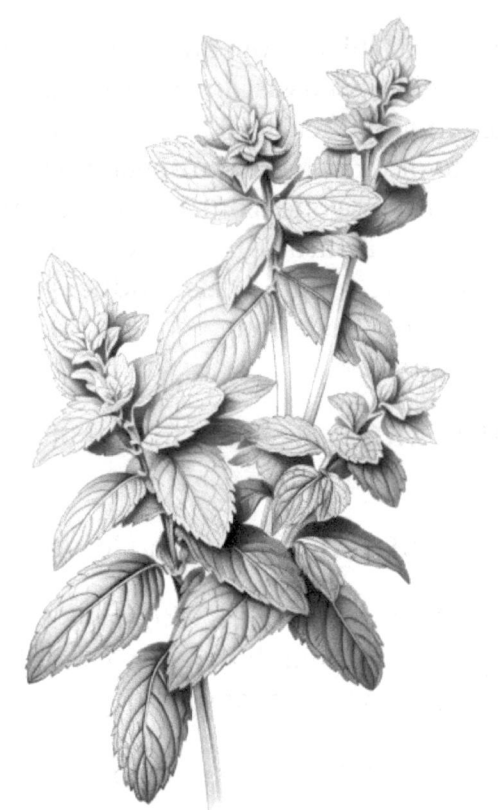

NATIVE AREA: Eurasia, North America, southern Africa, and Australia

MEDICINAL PART: Leaves and oils.

MEDICINAL USES: Digestive problems.

SCIENTIFIC NAME: Mentha

71.   MISTLETOE

Mistletoes are commonly found growing on trees in the winter, but they may also be found growing on other sorts of plants in warmer parts of the world, such as Japan, China, Africa, and India, and can easily be grown indoors if you don't have access to a tree. Because they are associated with the Greek Deity Pan, they are regarded the most powerful of all plants for good luck. Mistletoe was utilized to craft wands, kissers, and sacred things that were all employed for positive magic. Some cultures still utilize it today; for example, the Japanese think kissing under mistletoe or hanging it above your bed will bring you sweet dreams.

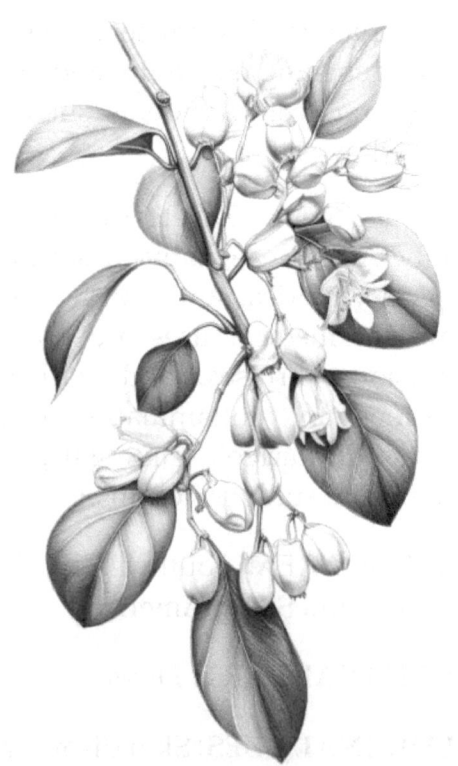

NATIVE AREA: Mexico.

MEDICINAL PART: Flower, fruit, leaf and stem.

MEDICINAL USES: Seizures, headaches and menopause symptoms.

SCIENTIFIC NAME: Viscum album.

72. MORNING GLORY

The common morning glory is known as a "Cupid's Darts" because of its pretty white flowers and the fact that it symbolizes love. Because of this, it is often given as a gift to someone because of their beauty or as a gesture to show that you love them.

For millennia, the morning glory has been used as a laxative in Asian and Mesoamerican cultures, and a tea made from its roots was sometimes employed as a diuretic and expectorant. Herbalists have also employed tea made from dried leaves to cure headaches.

NATIVE AREA: Central and South America.

MEDICINAL PART: Dry leaves and root.

MEDICINAL USES: Laxative, diuretic and expectorant.

SCIENTIFIC NAME: Convolvulus arvensis/calibrisiensis.

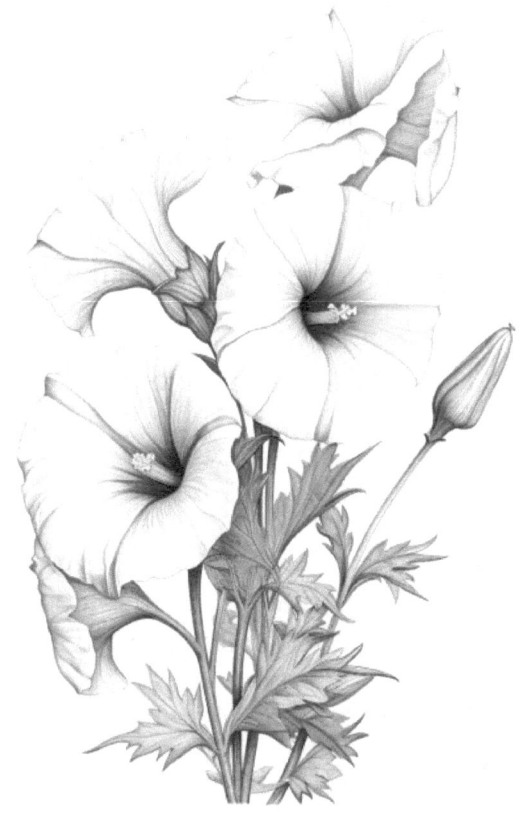

73.   MUGWORT

This herb, also known as Artemisia, has been utilized in Chinese culture for thousands of years and is widely used medicinally.

Mugwort is a popular name for numerous scented blooming plants of the Artemisia genus. In Europe, mugwort usually refers to the species Artemisia vulgaris, often known as common mugwort. While other species have more distinct common names, they are often referred to as "mugwort" in numerous settings.

NATIVE AREA: Europe and eastern Asia.

MEDICINAL PART: The plant parts that grow above the ground and the root.

MEDICINAL USES: For digestive problems, irregular menstruation, high blood pressure. Also used as a sedative, laxative, and liver tonic.

SCIENTIFIC NAME: Artemisia vulgaris.

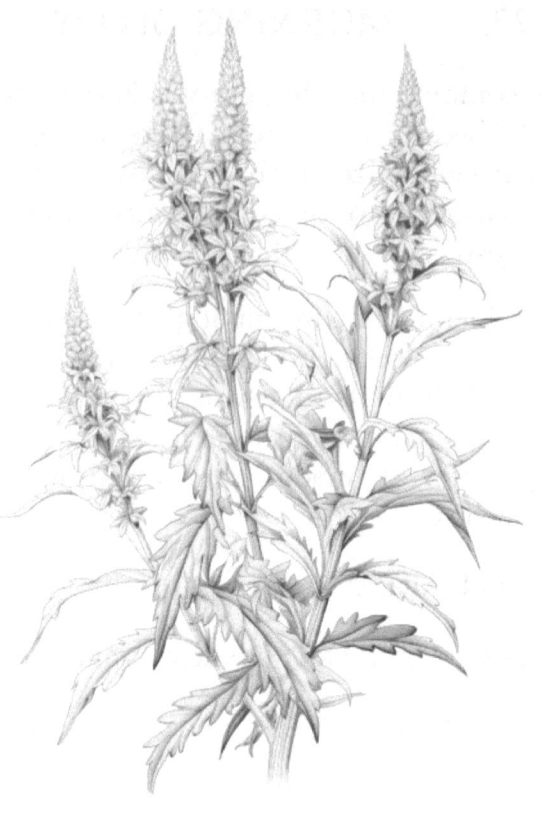

74.   NARCISSUS

The narcissus is thought to be a symbol of purity because it can grow from the seed of an old flower. It was also associated with resurrection since the bulb could be dug up after multiple years and returned to life.

NATIVE AREA: Southern Europe and North Africa.

MEDICINAL PART: The bulb, leaf, and flower.

MEDICINAL USES: For relieving catarrh and for epidemic dysentery.

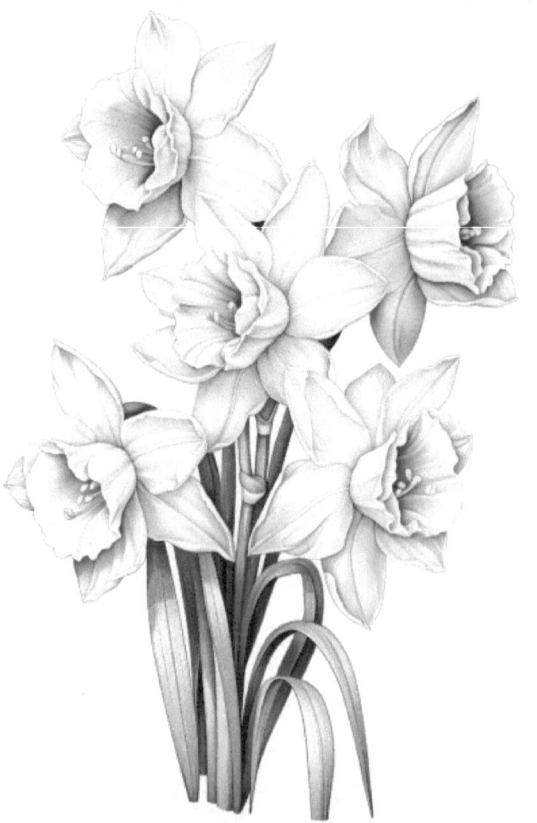

75.   OLIVE LEAF

Olive-leaf tea relieves coughs and clears the throat, making it useful in treating bronchitis. Because of its laxative impact on the colon, it can also be used to aid in weight loss.

Olive-leaf tea is useful against yeast infections and viral disorders such as herpes. Some studies suggest antioxidants may help treat tumors and malignancies like breast, liver, and prostate cancer. In these cases, Olive Leaf Tea is best known for its preventive function, which promotes normal DNA repair.

NATIVE AREA: Mediterranean Europe, Asia, and Africa.

MEDICINAL PART: Leaf.

MEDICINAL USES: Stronger Immune System.

SCIENTIFIC NAME: Olea europaea.

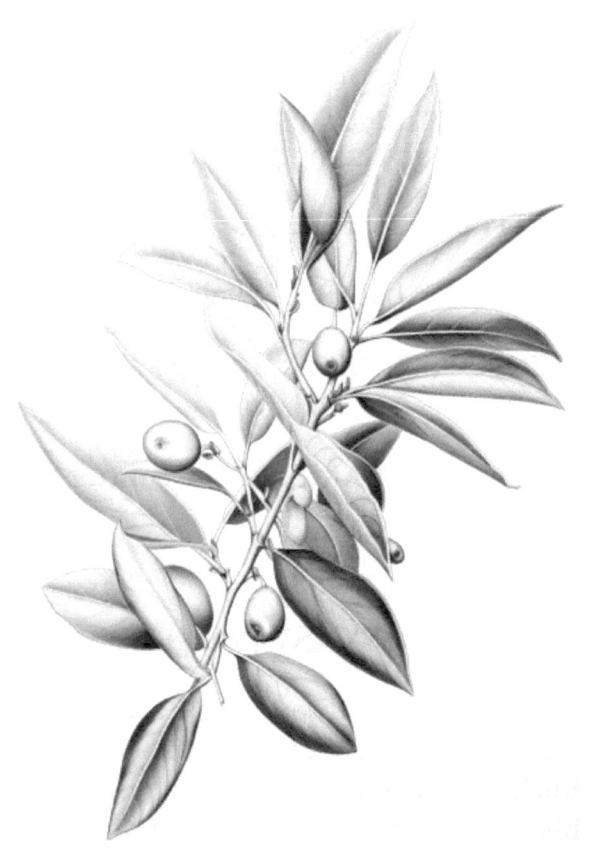

76. ORCHIDS

The Chinese were the first to discover the medicinal virtues of orchids. In his therapeutic works from the 28th century BC, Emperor Shen Nung, the "Father of Chinese Medicine," listed a dendrobium species and Bletilla striata. Orchids are still used for therapeutic purposes in China, most notably in the form of medicinal tea. Dried dendrobium is thought to have therapeutic characteristics that can aid in treating cancer, strengthen the immune system, and improve vision.

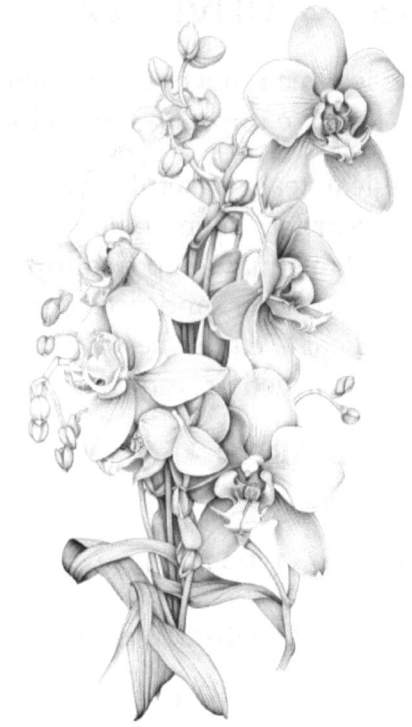

NATIVE AREA: China.

MEDICINAL PART: Whole plant, root.

MEDICINAL USES: It helps treat cancer, strengthen the immune system, and improve eyesight.

SCIENTIFIC NAME: Angraecum magdalenae, Phalaenopsis cornu-cervi.

77. PANSY (Viola tricolor.)

Many gardeners throughout Europe cultivated violas and wild pansies. We now call pansy plants started in Iver, Buckinghamshire, England. A curious Lord Gambier and his gardener William Thompson began crossing numerous Viola species in the early 1800s. Pansy has been a favorite flower since the Middle Ages and is currently thought to be an aphrodisiac, but there is no proof of this.

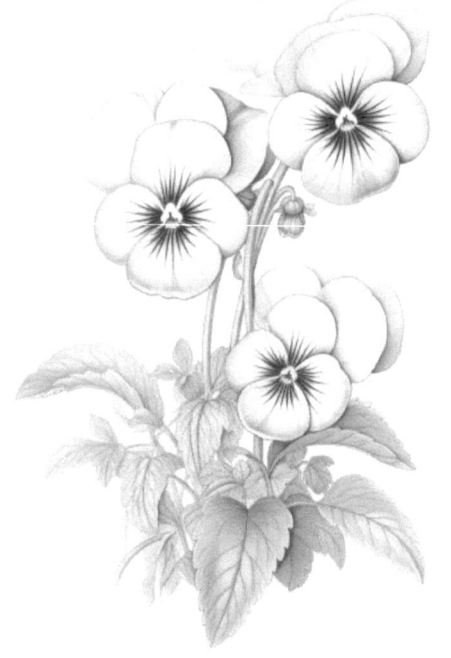

It includes mucilage, which has calming, antitussive, and anti-inflammatory qualities, effectively treating bronchitis and lung inflammation. It also contains analgesics like salicylic acid and salicylates, potent pain relievers. Externally, the flowering pansy herb treats mild seborrheic skin conditions such as dandruff, itching, cradle cap, and acne. Pansy is used to treat internal skin diseases. The plant is said to be able to purify the blood or promote metabolism in traditional medicine.

NATIVE AREA: Europe.

MEDICINAL PART: Whole plant.

MEDICINAL USES: Treat bronchitis and inflammation of the lungs.

78.   PASSION FLOWER

The Passion Flower is well-known for appearing in religious paintings, notably The Last Supper. It's also a popular ingredient in soaps and perfumes because it's supposed to smell like a mix of vanilla and honey. Passionflower (Passiflora incarnata) is a climbing vine that blooms in white and purple and contains compounds that are relaxing. The southeastern United States, as well as Central and South America, are native to this herb. It acts as a sedative and aids in the reduction of anxiety.

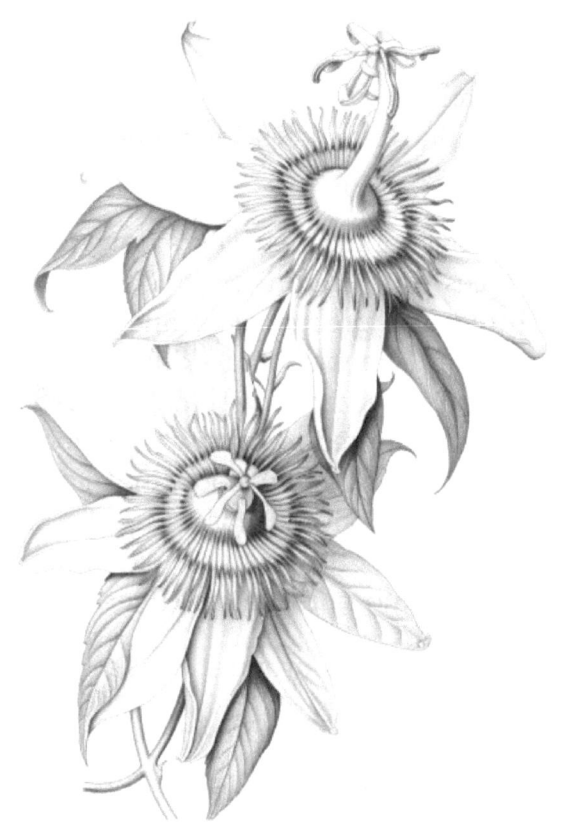

Passionflower is frequently used as an ingredient in teas that help to soothe the nervous system. It also relieves anxiety and provides a sense of calm to people who have insomnia. This allows patients to relax and sleep, which is a vital component of their daily recovery!

NATIVE AREA: Southeastern United States and Central and South America.

MEDICINAL PART: The above ground parts.

MEDICINAL USES: Dietary supplement for anxiety and sleep problems.

SCIENTIFIC NAME: Passiflora incarnata.

79.   PEPPERMINT

Peppermint oil is an effective treatment for sinusitis, loss of smell, nausea, vomiting and flatulence. It can also be used to treat headaches, toothaches caused by colds, flu and as a natural bug repellant.

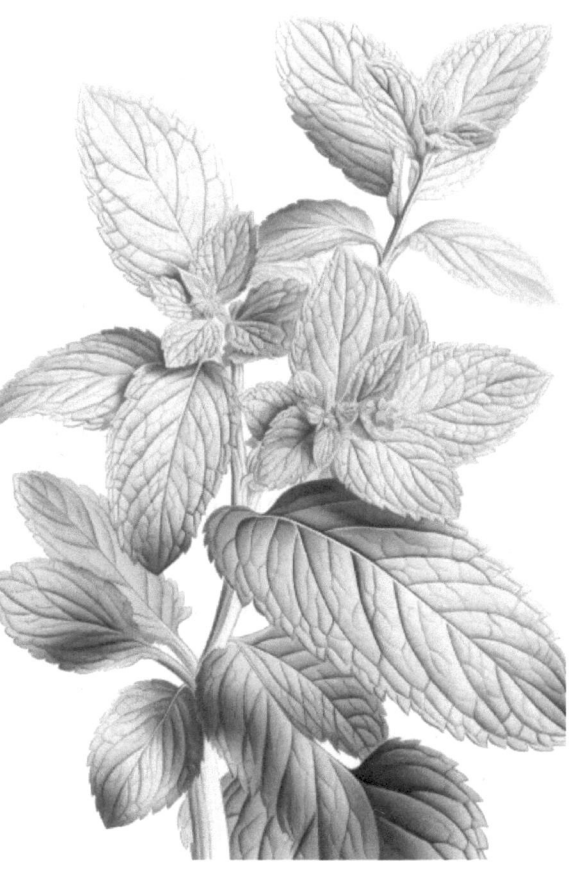

NATIVE AREA: Europe and Middle East.

MEDICINAL PART: Oil.

MEDICINAL USES: Digestive problems, sinus infections, headaches, the common cold.

SCIENTIFIC NAME: Mentha × piperita.

80. RED CLOVER

Red clover promotes bone density and reduces osteoporosis progression, effectively preventing or reducing bone loss. It can also be used to treat menopausal symptoms such as hot flashes and depression. It reduces inflammation in osteoarthritis patients.

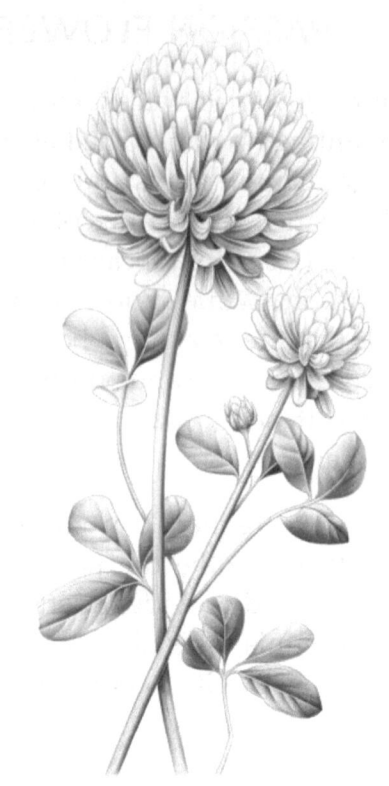

Red Clover increases blood flow to the uterus and enhances progesterone production, both of which are required for pregnancy. Cancer, whooping cough, respiratory illnesses and skin inflammations such as psoriasis and eczema have all been treated with it. Red clover is supposed to "purify" the blood by acting as a diuretic (assisting the body in getting rid of excess fluid) and expectorant (assisting the body in clearing phlegm from the lungs), as well as improving circulation and purifying the liver.

NATIVE AREA: Europe and Asia.

MEDICINAL PART: Flowers and leaves.

MEDICINAL USES: Hair and skin disorders.

SCIENTIFIC NAME: Trifolium pratense

81. RHODODENDRON

The Rhododendron is one of the most popular garden plants, but it has also been used as traditional medicine for ailments such as colds and headaches.

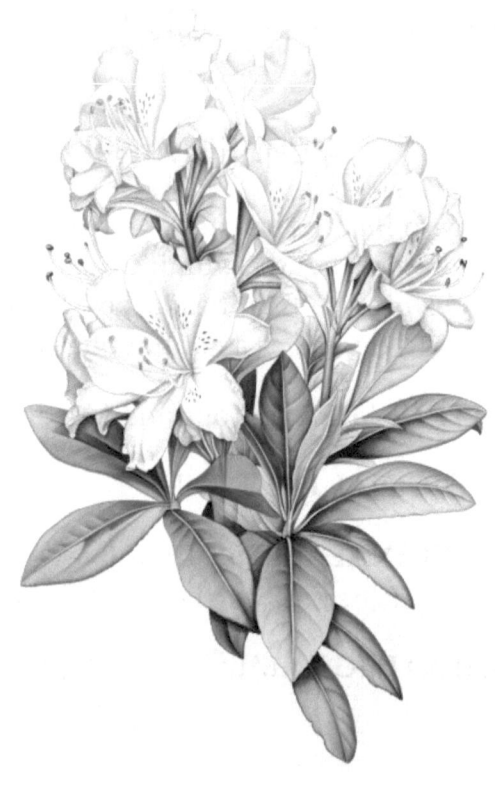

It is also used to treat fever and edema. Rhododendron arboretum is a woody plant of the Ericaceae family that grows in the North Temperate Zone, notably in the damp acid soil of Southeast Asia's Himalayas. The plant grows in Bhutan, China, Myanmar, Nepal, Sri Lanka, Pakistan, and Thailand, and can be found from Kashmir to Nagaland in the Himalayas.

Because of its wonderful flower tree plant, it is often used in gardens and plantations. It is used in traditional treatments for various diseases due to its phytochemical activity. This review focuses on the medicinal properties of several parts of the Rhododendron arboretum.

NATIVE AREA: Asia, North America, and Europe, as well as to the tropical regions of southeast Asia and northern Australia.

MEDICINAL PART: Leaves and twigs.

MEDICINAL USES: Heart disease prevention and therapy, detoxification, inflammation, dysentery, diarrhea, fever, constipation, bronchitis, and asthma

SCIENTIFIC NAME: Rhododendron 'Winter Rose'

82.   ROSE

The rose is one of the most popular flowers in history and has been used as a decorative piece since Roman times.

Throughout history, it has also been used as a symbol of love, victory, fame and death. In fact, the rose is so important that it's been used as a national symbol for countries such as England, Germany and Luxembourg.

Antibacterial, astringent, and tonic properties are all present in the petals. Colds, gastritis, diarrhea, bronchial infections, depression, and lethargy are all treated with them internally. They're used to treat eye infections, sore throats, minor injuries, and skin issues on the outside.

Many members of this genus produce fruit high in vitamins and minerals, including vitamins A, C, and E, and flavonoids and other bioactive substances.

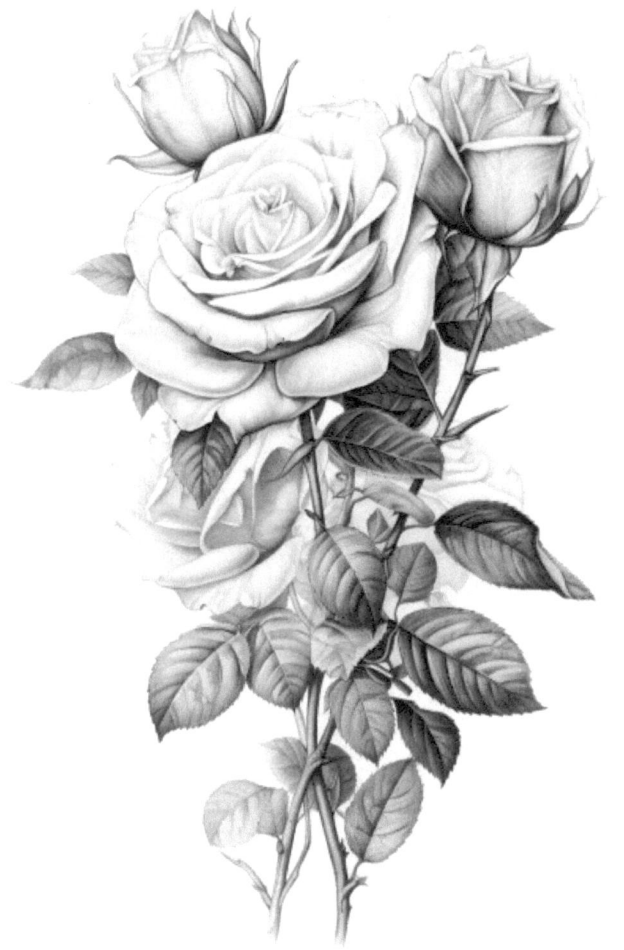

It also has a high concentration of essential fatty acids, which is unusual for a fruit. It's being studied as a cancer-prevention food and a way to slow or reverse the progression of tumors.

NATIVE AREA: New England.

MEDICINAL PART: Petals.

MEDICINAL USES: Colds, gastritis, diarrhea, bronchial infections, depression, and lethargy.

SCIENTIFIC NAME: Rosa gallica.

83.   ROSEMARY

For financial success, wealth, and abundance: It functions as a natural cleanser for wealth-related items.

Rosemary, often known as "The Herb of Remembrance," has long been associated with remembrance and utilized in commemorative rituals. This plant is frequently used to treat coughs, remove gas accumulation, promote digestion, and treat headaches.

It can also be used to treat wounds, cuts, scrapes, and other skin diseases as an antibacterial. When applied to the scalp, it increases blood circulation, which may aid in the growth of hair follicles.

Rosemary is commonly used in Italian cooking, but it can also be eaten raw as a plate garnish with dishes such as meatballs. Salvia Rosmarinus, sometimes known as rosemary, is a Mediterranean shrub with fragrant, evergreen needle-like leaves and white, pink, purple, or blue flowers.

It was previously known as Rosmarinus officinalis, which is now a synonym.

NATIVE AREA: Hills along Portugal, northwestern Spain and the Mediterranean

MEDICINAL PART: The leaf and its oil

MEDICINAL USES: Lower the risk of infections. Help the immune system fight off infections that occur.

SCIENTIFIC NAME: Salvia Rosmarinus

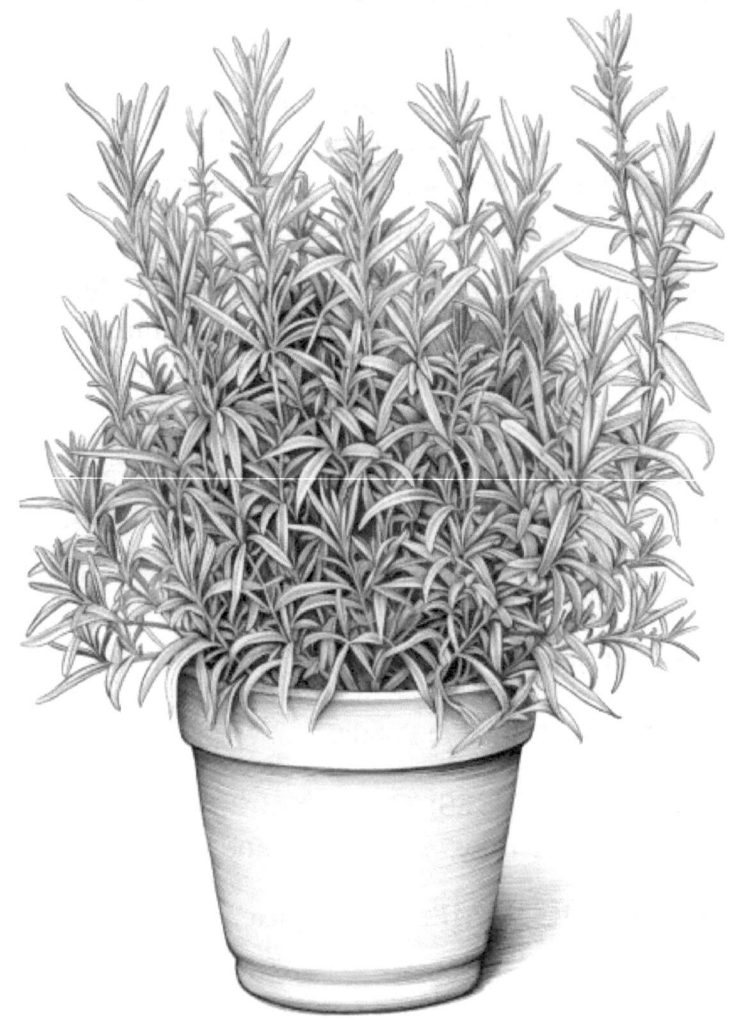

84. SAGE

Sage has a direct effect on your psychic senses, alerting you to knowledge that is being concealed from you. It is also used to help with meditation and gain access to the subconscious mind. This herb often treats various diseases, including sore throats, coughs, and respiratory problems. It can also be boiled with other herbs to treat digestive problems like gas, nausea, diarrhea, and cramps.

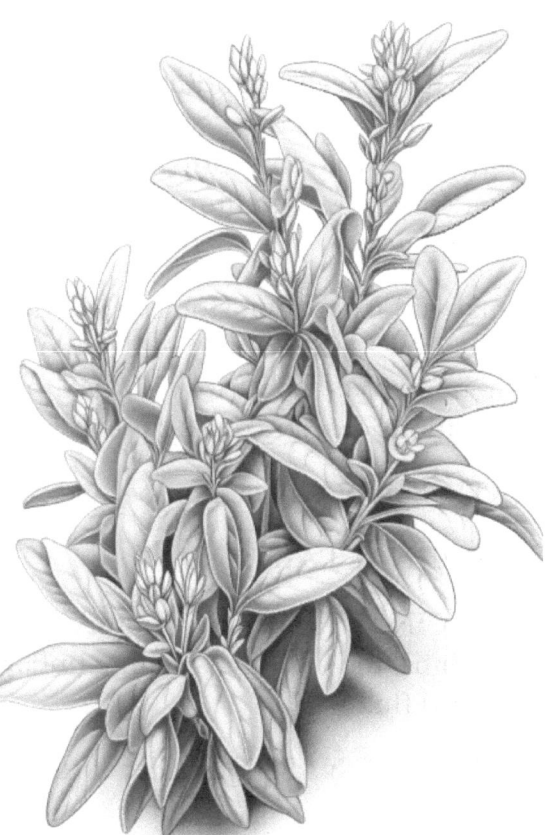

Salvia officinalis, also known as common sage or simply sage, is a woody-stemmed, evergreen subshrub with grayish leaves and blue to purplish flowers. It belongs to the mint family Lamiaceae.

NATIVE AREA: Mediterranean region

MEDICINAL PART: The leaf.

MEDICINAL USES: For digestive problems, for depression and memory loss

SCIENTIFIC NAME: Salvia officinalis.

85. SPIRULINA

As protein and iron-rich blue-green algae, Spirulina is well-known for its detoxifying qualities. It contains phycocyanins, which are antioxidants that have been found to attack malignant cells by flooding the immune system with killer T-cells.

Spirulina is a high-nutrient alga; It contains phycocyanin, a plant-based protein that is good for you. According to study, this possesses antioxidant, pain-relieving, anti-inflammatory, and brain-protective properties. Spirulina includes a high concentration of antioxidants, which have anti-inflammatory actions in the body.

NATIVE AREA: Mesoamerica.

MEDICINAL PART: Plant.

MEDICINAL USES: Pain-relieving, anti-inflammatory.

SCIENTIFIC NAME: Arthrospira platensis.

86. STAR ANISE

The magnolia family includes the star anise produced in Asia, Europe, and North America. Its strong licorice flavor makes it an excellent addition to certain herbal teas. Its star-shaped fruit was once considered a good luck symbol in China, but it is now primarily used to flavor meals and beverages. It's antifungal, antibacterial, and anti-inflammatory.

It may aid in treating stomach ulcers, blood sugar control, depression, and menopausal symptoms. Anise seed can help numerous aspects of your health when combined with a nutritious diet and a healthy lifestyle.

NATIVE AREA: Asia, Europe, and North America.

MEDICINAL PART: Oil.

MEDICINAL USES: Respiratory tract infections, cough, bronchitis, the flu, lung swelling (inflammation), swine flu, and bird flu.

SCIENTIFIC NAME: Illicium verum.

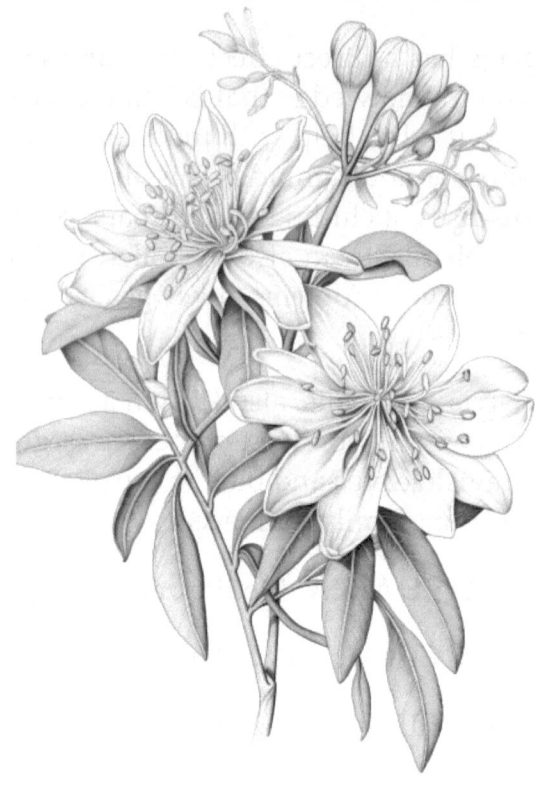

87. STRAWBERRIES

The strawberry is a blooming plant: the fruit is both edible and medicinal, and the leaves are used to make medications.
Strawberry is used to cure diabetes, high cholesterol, high blood pressure, osteoarthritis, and other conditions, however there is no scientific evidence to support these claims. Strawberries are also abundant in vitamin C and are considered a "super fruit" because of this. antioxidants, antioxidants, and fiber.

NATIVE AREA: North America

MEDICINAL PART: Fruits and leaves.

MEDICINAL USES: Diabetes, high cholesterol, high blood pressure, osteoarthritis

SCIENTIFIC NAME: Fragaria ananassa

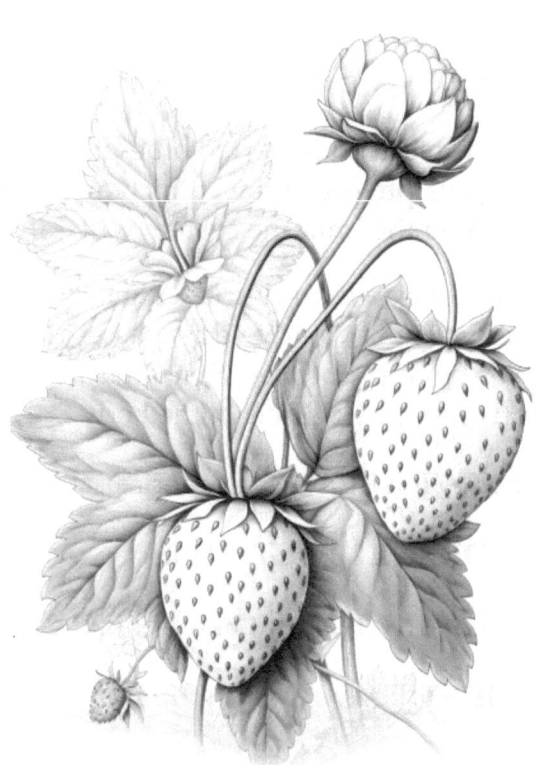

88. SUMAC

Sumac has been used as a medicinal herb and a spice for centuries. Among the medicinally active components are organic acids, phenolic acids, flavonoids, anthocyanins, hydrolyzable tannins, and terpenoids. This plant is the scientific name for the Anacardiaceae family, often known as the cashew or sumac family. The common names for this plant include blue glabrum, dwarf sumac, mountain sumac, Indian salt (the powder on the berries), Pennsylvania sumach, red sumac, sleek sumac, smooth sumac, and upland sumach.

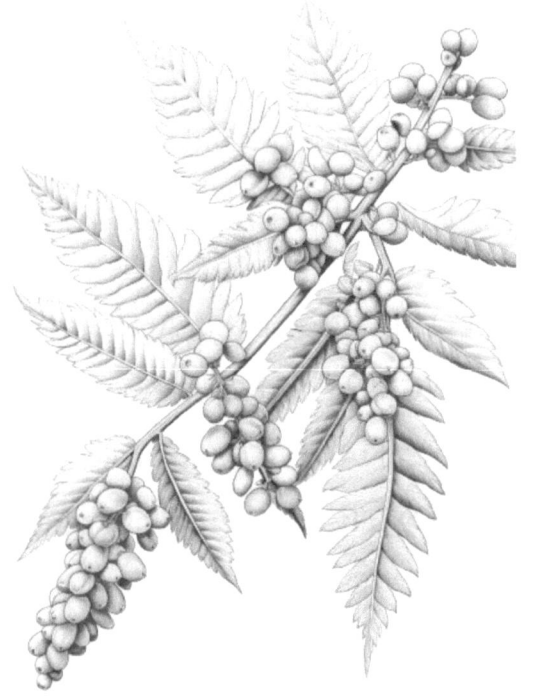

NATIVE AREA: Canada and North America.

MEDICINAL PART: The seeds and leaves.

MEDICINAL USES: Diarrhea.

SCIENTIFIC NAME: Rhus.

89. THYME

For good luck in business and a prosperous financial future: It strengthens the willpower of those who are immediately influenced by its use. This herb is available in tea form and can help relieve pain in various conditions, such as joint aches, tension headaches, and more. It can also be cooked with other herbs to help with digestion issues like flatulence or nausea. Thyme oil can also be used topically to treat wounds, scrapes, and other skin diseases such as burns. Thyme has an appealing aroma and flavor and is frequently used in French cuisine to cook meats such as beef, hog, or lamb. It is an aromatic perennial evergreen herb in the mint family Lamiaceae, belonging to the Thymus genus. Thymes are relatives of the Origanum genus: they have culinary, medicinal, and ornamental benefits, with Thymus vulgaris being the most extensively cultivated and utilized for culinary purposes.

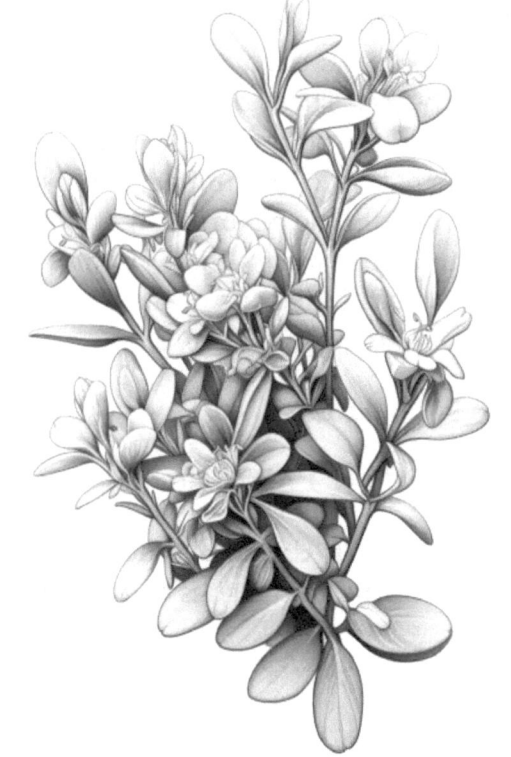

NATIVE AREA: Southern Europe.

MEDICINAL PART: Flowers, leaves and oil.

MEDICINAL USES: Combat bacterial and fungal diseases while also relieving coughs.

SCIENTIFIC NAME: Thymus vulgaris

90. TRILLIUM

Trillium is a tiny plant that blooms in late spring and early summer with lovely white flowers. They are a vital member of the trillium family, which also includes trilliums, muscari, and water lilies. Trillium species are native to temperate parts of North America and Asia, with the largest diversity of species found in the southeastern United States' southern Appalachian Mountains.

NATIVE AREA: North America and Asia.

MEDICINAL PART: The root.

MEDICINAL USES: Stimulates menstruation.

SCIENTIFIC NAME: Trillium grandiflorum

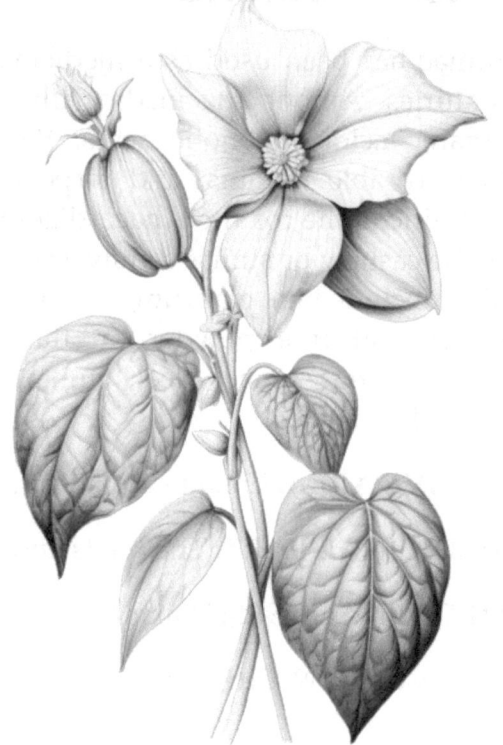

91. TULIP

Tulips, primarily valued for their ornamental beauty, have limited medicinal applications. In traditional herbal remedies, tulip bulbs were occasionally used to address respiratory, digestive, and skin conditions. However, these uses lack significant scientific support in modern herbal medicine.

Today, tulips are cherished for their vibrant colors and graceful form, enhancing gardens and floral arrangements worldwide. Their diverse varieties allow for captivating displays throughout the spring season. While their medicinal role is limited, tulips provide a fascinating glimpse into the historical intersection of plants and human health. Ultimately, they continue to inspire with their beauty, reminding us of the profound connection between nature and our well-being.

NATIVE AREA: Asia.

MEDICINAL PART: Flowers.

MEDICINAL USES: Excellent poultice for insect bites, bee stings, burns, and rashes on theskin.

SCIENTIFIC NAME: Tulipa.

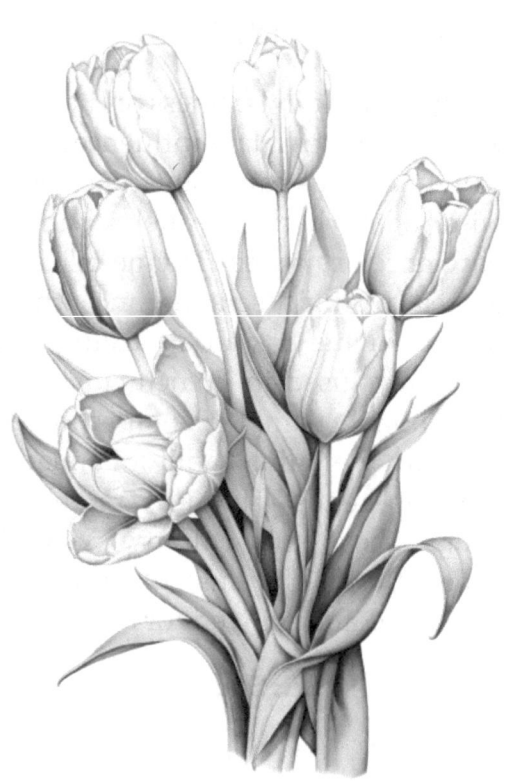

92. TURMERIC

Turmeric, scientifically known as Curcuma longa, is a golden-hued spice renowned for its potent medicinal properties. The key compound responsible for its health benefits is curcumin. Curcumin exhibits powerful anti-inflammatory and antioxidant effects, making turmeric a valuable herb in herbal medicine. It aids in reducing inflammation, easing pain, and supporting joint health. Turmeric also promotes digestive well-being, alleviating discomfort and promoting a healthy gut. Additionally, turmeric is believed to support cognitive function, enhancing memory and protecting against cognitive decline.

Beyond its medicinal uses, turmeric adds a distinctive flavor and vibrant color to culinary creations, being a staple in curries, sauces, and beverages. With its versatile applications and potential health benefits, turmeric holds a prominent place in both traditional remedies and modern wellness practices.

NATIVE AREA: South Asia.

MEDICINAL PART: Yellow powder and leaves.

MEDICINAL USES: relieves cold symptoms, jaundice, and intestinal worms, aids digestion, and can avoid bloating and abdominal discomfort. Turmeric powder treats conditions such as conjunctivitis, rheumatoid arthritis, chronic anterior uveitis, skin cancer, smallpox, wound healing, chicken pox, urinary tract infections, and liver problems.

SCIENTIFIC NAME: Curcuma longa

93. TURTLEHEAD

Turtlehead is a clump-forming perennial wildflower native to eastern North America. It bears hooded flowers like snapdragon blossoms. The flower gets its common name from its similarity to a turtle's beak.

On the other hand, the genus name Chelone refers to a mythological creature from ancient Greece. According to tradition, a nymph named Chelone refused to attend Zeus and Hera's wedding and was tossed into a river with her home; she transformed into a tortoise and took her back home.

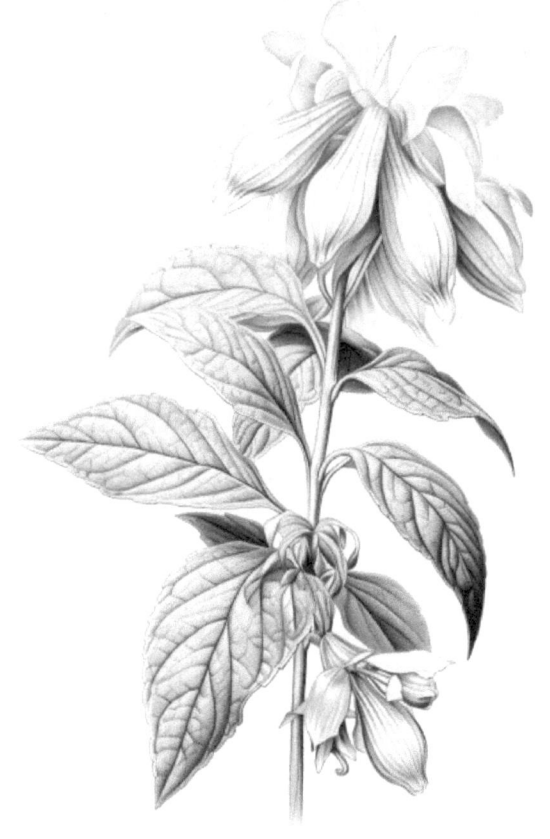

Turtlehead species thrive in similar environments but differ in size, appearance, bloom color and timing, and native distribution. The red turtlehead (Turtlehead oblique) blooms in late summer or early fall. It thrives in wetland environments but can also be grown in a moderately shaded home garden. Even while in bloom, the plant's opposing dark green, oval leaves are slightly serrated, and the stems remain upright.

NATIVE AREA: North America.

MEDICINAL PART: The part that grow above the ground.

MEDICINAL USES: Fever and jaundice.

94.   VALERIAN

This herb has been used to treat anxiety and despair for millions of years. It has soothing properties and can help reduce the frequency and length of panic attacks. It also helps with stress management, which is a key cause of chronic pain.

It naturally alleviates symptoms such as irritation, agitation, and sleep loss. Patients enjoy valerian tea because it relaxes the mind and body while reducing symptoms such as muscle aches and anxiety.

Valerian has traditionally been used to treat sleep disorders, migraines, lethargy, and stomach pains.

Today, Valerian treats insomnia, anxiety, sadness, PMS, menopause symptoms, and headaches. Valerian roots and rhizomes (underground stems) are used to treat various diseases.

NATIVE AREA: North America.

MEDICINAL PART: The roots and rhizomes.

MEDICINAL USES: Insomnia, anxiety, melancholy, menopause symptoms and headaches.

SCIENTIFIC NAME: Valeriana officinalis.

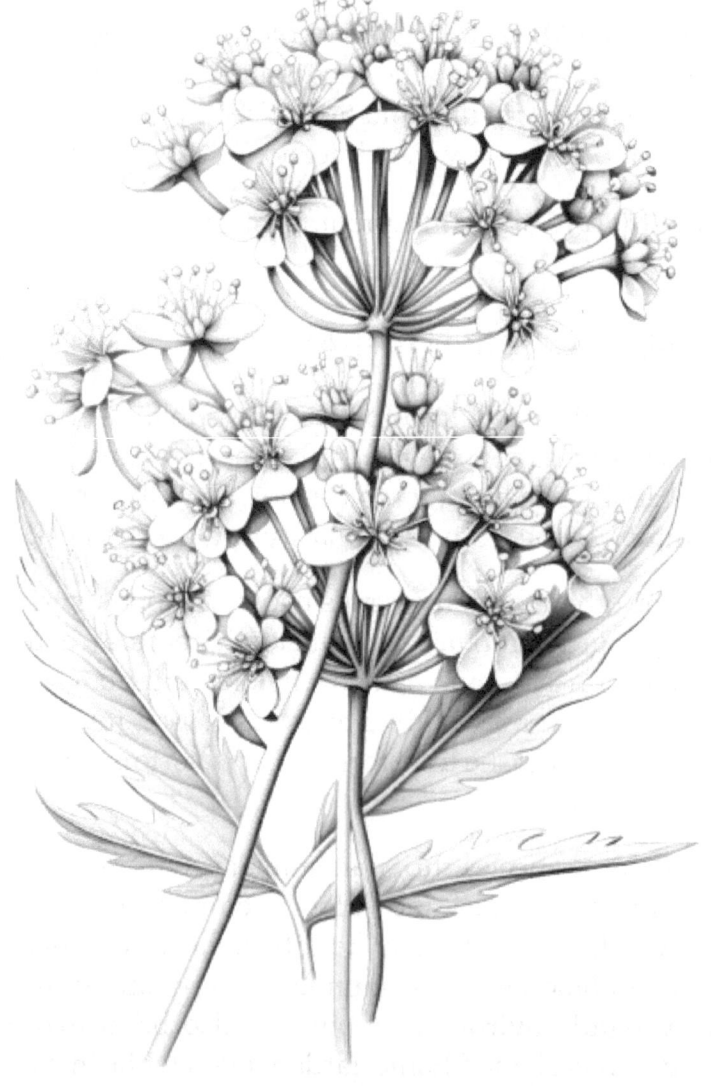

194

95.   VERBENA

Verbena, a perennial herb with slender stems and toothed leaves, is a valuable herb with diverse applications in herbal medicine. It is cultivated worldwide for its medicinal properties and plays a significant role in the realm of natural remedies.

Native to Europe and North America, Verbena's lance-shaped leaves possess remarkable healing potential. When crushed, they release a refreshing lemony scent, indicating the presence of beneficial compounds.

Verbena's clusters of small, vibrant flowers in shades of purple, pink, blue, or white not only add beauty to gardens but also attract essential pollinators.

In herbal medicine, Verbena is highly regarded for its antispasmodic, anti-inflammatory, and diuretic properties.

Its leaves contain essential oils, tannins, and flavonoids, which contribute to its therapeutic efficacy. Verbena is frequently employed in the treatment of various digestive disorders, including indigestion, bloating, and cramps.

Additionally, it is known to have a calming effect on the nervous system, making it a valuable herb for reducing anxiety and promoting relaxation

NATIVE AREA: Europe.

MEDICINAL PART: Parts above the ground.

MEDICINAL USES: Chest pain and related conditions.

SCIENTIFIC NAME: Verbena Officinalis.

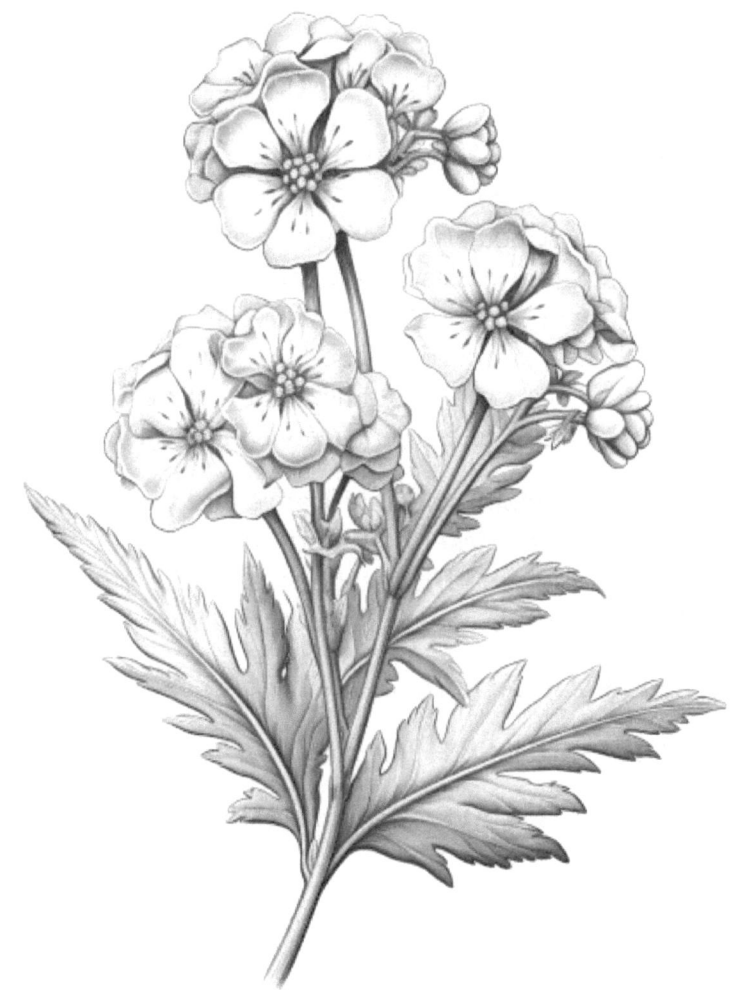

96.   VIOLETS

Violets have been used as a natural remedy for ailments such as sore throats and colds since the 9th century. It can also be used to treat asthma, hay fever, coughs, bronchitis, sinusitis, and other respiratory illnesses as an anti-inflammatory. Violet is moist and cooling, and when applied externally, the leaves alleviate inflammation and soothe skin irritations and swelling. It has a lymphatic affinity and can aid in maintaining healthy lymphatic function, and its antibacterial properties are currently being studied in modern research.

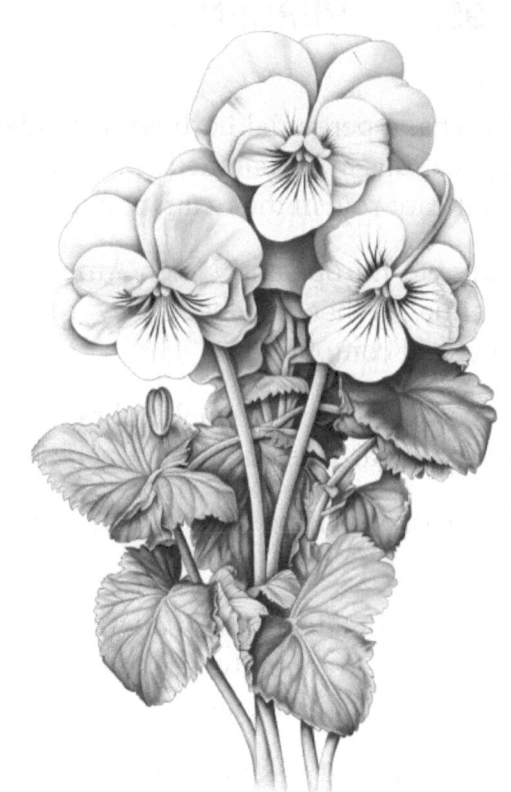

NATIVE AREA: North America.

MEDICINAL PART: Leaves.

MEDICINAL USES: Reduce inflammation and skin irritations.

SCIENTIFIC NAME: Viola.

97.   WHITE WILLOW

White Willow is a tree that grows to a height of 10-30 meters and possesses a large, domed crown. Its bark is rough and scaled, typically grey-brown. It has narrow, finely serrated leaves and small flowers that appear as yellow-green catkins.White Willow is a plant known for its medicinal properties. The bark can be used to create remedies because it contains a compound called salicin, which is similar to aspirin (acetylsalicylic acid).

The tree has historical significance and was once used to create baskets, cricket bats, and other wooden items due to its flexible wood.The catkins of white willow are an important source of early spring pollen for bees.

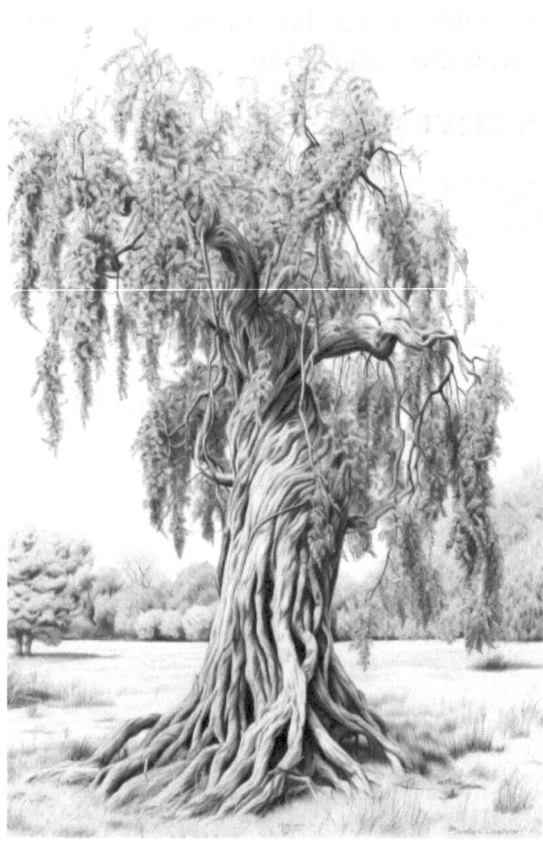

NATIVE AREA: Europe and Western and Central Asia.

MEDICINAL PART: The bark.

MEDICINAL USES: Treating pain, inflammation, and fever.

SCIENTIFIC NAME: Salix alba.

98.   WILD GERANIUM

Wild Geranium helps to balance female hormones and makes a pregnant woman feel better physiologically. Women who do not have correct hormone balance may have exhaustion after delivery, therefore this is an excellent herb for postpartum healing as well as fertility difficulties.

Wild geranium has been used as a natural cure for menstruation disorders such as irregular and painful periods for hundreds of years.

NATIVE AREA: North America.

MEDICINAL PART: Roots.

MEDICINAL USES: Treat burns and hemorrhoids.

SCIENTIFIC NAME: Geranium maculatum.

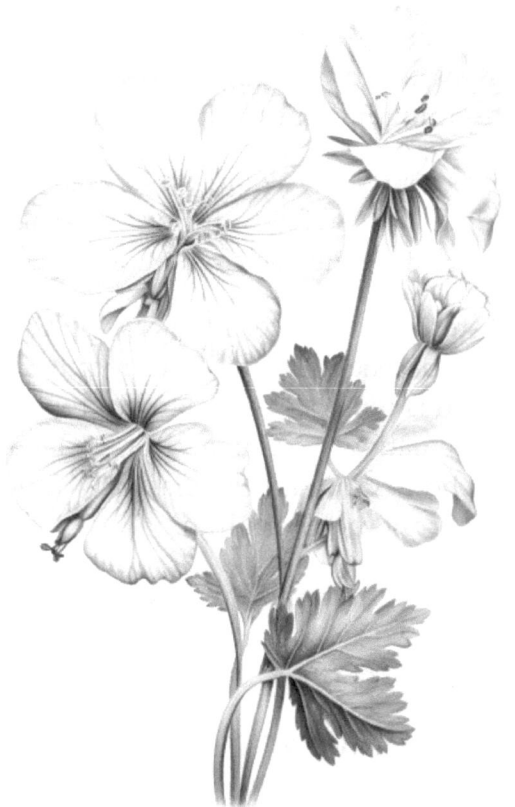

99.   WITHC HAZEL

Witch Hazel is an autumn-flowering shrub that grows to a height of 3-4.5 meters and has the potential to grow into a big tree. It has radially symmetrical flowers with narrow, long folded petals mature to a beautiful golden color, while the leaves are long and have wavy edges.

Witch hazel is a plant with medicinal effects. The bark and leaves can be used to make a topical astringent.

Dowsers have long utilized witch hazel branches to find water.

The petals of witch hazel are temperature sensitive, reflexing when cold and unfurling when warm.

NATIVE AREA: North America.

MEDICINAL PART: The bark and twig.

MEDICINAL USES: Treating skin inflammations and itchy skin.

SCIENTIFIC NAME: Hamamelis.

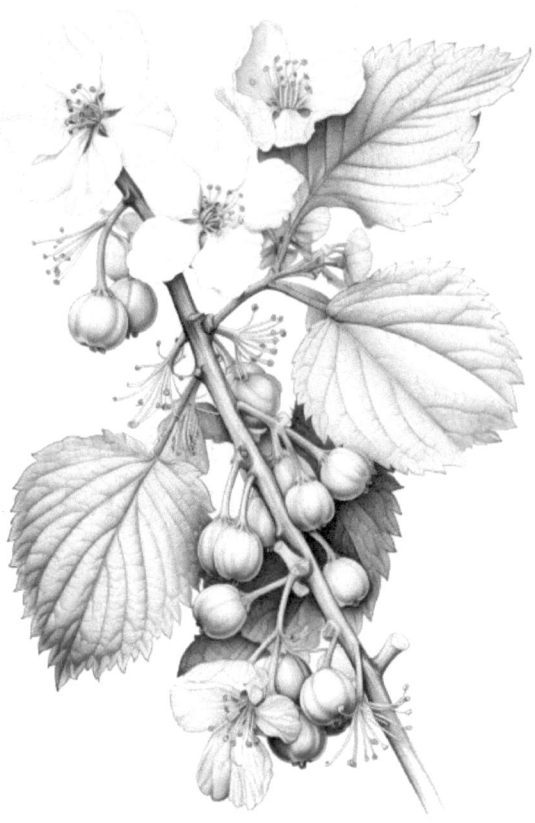

100. WISTERIA

Chinese Wisteria is claimed to confer longevity to its devotees while also providing inflammation treatment.

It has also been hypothesized that it can reduce miscarriages during pregnancy by boosting uterine circulation.

Wisteria is a flowering plant genus in the Fabaceae (Leguminosae) family that includes ten species of woody twining vines native to China, Korea, Japan, Southern Canada, the Eastern United States, and northern Iran.

NATIVE AREA: China, Korea, Japan, Southern Canada, the Eastern United States and northof Iran.

MEDICINAL PART: Seeds

MEDICINAL USES: Used in the treatment of cardiac disorders and as a diuretic.

SCIENTIFIC NAME: Wisteria sinensis.

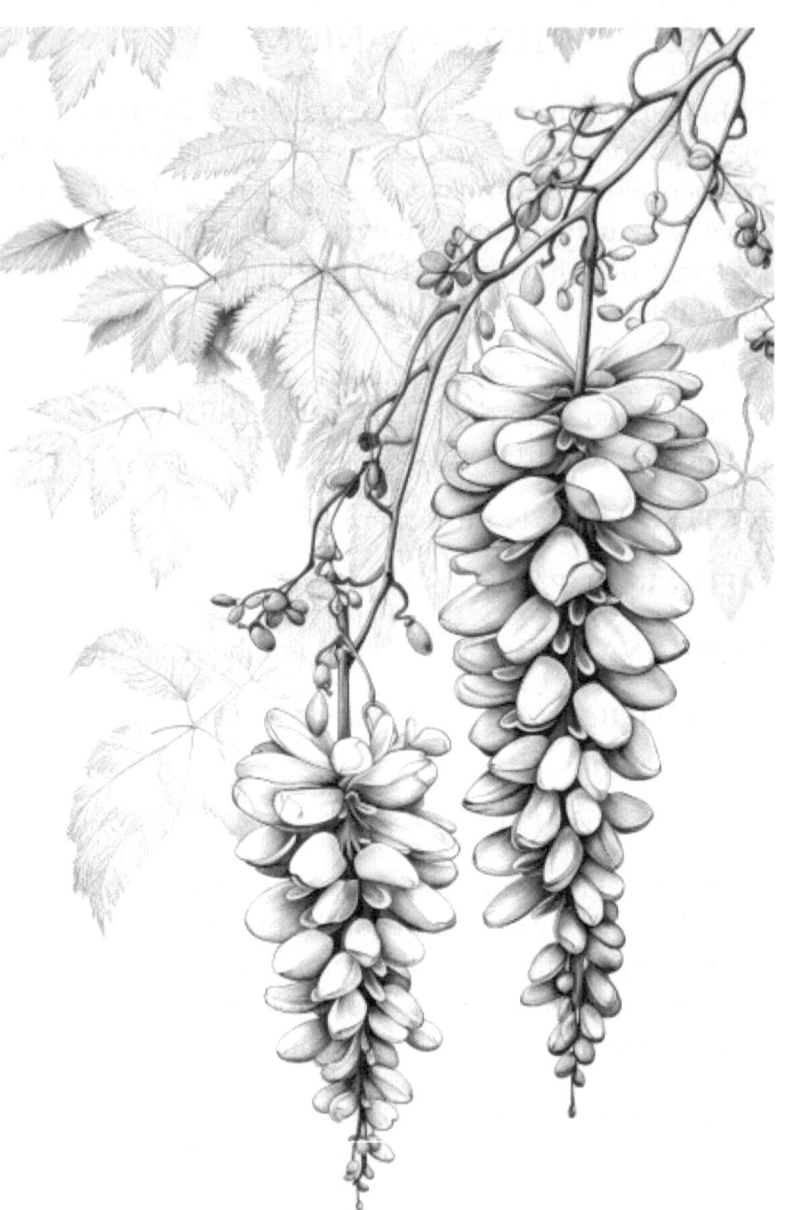

SCAN THE QR CODE TO DISCOVER ANOTHER 50 MEDICINAL PLANTS!

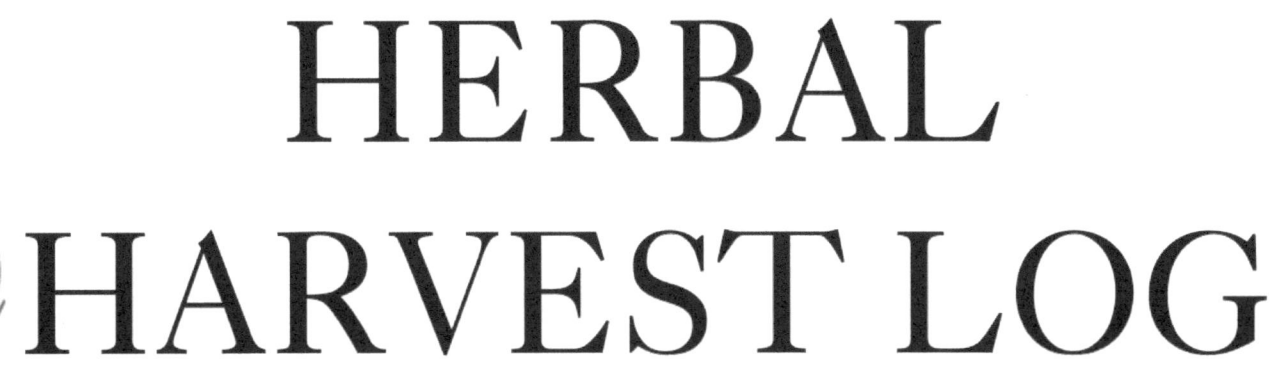

HERBAL HARVEST LOG

Welcome to the Herbal Harvest Logbook, a vital tool crafted with the avid herbalist in mind. As you traverse the enriching journey laid out in this book, you'll find that keeping a detailed record of your herbal harvests can be both rewarding and enlightening.

This logbook is designed to help you track various details of your harvests, from the type and quantity of herbs gathered to the harvesting location and conditions.

By utilizing this logbook, you will not only foster a deeper connection with the earth and the bounty it offers but also streamline your herbal preparation endeavors. This hands-on approach encourages you to become a more mindful and informed herbalist, enhancing your experience and expertise with each entry.

As an added bonus, by scanning the accompanying QR code, you will gain access to an additional 100 pages, providing you with even more space to document your herbal adventures.

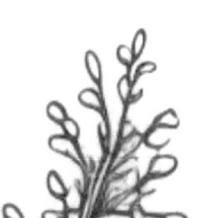
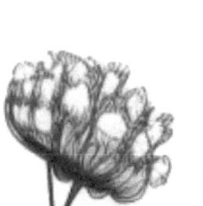
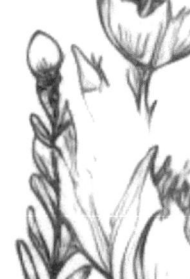
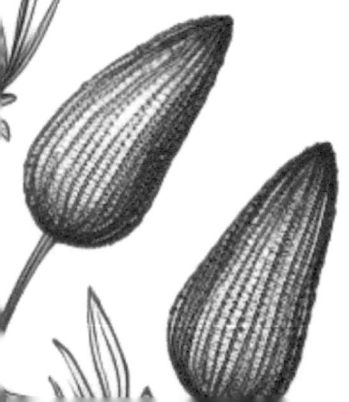

HERBAL HARVEST LOG

Date: /   /

Harvest Location

_____

_____

_____

Herb Type	Qty Harvested	Notes

Recipes/Tips

_____

_____

_____

_____

_____

Photo

attach photos of
the harvested herbs

HERBAL HARVEST LOG

Date: /   /

Harvest Location

_____

_____

_____

Herb Type	Qty Harvested	Notes

Recipes/Tips

_____

_____

_____

_____

_____

Photo

attach photos of
the harvested herbs

HERBAL HARVEST LOG

Date: /   /

Harvest Location

_____
_____
_____

Herb Type	Qty Harvested	Notes

Recipes/Tips

_____
_____
_____
_____
_____

Photo

attach photos of
the harvested herbs

NATIVE AMERICAN HERBAL RECIPES VOL. I

My Favorite Recipes

_____

_____

_____

_____

_____

_____

_____

INTRODUCTION

Essential oils are aromatic, all-natural plant-derived compounds derived from bark, flowers, fruit peel, roots, or other plant elements. They offer several health and wellness advantages and can be easily found in your area.For millennia, people have used these strong-smelling compounds without fully realizing their potential for healing or relaxation. However, clinical studies now reveal that essential oils are more than just a passing fad. They are being utilized to help people suffering from anxiety issues achieve better sleep. In fact, essential oils may help you relax and fall asleep faster than other options, as they have a long history of relieving stress.

Additionally, essential oils can serve as a natural remedy for insomnia by helping your body relax and quiet down. Some individuals suggest using a vaporizer to distribute the aroma into the air, while others recommend adding the oil to bathwater or dabbing it on your pillowcase before going to bed.Each essential oil comprises distinct components that have different effects on the body. For example, lavender essential oil contains linalool, which helps to improve your mood. Vetiver essential oil is known to reduce the effects of stress and anxiety due to its calming impact on neurotransmitters.

Moreover, essential oils can also assist with skin issues. Chamomile extracts are used to relieve skin irritations and disorders such as eczema and acne. Rose essential oil, commonly used to heal wounds, may also aid with insomnia, making it a potential natural remedy for falling asleep faster at night.Beyond health reasons, essential oils can help you eliminate domestic pests. The oil's soothing aroma can repel moths and other insects that may be drawn to your home.

Although essential oils and their use have been around for centuries and have gained popularity, the scientific understanding of these oils is relatively recent. The ability to extract compounds from plants and flowers that can alter our sense of smell, taste, mood, energy levels, sleep regulation, and disease-fighting abilities is truly amazing. Essential oils are excellent for therapeutic uses, such as boosting the immune system to help fight colds and healing minor skin wounds. They can stimulate or calm you, offering a contrast to stress-induced cortisol, making them wonderful for relaxation after a long day at work.

However, it's important to understand how your body reacts to essential oils to use them effectively for your health. While most people have at least one type of essential oil in their homes, many are unaware of their benefits. Questions may arise regarding the "natural" status of essential oils and whether they contain manufactured chemicals or chemical toxins. Safety concerns may also arise, such as the FDA approval of their use, their potential for aiding weight loss, their safety during pregnancy or breastfeeding, and their connection to cancer or congenital disabilities. It is crucial to seek scientific evidence and gain a comprehensive understanding of essential oils to use them safely and effectively.

DIY HERBAL RECIPES

Tea Recipes

1. Refreshing Kidney Cleansing tea

Preparation Time: 5 minutes**Cooking Time:** 0 minutes **Servings:** 1
Nutrition: 132 Calories; 1.6 g Fats; 4 g Protein; 27 g Carbohydrates; 3 g Fiber;
Ingredients:

- 1 teaspoon Prodigiosa powder
- 1 teaspoon burdock root powder
- 1 cup spring water

Directions:
1. Combine all ingredients in a tea kettle.
2. Boil for 10 minutes, then remove from heat, cover, and let for another 10 minutes.
3. Remove from heat and serve

2. Colon-Gallbladder Tea

Preparation Time: 5 minutes**Cooking Time:** 0 minutes **Servings:** 2
Nutrition: 130 Calories; 2.5 g Fats; 5 g Protein; 24 g Carbohydrates; 4 g Fiber;
Ingredients:

- 1 teaspoon Cascara powder
- 1 teaspoon Chaparral
- 1 cup spring water

Directions:
1. Combine all of the ingredients in a tea pot.
2. Boil for 10 minutes, then remove from heat, cover, and set aside for another 10 minutes.
3. Remove from heat and serve

3. Mucus Liver Cleansing Tea

Preparation Time: 5 minutes**Cooking Time:** 0 minutes **Servings:** 1
Nutrition: 140 Calories; 1.5 g Fats; 4g Protein; 16 g Carbohydrates; 6 g Fiber;
Ingredients:

- 1 teaspoon dandelion root powder
- 1 teaspoon Prodigiosa powder
- 1 cup spring water

Directions:
1. Combine all of the ingredients in a tea pot.
2. Boil for 10 minutes, then remove from heat, cover, and set aside for another 10 minutes.
3. Remove from heat and serve

4. Liver-Kidney Cleansing Tea

Preparation Time: 5 minutes
Cooking Time: 0 minutes
Nutrition: 120 Calories; 1.4 g Fats; 6 g Protein; 28 g Carbohydrates; 5 g Fiber;
Ingredients:

- 1 teaspoon dandelion root powder
- 1 teaspoon burdock root powder
- 1 cup spring water

Directions:
1. Combine all of the ingredients in a tea pot.
2. Boil for 10 minutes, then remove from heat, cover, and set aside for another 10 minutes.
3. Remove from heat and serve

5. Colon-Gallbladder Cleansing Tea

Preparation Time: 5 minutes**Cooking Time:** 0 minutes **Servings:** 1
Nutrition: 113 Calories; 1.5 g Fats; 6 g Protein; 22 g Carbohydrates; 3 g Fiber;
Ingredients:

- 1 teaspoon Cascara powder
- 1 teaspoon Rhubard root powder

- 1 cup spring water

Directions:
2. Combine all of the ingredients in a tea pot.

3. Boil for 10 minutes, then remove from heat, cover, and set aside for another 10 minutes.
4. Remove from heat and serve

Popsicles

1. Blueberry White Chocolate Popsicle Recipe

You will require the following items:

- 2 cups frozen organic blueberries
- 1/2 cup white chocolate chips (not sugar-free)
- 1 tablespoon pure maple syrup or raw honey

Directions: Blend all of the ingredients in a blender until smooth. Fill popsicle molds halfway with the mixture. Fill a cup halfway with the mixture, place it in the freezer for about 5 minutes to firm, and then turn it out.

2. Mango Papaya Popsicle Recipe

You will require the following items:

- 2 cups 100% orange or apple juice
- 1 cup mango or papaya chunks
- 1/2 lime, juiced
- 2 tablespoons shredded coconut

Directions: In a blender, combine all of the ingredients and blend until smooth. Fill popsicle molds halfway with the mixture. Fill a cup halfway with the mixture, place it in the freezer for about 5 minutes to firm, and then turn it out.

3. Cherry Limeade Popsicle Recipe

What you'll need:

- 12 ounces frozen organic cherries
- 6 ounces frozen limeade concentrate
- 6 ounces 100% white grape juice (or any other non-dairy juice you'd like)

- 2 tablespoons sugar (optional) or 1 tablespoon honey (or pure maple syrup if vegan)

Directions: In a blender, combine all of the ingredients and blend until smooth. Fill your popsicle molds with the mixture. Fill a cup halfway with the mixture, place it in the freezer for about 5 minutes to firm, and then turn it out.

4. Strawberry Basil Popsicle Recipe

You will require the following items::

- 2 cups fresh or frozen strawberries
- ½ cup 100% unsweetened orange juice without vitamin A
- ¼ cup almond milk (or any other non-dairy milk)
- 1 tablespoon finely chopped basil leaves
- 1 tablespoon honey (or pure maple syrup if vegan)
- 4 or 5 ice cubes

Directions: In a blender, combine all of the ingredients and blend until smooth. Fill your popsicle molds with the mixture. Fill a cup halfway with the mixture, place it in the freezer for about 5 minutes to firm, and then turn it out.

5. Mint Lemonade Popsicle Recipe

You will require the following items:

- 1/4 cup fresh mint leaves
- 1/2 cup fresh lemon juice
- 3 tablespoons cane sugar (or any other sweetener of your choice)

Directions: In a blender, combine all of the ingredients and blend until smooth. Fill popsicle molds halfway with the mixture. Fill a cup halfway with the mixture, place it in the freezer for about 5 minutes to firm, and then turn it out.

Washcloths

Even the most ordered family might struggle with washcloths. Nobody enjoys waking up with a runny eye and having to search for one in a pile of towels or wandering around their bathroom. You'll never have that problem again with these simple herbal recipes!

Soothing Diaper Rash Washcloth: Soak an old washcloth in 1 teaspoon aloe vera gel overnight. Add it to your wash with your diapers the next day.

Sinus Relief Washcloth: Soak a washcloth in a bowl of water with 2 tablespoons of Vick's Vapor Rub for about an hour. If you have allergies, you can substitute Vicks Vapo-rub for the aloe vera gel. Then put it in the washer with your towels and linens. This washcloth can provide immediate relief from sinus strain and congestion.

Anti-fungal Towel: combine 8 drops oregano oil and 4 drops tea tree oil on an old washcloth and let it overnight. Drop it in the washer with your towels the next day and run it through the wash cycle. This will aid in the treatment of any fungal infections you may have.

Sudsy Washcloth: For a freshly perfumed wash, add 2 drops of lemon essential oil to any liquid laundry soap when adding it to the wash. If you're using powdered detergent, you'll need to dissolve some of it in water first before adding the oil.

Washcloth with Herbal Extracts: Pour 1 tablespoon of Dr. Bronner's Castile Soap into a bowl of water and soak a washcloth in it overnight. The next day, rinse it and hang it to dry before using it again.

Compresses

Headache: In several glasses of boiling water, steep an equal number of lavender flowers (Lavandula angustifolia) and sage leaves (Salvia officinalis) for 10 minutes. Strain and apply to your brow.

Tension headaches: For about 10 minutes, steep a handful of mugwort (Artemesia Vulgaris) in a cup of water. Then drain the leaves from the water, load the jar or bowl with a clean cloth, fill with hot water, and place on your forehead.
To keep the heat in, cover with a cloth.

Earache: In a quart of boiling water, steep a tablespoon of chamomile flowers (Matricaria recutita) and an equal amount of mullein leaves (Verbascum thapsus) for 10 minutes. Pour the herbs from the water into a pan large enough to contain a pillowcase; pack the herbs in the pan with a clean towel and fill it with hot water. Squeeze the excess water from the pillowcase and compress it.

Stress: Add a few slices of ginger (Zingiber zerumbet) to 4 cups of boiling water to relieve stress. Lay on your left side for 20 minutes with a cloth over your head.

Tinea pedis (athlete's foot): In a dish, combine a few drops or a capful of organic tea tree essential oil (Melaleuca alternifolia) with white vinegar. Before going to bed, soak your feet for 15 to 20 minutes.

Insomnia: Drink an infusion of your choice of herbs. Chamomile and valerian teas, which can be obtained at the grocery store, are very beneficial for insomnia. Passionflower (Passiflora incarnata), skullcap (Scutellaria lateriflora), and chamomile are examples of herbs that have a slight sedative effect. Try to keep your eyes closed while sipping the tea, as reading or watching TV afterward may make it difficult to go asleep.

Ice Cubes

1. Blueberry Ice Cubes

Ingredients:

- 5 blueberries
- 2 tablespoons honey
- ¼ cup water.

Directions: Blueberries should be steeped for around 10 minutes. Fill ice cube trays or freezer bags halfway with the mixture. To taste, add honey and water, then freeze until your next fruit smoothie!

2. Relaxation Tea Ice Cubes

Ingredients:

- 3 chamomile tea bags
- ¼ cup boiling water
- 2 tablespoons lemon juice.

3. Chamomile Ice Cubes

For 5-10 minutes, steep three chamomile tea bags in boiling water. Remove the leaves and discard them. Allow the tea to cool completely before transferring it to ice cube trays or freezer bags. To taste, add lemon juice.

4. Cinnamon Apple Ice Cubes

Ingredients:

- 1 cup apple juice
- ½ teaspoon cinnamon powder
- 4 slices of apple.

Directions: Freeze for at least 6 hours after combining all ingredients in a plastic bag or airtight container. Remove from the freezer 5-10 minutes before using to make them easier to handle. To taste, add freshly squeezed lemon juice.

5. Lavender Ice Cubes

For 10 minutes, steep two tablespoons dried lavender in boiling water. Pour into ice cube trays or airtight freezer bags, then add lemon juice to taste.

Tinctures

Basic Tincture Recipe

- 1/4 Cup Alcohol (either vodka or brandy can be used)
- 1/8 Cup water

- **Herbal Treatments for Cold Symptoms**: Feverfew can be used as a natural antihistamine, lowering body temperature and alleviating common cold symptoms such as congestion and headache. It is also used as a complementary medicine to treat colds and flu. It is employed in

- **Herbal remedies for warmer weather**: include wintergreen, winter savory, and horehound.

Passionflower and other herbs can help cure cold symptoms like chest congestion.

- **Herbal Treatments for Chest Congestion**: When you brew your own herbal tinctures to keep in your medical cabinet, anise, licorice root, and wild cherry bark will help relieve chest congestion. Simply combine tea bags from the plants with vodka to create your own chest-relieving solution. To ease chest congestion, consider drinking peppermint tea with spearmint or preparing poultices with fresh aloe leaves.

- **Herbal Anxiety Treatments**: Tensions are most likely at their peak during the winter months, which is why cinnamon bark, hops, and wintergreen are excellent anxiety-relieving herbs. If you want to get your anxieties out of your system, garnishing tequila with fresh lemon peel garnished with spearmint is an excellent way to do so.

- **Herbal Treatments for Flu Symptoms:** To cure influenza, people make tinctures or teas from goldenseal, echinacea, and elderberry. When you're feeling under the weather, consider sipping ginger tea or eating candied ginger with orange juice.

- **Herbal Cold treatments:** Consider the following ingredients for cold treatments this winter: anise, hops, cinnamon bark, or tinctures produced from sweet woodruff or ginger. During the winter months of the year, dried angelica root can also be used to treat coughs and sore throats.

Poultices

Poultice made from Blue Vervain for Ear Pain

Ingredients:

- 1 cup of water
- 2 teaspoons dried blue vervain

Directions:

1. Bring the water to a boil in a saucepan.
2. After adding the herbs, cover the pan for a few minutes.
3. Using a cheesecloth, strain the infused water into a mug.
4. Dip a cotton swab in the poultice before rubbing it on your child's ear.
5. You will feel out-of-the-ordinary results.

For Sprains and Strains:

1. Combine 1 part yarrow, 1 part plantain leaves, and 1 part lavender flower petals for sprains and strains.
2. Optionally, add 6 drops lavender essential oil.
3. Pillow yourself with the mixture at night. If necessary, cover with a dry cloth or a denim shirt.
4. Change your pillowcases on a regular basis.

For Inflammation:

2. Combine one part yarrow and one part mullein leaves or flower petals.
3. Optionally, add 6 drops lavender essential oil.
4. Pillow yourself with the mixture at night. If necessary, cover with a dry cloth or a denim shirt.

For Bruises:

1. Combine 1/2 cup dried nettles leaves with 1/2 cup water to make a thick paste (wear gloves while handling nettles - they can sting!).
2. Apply with a towel (avoid getting it in your eyes!).
3. If necessary, cover with a dry cloth or a

denim shirt.

Plantain Leaf Poultice:

1. Combine 1 part plantain leaves and 4 parts mullein leaves or flower petals (dry somewhat).
2. Optionally, add 5 drops lavender essential oil.
3. Pillow yourself with the mixture at night. If necessary, cover with a dry cloth or a denim shirt.
4. Change your pillowcases on a regular basis.

For Swelling:

1. Combine one part yarrow and one part mullein leaves or flower petals.
2. Optionally, add 5 drops lavender essential oil.
3. Pillow yourself with the mixture at night. If necessary, cover with a dry cloth or a denim shirt.

For Sore Joints:

1. Combine 1/2 cup dried plantain leaves with water to make a thick paste (handle plantain leaves with gloves - they can sting!).
2. Apply with a towel (avoid getting it in your eyes!). If necessary, cover with a dry cloth or a denim shirt.

For Aching Muscles:

1. Combine 1 part catmint, 1 part plantain leaves, and 1 part mullein leaves or flower petals (allowing them to dry slightly) for aching muscles.
2. Optionally, add 5 drops lavender essential oil.
3. Pillow yourself with the mixture at night. If necessary, cover with a dry cloth or a denim shirt.
4. Change your pillowcases on a regular basis.

Bath

1. Peppermint Soak Off

This is an excellent treatment for aching bones and fatigued feet.

You will require:
- ½ cup of olive oil
- 4 Drops of Peppermint essential oil

Combine the oils and pour them into a hot tub.

2. Lemon Up Bath Oil

With this surprisingly delicious addition, you can add some flavor to your bath. It's ideal for a night of pampering yourself with a little pick-me-up power.

You will need:
- ½ cup of jojoba oil
- 6 Drops of Lemon essential oil

Simply combine the ingredients and pour into a hot tub of water. Make extra to store in an airtight glass bottle for further use.

3. Lavender Luxury Soak

Sometimes we just need to soak... for fun! Play some soothing music, dim the lights and light a candle. This soak is really amazing; the recipe allows for multiple soaks because you will undoubtedly want more.

You will require:
- 1 cup of Epsom salts
- 1 cup of baking soda
- 5-10 Drops of Lavender essential oil

Combine the ingredients and place them in a glass jar. Place a heaping pinch in each bath for a fantastic soak that will leave you wanting to stay in the tub forever.

4. Roses Bath Soak

Roses are lovely and calming, so it stands to reason that the essential oil generated from them is also beneficial. Rose essential oil has anti-anxiety properties and is a powerful antioxidant. When you're up to your shoulders in tension, this will help.

You will require:
- 1 cup of Epsom salts
- 6 Drops of Rose essential oil
- Rose petals

Combine the essential oil and salts in an airtight glass jar. Fill a tub with rose petals and a large pinch of the salt and oil mixture. You can store the rest of the mixture for another time, so keep some fresh rose petals on hand.

5. Pep Me up Soak

While most bath soaks are intended to soothe you and prepare you for a good night's sleep, this one is ideal for when you just want to unwind before a night out. When you emerge from this bath, you will feel revitalized and ready to go.

You will need:
- 1 cup of sea salt
- 5 Drops of Lime essential oil
- 3 Drops of Peppermint essential oil

Combine the ingredients for later use in a glass jar. Enjoy about a spoonful in a hot to warm bath!

Breast Milk

1. Breastmilk with Honey and Cinnamon Recipe
- Honey
- 1 cup warm water
- Cinnamon powder

Preparation Time: 10 minutes

Allow the teaspoon cinnamon powder to steep for five minutes in a cup of heated water before adding honey to taste instead of sugar. Stir everything together, then drink while it's still warm.

2. Breast Milk Steamed Quinoa Herbal Tea Recipe
- Steamed Quinoa

Blend all of the ingredients in a blender until smooth. Adjust the sweetness as required. Pour into a glass and top with additional coconut if desired. Use half of the coconut milk if you

- 1 cup of quinoa (rinsed)
- 1-2 tablespoons of sesame seeds
- Salt to taste

In a skillet, combine the quinoa, sesame seeds, and salt. Add enough water to cover the quinoa by about one inch. Cook for about 10 minutes, covered, over medium heat, or until all liquid has evaporated.

3. Breastmilk Papaya Drink Recipe
- Papaya Shake
- 1 peeled and seeded papaya
- 1/2 teaspoon ginger powder
- 1 cup of water

Preparation Time: 10 minutes

want a less creamy flavor.

4. Breastmilk Tea Recipe
- 2 tablespoons of fenugreek seeds

- 2 cups of water

For two hours, soak the fenugreek seeds in water. If feasible, strain and drink up to three times each day.

5. Breastmilk Ginger Tea Recipe
- 2 teaspoons of fresh ginger juice
- 2 cups of water

Preparation Time: 10 minutes

2 cups boiling water should be poured over the ginger juice, strain and allow to cool before drinking. Sweeten with honey if desired.

If you like hot ginger tea rather than cold, heat the ginger juice first before adding the water. During the first trimester, take it twice a day. This amount consumed every day is reported to improve breast milk production by up to 30%. During the lactation period, this plant aids in the prevention of morning sickness and nausea.

6. Breastmilk with Fenugreek Recipe
- 2 tablespoons of fenugreek seeds
- 2 cups of water

For two hours, soak the fenugreek seeds in water. If possible, strain the tea and drink it up to three times a day.

7. Breastmilk with Cinnamon Recipe
- 2 tablespoons of cinnamon powder
- 1 cup of milk

Preparation Time: 10 minutes

Fill a glass halfway with cinnamon powder. Taste and adjust with extra cinnamon powder if necessary.

8. Breastmilk Honey Tea Recipe
- 1 teaspoon of lemon juice
- 1 cup of water

Allow the lemon juice to steep in boiling water for 5 minutes before adding honey to taste. Instead of lemon juice, you can substitute fresh ginger juice or grated orange peel.

DOSAGE AND ENCAPSULATION

For some people, encapsulating plants is preferable to consuming herbs directly. When herbs are encapsulated, the body absorbs them more easily.

The herbs are packaged in capsules or hard shells, making them convenient to transport and dispose of after use. The ordinary human tongue cannot hold enough liquid to fully disperse the herbs, but encapsulating plants overcomes this limitation. As a result, many health food stores sell empty capsules. When purchasing empty capsules, ensure they are of excellent quality and free from lead or other dangerous chemicals that could contaminate the herbal contents. Ingesting lead capsules can have hazardous effects (Hoffman, 2011).

Dosage Recommendations Based on Common Sense

Using these products in smaller quantities will help minimize adverse effects while maintaining their effectiveness. Here are some common rules to follow when using herbal products:

- One dropper of liquid herbal extract is sufficient for one day's use. Taking smaller amounts regularly provides greater benefits than taking larger amounts occasionally.

- For children, a few drops of liquid herbal extract are sufficient.

- Liquid herbal extracts can be used as solutions for other formulations that can be added to your bath, sauna, or shower.

- Due to the potency of herbs and their potential negative effects, it is advisable to use lower daily amounts. However, there may be exceptions, as individual needs vary and your body will signal its requirements.

Capsule Varieties

Capsules of various sorts

Enteric-coated capsules are made to disintegrate in high-pH environments, such as the stomach. They are often produced from an ethylcellulose and shellac emulsion blend or a non-toxic FDA-approved polymer called Eudragit S 100. Eudragit S 100 is absorbed on the surface of enteric-coated capsules, where it acts as a protective coating, sealing the capsule and preventing premature disintegration.

The capsule's minuscule particles comprise some coating material, active substances, and fillers. Depending on the product, they can be packed in either a fluid or powdered form. Because these capsules must tolerate pH levels of up to 4, they are typically stored in acid-resistant bottles, such as amber glass. The acid-resistant bottles will keep the capsules intact when stored at room temperature for up to 30 days.

The size of enteric-coated capsules varies depending on the manufacturer. They differ in shape and size as well. The active component, strength and required dosage determine the size.

Gelatin capsules have a gelatin shell containing an active substance, such as sodium chloride or calcium acetate. These capsules must be safeguarded from temperature changes and cooking heat, which can induce capsule wall deterioration and active content release. Because of their greater melting point and stability at high temperatures, capsules containing amino acids such as L-lysine or L-methionine are recommended for sensitive people.

Gelatin capsule filling ingredients range from ethylcellulose to granulated sugar. Organic acids and fibers such as carboxymethylcellulose and methylcellulose are used by some producers.

The #00 size is the most frequent (a little more than 200 mg of powdered pharmaceutical ingredient, or PAPI).

Time-release capsules are used to gradually deliver medication into the body for many hours. These capsules utilize a specific coating (often polymers such as hydroxypropylmethylcellulose) that prevents the capsule from disintegrating prematurely in the stomach. Depending on the patient's demands, these coatings can be made to dissolve in water or fat-based solutions. The enteric-coated capsule is one of the most often utilized time-release capsules. Patients who take time-release capsules frequently request that they be delivered in liquid form to be absorbed faster and cause less discomfort.

Capsules Vs Tablets

1. Capsules are more convenient as they can be taken without water and leave no residue. However, if

you need to take your medication while traveling, tablets are the preferred option. Most pharmacies and supermarkets sell over-the-counter (OTC) tablets for $5-$20 per bottle. This cost can quickly accumulate if you require multiple prescription doses daily.

2. Tablets are often manufactured in a solid form as they are easier to swallow than capsules. This means that tablet therapy may be preferable for chronic diseases if a medication is ineffective. Capsules can also dissolve under the tongue, but precision is challenging, increasing the risk of overdose.

3. Tablets undergo constant evaluation for bioequivalence. This ensures that an OTC tablet delivers the same amount of active substance into your system as a prescription-strength tablet over time. However, capsules are not subject to the same FDA requirements.

4. Tablets can be used in recipes, consumed whole or crushed, and blended with other foods. Capsules are difficult to incorporate into food or consume independently.

5. Many foods and beverages can interfere with pill absorption. However, capsules can be easily consumed without the need for water.

6. Capsules are the recommended choice if you prefer chewable medication that is easy to swallow or if you want flavors to mask an unpleasant taste. Tablets do not have flavors (or colors like red or yellow), but they can contain additional calcium and other nutrients.

7. Capsules are more challenging to divide into smaller doses compared to tablets. If very small doses are required or precise dosing is desired, oral syringes may be the best option.

8. Capsules can be made with gelatin, starch, or vegetable oils (including MCT oil), making them suitable for vegans and people with dietary requirements such as gluten sensitivity. They also do not contain additional fillers or coatings that could trigger an allergic reaction.

9. While tablets can get stuck in the throat or cause choking if not swallowed quickly enough, capsules are less likely to cause choking since they are tightly sealed and do not expand when moist.

10. Capsules can be taken with various beverages, including coffee, orange juice, whole milk, and water (but check the label first). Tablets, on the other hand, are typically only taken with water.

11. Pharmaceutical companies are increasingly using softgels instead of tablets due to their lower production cost. Softgels do not require coating (if your tablet is composed of gelatin, it may actually be a hard plastic shell with a colored coating).

Herb Encapsulation Techniques

To begin, cut small portions of the plant that can be easily gathered; these will serve as the stems for your container. Then, using a knife, slice open any leaves clinging to the stems to reveal the underlying woody material known as "bark"; this will provide additional support for your liquid herb blend.

Next, using a cup or bowl is easier, but there's no reason not to use a real cooking pot; after all, herbs are meant to be cooked. Start by filling the cooking vessel about two-thirds full with water, then add the bark (as mentioned above), herb stems, and any leaves you want to use. Place it on the cooktop on the lowest heat setting and leave it overnight.

When you return in the morning, your herb mixture will have a grassy (blue) color with some orange tips. This is excellent! It means that if you did not use all of the plant material, there would be insufficient liquid for the container mix to absorb. So, discard what isn't used (mainly the leaves), set the mixture aside for a few hours, and strain it into your preferred storage vessel. Allow your creation to sit at room temperature for several days; the herbs will begin to flavor the water after a week or so.

Take a look at this unique process and consider how easy it is to preserve the fragrance and flavor of fresh herbs—it's actually easier than most people believe!

I always keep several containers running and only fill them up when I'm ready to cook with them. They have already been sitting for weeks at that point, allowing the herbs to marinate in the liquid from their prior use.

Remember that some herbs will take longer to infuse than others, and some herbs require regular exposure to the liquid to prevent drying out. This is one of the reasons I prefer glass containers; it's easy for me to see any changes in the mixture after weeks of sitting around.

If you want to experiment with aluminum or plastic, place your blend in something that will receive regular sunlight (a glass jar with aluminum foil on top works great).

The same holds true for potted plants; if you don't mind removing them from the pot (e.g., basil), exposing them to direct sunlight several times a week will help speed up the infusion process.

How Much Cleansing Herbs Should I Take?

The solution to this question depends entirely on your individual needs. While most people recommend taking 1-2 tablespoons of herbal tea with each meal, your consumption will vary based on how frequently you consume solid foods. If you regularly eat solid foods, 2 tablespoons per meal should be sufficient. However, for those who rarely or never eat solid food, increasing the dosage may be beneficial.

It's important to remember that everyone's body is unique, and what works for one person may work differently for another. It is always advisable to start with a lower dose and gradually increase it until you find the right amount that meets your needs without causing any side effects or adverse reactions.

For individuals who are currently using a herbally-based formula diet as part of a cleansing regimen for a specific condition, the frequency of herb intake may be different from solid food. This is because the body naturally detoxes and reduces toxin levels during the cleansing process. As a result, the herbs may or may not be necessary to aid in the body's cleansing. In fact, if you're not eating well at all, it may be wise to discontinue using these herbs until your system returns to a healthy state.

Remember that everyone's system is different, and it may take some trial and error to find the right herb dosage for you. Starting with a modest dose and gradually increasing it as needed is recommended.

NATIVE AMERICAN HERBAL RECIPES VOL. II

My Favorite Recipes

_____

_____

_____

_____

_____

_____

_____

1. ALGONQUIN NUT SOUP

Preparation time: 20 minutes Cooking time: 1 hour 30 minutes Difficulty Level: Medium Servings: 6

Ingredients:

- 1 cup wild rice
- 1 cup mixed nuts (such as walnuts, pecans, and almonds), chopped
- 1 onion, finely chopped
- 2 cloves garlic, minced
- 3 carrots, diced
- 3 celery stalks, diced
- 4 cups vegetable broth
- 1 cup coconut milk
- 2 tablespoons olive oil
- 1 teaspoon dried thyme
- Salt and pepper to taste
- Fresh parsley, chopped (for garnish)

Directions:

- Rinse the wild rice thoroughly under cold water. In a large pot, bring 4 cups of water to a boil. Add the wild rice and cook for 45 minutes or until tender. Drain any excess water and set aside.
- In a separate large pot, heat the olive oil over medium heat. Add the onion and garlic, and sauté until they become translucent.
- Add the chopped mixed nuts, carrots, and celery to the pot. Stir and cook for about 5 minutes until the vegetables start to soften.
- Pour in the vegetable broth and coconut milk. Stir in the dried thyme, salt, and pepper. Bring the mixture to a boil, then reduce the heat to low and let it simmer for 1 hour.
- Add the cooked wild rice to the pot and stir well. Simmer for an additional 15 minutes to allow the flavors to meld together.
- Taste and adjust the seasonings if needed.
- Serve the Algonquin Nut Soup hot, garnished with freshly chopped parsley.

Nutritional Information (per serving):

Calories: 320 kcal, Carbohydrates: 29 g, Protein: 9 g, Fat: 20 g, Fiber: 6 g, Sodium: 600 mg, Sugar: 6 g

2. APACHE STEW

Cooking time: 6 hrs, Difficulty Level: Hard, Servings: 8

Ingredients

- Red peppers 2
- Chilies 4 oz
- Oil 1 tbsp
- venison roast 1 lb
- onion 1
- Garlic 3 cloves
- Carrots 2
- Hominy 3 cups
- Water 3 cups
- Beef broth 3 cups
- salt plus pepper as required
- chopped endive 1 cup
- Coriander

Directions

- Combine in a pot all the ingredients, except theendive
- Cook for 6 hours on low heat.
- Finish with endive and coriander.

Nutritional information

Calories: 294 kcal, Carbohydrates:15 g,Protein: 17 g, Fats: 18 g

3. BANAHA

Cooking time: 40 minutes Difficulty Level: Medium Servings: 4

Ingredients:

- 2 cups Cornmeal
- 1 tsp Baking soda
- 1 ½ cups Hot water
- 1 tsp Salt
- Boiled corn shucks

Directions:

1. In a mixing bowl, combine the cornmeal, baking soda, and salt.
2. Gradually add hot water to the dry ingredients while stirring continuously. Mix until a smooth batter is formed.
3. Let the batter rest for 10 minutes to allow the cornmeal to absorb the moisture.
4. Take a boiled corn shuck and lay it flat on a clean surface.
5. Scoop a spoonful of the batter onto the

center of the corn shuck.

6. Fold the sides of the corn shuck inward, wrapping the batter completely.
7. Repeat the process with the remaining batter and corn shucks.
8. Fill a large pot with water and bring it to a boil.
9. Gently place the wrapped Banaha into the boiling water.
10. Cook the Banaha for 30 minutes or until they are firm and cooked through.
11. Remove the Banaha from the water and let them cool slightly before serving.

Nutritional Information (per serving):
Calories: 220 kcal, Carbohydrates: 48 g, Protein: 4 g, Fat: 1 g, Fiber: 4 g, Sugar: 1 g, Sodium: 400 mg

4. BANNOCK

Cooking time: 12 min, Difficulty Level: Easy, Servings:6

Ingredients
- Cornmeal 2 cups
- Berries ½ cup
- Water ¾ cup
- Oil ¼ cup

Directions
- In a blender, combine cornmeal, water, and 5 tablespoons oil. Add the berries and mix well.
- Heat the oil in a big skillet. In little spoonful's, drop the batter into the oil.
- Fry one side until golden brown, then flip and cook for another 5 minutes.

Nutritional information
Calories: 256 kcal, Carbohydrates: 33 g, Protein: 3 g, Fats: 13 g

5. BEEF CASSEROLE

Cooking time: 2 hours 30 minutes Difficulty Level: Intermediate Servings: 6

Ingredients:
- 2 pounds beef stew meat, cubed
- 2 tablespoons all-purpose flour
- 2 tablespoons vegetable oil
- 1 onion, diced

- 2 cloves garlic, minced
- 2 carrots, sliced
- 2 celery stalks, sliced
- 1 cup mushrooms, sliced
- 2 cups beef broth
- 1 cup red wine
- 2 tablespoons tomato paste
- 1 teaspoon dried thyme
- 1 bay leaf
- Salt and pepper to taste
- Fresh parsley, chopped (for garnish)

Directions:
- Preheat the oven to 325°F (165°C).
- In a large bowl, toss the beef stew meat with the flour until well coated.
- Heat the vegetable oil in a large Dutch oven or oven-safe pot over medium-high heat. Add the beef cubes and cook until browned on all sides. Remove the beef from the pot and set aside.
- In the same pot, add the diced onion and minced garlic. Sauté until the onion becomes translucent and the garlic is fragrant.
- Add the sliced carrots, celery, and mushrooms to the pot. Cook for a few minutes until the vegetables start to soften.
- Return the browned beef cubes to the pot. Pour in the beef broth and red wine. Stir in the tomato paste, dried thyme, bay leaf, salt, and pepper.
- Bring the mixture to a simmer. Cover the pot with a lid and transfer it to the preheated oven.
- Bake for approximately 2 hours or until the beef is tender and the flavors have melded together.
- Remove the casserole from the oven and discard the bay leaf.
- Garnish with fresh chopped parsley before serving.

Nutritional Information (per serving):
Calories: 400 kcal, Carbohydrates: 12 g, Protein: 32 g, Fat: 25 g, Fiber: 3 g, Sugar: 4 g, Sodium: 700 mg

6. BISON CHILI

Preparation time: 15 minutes Cooking time: 2 hours Difficulty Level: Medium Servings: 6

Ingredients:

* 1 pound (450g) ground bison
* 1 tablespoon olive oil
* 1 large onion, chopped
* 2 cloves garlic, minced
* 1 red bell pepper, chopped
* 1 green bell pepper, chopped
* 1 jalapeño pepper, seeded and minced
* 2 cans (14 ounces/400g each) diced tomatoes
* 1 can (15 ounces/425g) kidney beans, drained and rinsed
* 1 can (15 ounces/425g) black beans, drained and rinsed
* 2 tablespoons chili powder
* 1 tablespoon ground cumin
* 1 teaspoon paprika
* 1 teaspoon dried oregano
* Salt and pepper to taste
* Optional toppings: shredded cheese, sour cream, chopped green onions, cilantro

Directions:

* In a large pot or Dutch oven, heat the olive oil over medium heat.
* Add the ground bison and cook until browned, breaking it up into crumbles.
* Add the chopped onion, minced garlic, chopped red bell pepper, chopped green bell pepper, and minced jalapeño pepper. Cook until the vegetables are softened.
* Add the diced tomatoes, kidney beans, black beans, chili powder, ground cumin, paprika, dried oregano, salt, and pepper. Stir well to combine.
* Bring the chili to a boil, then reduce the heat to low. Cover the pot and let it simmer for about 2 hours, stirring occasionally.
* Adjust the seasoning with salt and pepper according to your taste preferences.
* Serve the bison chili hot in bowls. Top with shredded cheese, sour cream, chopped green onions, or cilantro if desired.

Nutritional Information (per serving):

Calories: 350 kcal, Carbohydrates: 34 g, Protein: 32 g, Fat: 10 g, Fiber: 10 g, Sodium: 600 mg

7. BLUEBERRIES AND PEACH SALSA

Preparation time: 15 minutes Difficulty Level: Easy Servings: 4

Ingredients:

* 1 cup fresh blueberries
* 2 ripe peaches, peeled, pitted, and diced
* 1 small red onion, finely chopped
* 1 jalapeño pepper, seeded and minced
* 1/4 cup fresh cilantro, chopped
* Juice of 1 lime
* 1 tablespoon honey
* Salt and pepper to taste
* Tortilla chips, for serving

Directions:

* In a medium bowl, combine the fresh blueberries, diced peaches, chopped red onion, minced jalapeño pepper, and chopped cilantro.
* In a small bowl, whisk together the lime juice and honey until well combined.
* Pour the lime-honey mixture over the fruit mixture and gently toss to coat.
* Season with salt and pepper to taste. Adjust the seasoning and sweetness by adding more honey if desired.
* Let the salsa sit at room temperature for about 10 minutes to allow the flavors to meld together.
* Serve the Blueberries and Peach Salsa with tortilla chips or as a topping for grilled chicken, fish, or tacos.

Nutritional Information (per serving):

Calories: 80 kcal, Carbohydrates: 20 g, Fiber: 3 g, Sugar: 15 g, Protein: 1 g, Fat: 0.5 g, Sodium: 5 mg

8. BLUE BREAD

Cooking time: 12 min, Difficulty Level: Easy, Servings: 30

Ingredients

* Juniper ash 1 cup
* Boiling water 1 cup

- Water 2 cups
- Boiling water 3 ½ cups
- Cornmeal 6 cups
- Salt ½ tsp

Directions

- Bring water and juniper ash to a boil in a saucepan.
- Half-fill a saucepan with juniper water.
- Stir in the blue cornmeal. Knead the dough until it is soft and firm.
- Form the ingredients into 30 small patties.
- Place in a hot skillet. Cook till golden brown on both sides.
- In a mixing bowl, combine the salt and 2 cups of water. Dip the loaves in a dish of salted water.

Nutritional information

Calories: 53 kcal, Carbohydrates: 19 g, Protein: 2 g, Fats: 1 g

9. BLUE CORN BREAD

Cooking time: 1 hr, Difficulty Level: Medium, Servings: 30

Ingredients

- Juniper ash 1 cup
- Boiling water 4 1/2 cup
- Water 2 cups
- Cornmeal 6 cups
- Salt1/2 tsp

Directions

- Boiling water with juniper ash.
- Stir in the blue cornmeal thoroughly.
- Knead the dough until it is soft but firm. Make two or three loaves. Bake in hot ashes for 1 hour.
- Brush the ashes away and serve warm.

Nutritional information

Calories: 86 kcal, Carbohydrates: 19 g, Protein: 2 g, Fats: 1 g

10. BLUE CORN FLAP JACKS

Preparation time: 10 minutes Cooking time: 15 minutes Difficulty Level: Easy Servings: 4

Ingredients:

- 1 cup blue cornmeal

- 1 cup all-purpose flour
- 2 tablespoons sugar
- 2 teaspoons baking powder
- 1/2 teaspoon salt
- 1 1/2 cups buttermilk
- 2 large eggs
- 2 tablespoons melted butter
- Cooking spray or additional melted butter for greasing the skillet
- Optional toppings: maple syrup, fresh berries, powdered sugar

Directions:

- In a large mixing bowl, whisk together the blue cornmeal, all-purpose flour, sugar, baking powder, and salt.
- In a separate bowl, whisk together the buttermilk, eggs, and melted butter.
- Pour the wet ingredients into the dry ingredients and stir until just combined. Be careful not to overmix; a few lumps are okay.
- Preheat a griddle or skillet over medium heat. If using a skillet, grease it with cooking spray or melted butter.
- Ladle about 1/4 cup of batter onto the griddle for each flapjack. Cook until bubbles form on the surface, then flip and cook for another 1-2 minutes until golden brown.
- Repeat with the remaining batter, greasing the griddle or skillet as needed.
- Serve the Blue Corn Flap Jacks hot, stacked on a plate. Top with maple syrup, fresh berries, or powdered sugar if desired.

Nutritional Information (per serving):

Calories: 320 kcal, Carbohydrates: 54 g, Protein: 10 g, Fat: 8 g, Fiber: 4 g, Sodium: 520 mg, Sugar: 9 g

11. BLUE CORN MEAL DUMPLINGS

Cooking time: 30 min, Difficulty Level: Medium, Servings: 30

Ingredients

- Juniper ash 1 cup
- Boiling water 4 ½ cup
- Ground blue cornmeal 6 cups

- Three cups water in a spare pot

Directions

- Combine juniper ash and water in a cup and pour to boiling water.
- Turn off the heat and add the blue cornmeal. Knead the dough until it is soft but firm. Form the dough into small balls the size of your thumb.
- Bring 3 cups of water to a boil. Incorporate the dough balls into the heated water. The dough will naturally produce its own gravy. Serve right away.

Nutritional information

Calories: 101 kcal, Carbohydrates: 21 g, Protein: 2 g, Fats: 1 g

12. BLUE CORN MUSH

Cooking time: 30 min, Difficulty Level: Medium, Servings: 16

Ingredients

- 1 cup juniper in 1 cup of water
- Boiling water 3 cups
- Blue cornmeal 4 cups

Directions

- Bring water to a boil with juniper ash.
- Stir in the blue cornmeal thoroughly.
- Cook for 30 minutes, stirring often. Take off the heat and serve.

Nutritional information

Calories: 101 kcal, Carbohydrates: 21 g, Protein: 2 g, Fats: 1 g

13. BLUE CORN NOODLES

Cooking time: 45-47 min, Difficulty Level: Medium, Servings: 20

Ingredients

- Blue cornmeal 16 cups
- Juniper ash ½ cup
- Boiling water 4 cups

Directions

- Combine juniper ash and hot water in a large mixing bowl. Make a soft dough out of the blue cornmeal.
- Roll the dough into little balls about 12 inches in diameter. Fill a kettle halfway with

boiling water. Cook at a low heat for 45 minutes.

Nutritional information

Calories: 156 kcal, Carbohydrates: 30 g, Protein: 3 g, Fats: 2 g

14. BLUE CORN TORTILLA WITH KALE

Preparation time: 20 minutes Cooking time: 15 minutes Difficulty Level: Easy Servings: 4

Ingredients:

- 4 blue corn tortillas
- 2 cups kale, chopped
- 1 red bell pepper, sliced
- 1 small red onion, sliced
- 2 cloves garlic, minced
- 1 tablespoon olive oil
- 1 teaspoon ground cumin
- Salt and pepper to taste
- Sliced avocado, for garnish
- Fresh cilantro, chopped (for garnish)

Directions:

- Heat olive oil in a large skillet over medium heat. Add the minced garlic and sauté for about 1 minute until fragrant.
- Add the sliced red onion and red bell pepper to the skillet. Sauté for 3-4 minutes until the vegetables start to soften.
- Add the chopped kale to the skillet. Cook for another 3-4 minutes until the kale wilts.
- Sprinkle ground cumin, salt, and pepper over the vegetables. Stir well to combine.
- Warm the blue corn tortillas in a separate dry skillet over medium heat for about 1 minute on each side until pliable.
- Divide the sautéed kale and vegetable mixture evenly among the tortillas.
- Garnish with sliced avocado and chopped cilantro.
- Serve the Blue Corn Tortilla with Kale warm and enjoy!

Nutritional Information (per serving):

Calories: 180 kcal, Carbohydrates: 26 g, Protein: 4 g, Fat: 8 g, Fiber: 5 g, Sodium: 220, mg, Sugar: 4 g

15. BOILED PUMPKIN

Preparation time: 10 minutes Cooking time: 20 minutes Difficulty Level: Easy Servings: 4

Ingredients:

- 1 medium-sized pumpkin
- Water, enough to cover the pumpkin
- Salt, to taste
- Butter or olive oil (optional, for serving)

Directions:

- Start by preparing the pumpkin. Wash the pumpkin thoroughly, then cut it in half. Remove the seeds and stringy pulp.
- Cut the pumpkin into manageable-sized pieces, about 2-inch cubes.
- In a large pot, add enough water to cover the pumpkin pieces. Bring the water to a boil over medium-high heat.
- Once the water is boiling, add a pinch of salt to enhance the flavor. Stir to dissolve the salt.
- Carefully place the pumpkin pieces into the boiling water. Reduce the heat to medium-low and cover the pot.
- Allow the pumpkin to simmer for about 20 minutes or until it becomes tender. Test with a fork to ensure it's cooked through.
- Once the pumpkin is soft and easily mashed with a fork, remove the pot from the heat and drain the water.
- Transfer the boiled pumpkin to a serving dish. Serve it as a side dish or use it as an ingredient in other recipes.
- For added flavor, you can drizzle some melted butter or olive oil over the boiled pumpkin before serving.

Nutritional Information (per serving):
Calories: 50 kcal, Carbohydrates: 12 g, Protein: 2 g, Fat: 0 g, Fiber: 2 g, Sodium: 150 mg, Sugar: 4 g

16. CACTUS FRUIT

Cooking time: 0 min, Difficulty Level: Easy, Servings: 2

Ingredients

- Cactus fruit 2

Directions

- Select extremely ripe fruit, such as bright red, plump prickly pears. Fruit that isn't fully ripe

tastes bitter. Rub the bristles with grass to remove them. They can be eaten raw, but the skin should be removed.

Nutritional information
Calories: 4 kcal, Carbohydrates: 1 g, Protein: < 1 g, Fat: 0 g

17. CACTUS PADS

Preparation time: 15 minutes Cooking time: 20 minutes Difficulty Level: Easy Servings: 4

Ingredients:

- 4 cactus pads (nopales)
- 1 tablespoon olive oil
- 1 small onion, finely chopped
- 2 cloves garlic, minced
- 1 jalapeno pepper, seeds removed and finely chopped
- 1 tomato, diced
- Salt and pepper to taste
- Fresh cilantro, for garnish (optional)
- Lime wedges, for serving

Directions:

- Start by carefully cleaning the cactus pads. Use a sharp knife to trim the edges and remove any thorns. Rinse them under cold water to remove any remaining debris.
- Cut the cactus pads into small strips or bite-sized pieces.
- In a large skillet, heat the olive oil over medium heat. Add the chopped onion, minced garlic, and jalapeno pepper. Sauté until the onions are translucent and fragrant.
- Add the diced tomato to the skillet and cook for a few minutes until the tomato softens.
- Add the cactus pads to the skillet and season with salt and pepper. Stir well to combine all the ingredients.
- Reduce the heat to low and cover the skillet. Allow the cactus pads to simmer for about 15-20 minutes or until they are tender.
- Stir occasionally to ensure even cooking and prevent sticking.
- Once the cactus pads are cooked to your desired tenderness, remove from heat.
- Garnish with fresh cilantro, if desired.

- Serve the Cactus Pads as a side dish or as a topping for tacos, salads, or other Mexican-inspired dishes.
- Squeeze fresh lime juice over the cactus pads before serving for added zestiness.

Nutritional information

Calories: 70, Total Fat: 4g, Saturated Fat: 0.5g, Cholesterol: 0mg, Sodium: 190mg, Carbohydrates: 8g, Fiber: 4g, Sugar: 4g, Protein: 2g

18. CACTUS PAD SALAD WITH JALAPENO DRESSING

Cooking time: 2-3 min, Difficulty Level: Easy, Servings: 6

Ingredients

- Oranges 3
- Cactus pads 6 large
- Red bell peppers 2
- Pumpkin seeds ¼ cupJalapeno Dressing
- Balsamic vinegar 3 tbsp
- Organic raspberry jam 2 tbsp
- Dijon mustard 1 tsp
- Salt ½ tsp
- Black pepper ¼ tsp
- Red chile powder ½ tsp
- Jalapeño pepper 1

Directions

- Peel oranges blanch cactus in salted water for about a minute. Cactus padswill turn a vivid green color.
- In a mixing bowl, combine the oranges, red pepper strips, cactus pad strips, and pumpkin seeds.
- In a mixing bowl, combine all of the ingredients for the dressing.
- To serve, toss the salad with the dressing.

Nutritional information

Calories: 169 kcal, Carbohydrates:31 g,Protein: 5 g, Fats: 4 g

19. CACTUS SEEDS

Cooking time: 3-4 min, Difficulty Level: Easy, Servings: 5

Ingredients

- Cactus seeds 1/2 cup
- Flour 1 cup

Directions

- Dry the seeds before grinding them into flour. This flour is used to thicken stews, soups, puddings, and fruit dishes.

Nutritional information

Calories: 4 kcal, Carbohydrates: 1 g,Protein: < 1 g, Fat: 1 g

20. CANAIGRE (RUMEX HYMENOSEPHALUS)

Preparation time: 10 minutes, Cooking time: 30 minutes, Difficulty Level: Intermediate, Servings: 6

Ingredients:

- 2 cups canaigre roots, peeled and diced
- 4 cups vegetable broth
- 1 tablespoon olive oil
- 1 onion, chopped
- 2 cloves garlic, minced
- 1 carrot, diced
- 1 celery stalk, diced
- 1 teaspoon dried thyme
- Salt and pepper to taste
- Fresh parsley, for garnish (optional)

Directions:

- In a large pot, heat the olive oil over medium heat. Add the chopped onion, minced garlic, carrot, and celery. Sauté for 5 minutes or until the vegetables are softened.
- Add the canaigre roots to the pot and stir to combine with the vegetables.
- Pour in the vegetable broth and add the dried thyme. Season with salt and pepper to taste.
- Bring the mixture to a boil, then reduce the heat to low. Cover the pot and simmer for 25 minutes or until the canaigre roots are tender.
- Remove the pot from heat and let the mixture cool slightly.
- Using an immersion blender or a countertop blender, blend the soup until smooth and creamy.

- Return the soup to the pot and heat over low heat until warmed through.
- Ladle the canaigre soup into serving bowls and garnish with fresh parsley, if desired.
- Serve hot and enjoy!

Nutritional Information (per serving):

Calories: 120 Carbohydrates: 25g Protein: 3g Fat: 2g Sodium: 400mg Fiber: 6g

21. CARROT CURRY

Cooking time: 10 min, Difficulty Level: Easy, Servings: 4

Ingredients

- Dry Spices
- Mustard Seeds 1/2 tsp
- Split chickpeas 1/2 tsp
- White lentil 1/2 tsp
- Hing Asofoetida Powder 1/4 tsp
- Cumin seeds 1/2 tsp
- Red Chilies Dried 5Vegetables
- Carrot Seven large 2 cup
- Ginger Diced Fine 1/4 tsp
- Green peas Dried, soaked overnight1/4 cup
- Cilantro Few
- Coconut Shredded 3 tbsp
- Green Chili pepper 1
- Curry leaves FewOther
- Salt to taste 1 tsp
- Vegetable oil 2 tsp

Directions

- Cut your carrots into small bits. Cut your green chiles into small pieces.
- Fill an instant pot with 1.5 mL of water. Place the diced carrots and green peas in the instant pot's steamer basket.
- Select the steam option and cook for about one minute. When the steam cycle is complete, simply release the pressure.
- Heat the oil in a nonstick skillet and add the dried spices.
- When you hear the popping sound, add your curry leaves and green chilies.
- Put the carrots and peas in the pan and spread them out evenly.

- Season with salt and continue to sauté your carrots with a spatula until your spices are combined.
- Finally, add your shredded coconut and toss to combine evenly.
- To finish, scatter cilantro leaves on top.

Nutritional information

Calories: 65 kcal, Carbohydrates: 6.8 g,Protein: 1.3 g, Fat: 3.8 g

22. CARROT & SWEETCORN BAKRO

Cooking time: 30 min, Difficulty Level: Easy, Servings: 16

Ingredients

- Sweetcorn kernels drained 40 g can
- Besan (chickpea flour) 75 g
- Fine semolina 90 g
- Vegetable oil 60 ml
- Plain flour 75 g
- Onion, finely chopped 1
- Grated carrot ½ cup
- Natural greek yogurt 1 cup
- Ground turmeric ¼ tsp
- Grated zucchini ½ cup
- Ground cumin ½ tsp
- Ground coriander ½ tsp
- Garlic, finely chopped ½ tsp
- Ginger, finely chopped ½ tsp
- Fine salt 2 tsp
- Green chili chopped ½ tsp
- Bicarbonate of soda ¼ tsp
- Baking powder 2 tsp
- Sesame seeds sauce 2 tsp

Directions

- Preheat your oven to 200°F.
- Using a wooden spoon, combine all of the remaining ingredients in one bowl, excluding the bicarb soda and sesame seeds.
- To make a fluffier bakro, mix in the bicarb soda last, then spoon into a greased 20 cm × 4 cm baking tray. Sesame seeds are strewn on top.
- Bake for 30 minutes at 350°F. Remove from oven and put aside to cool before slicing.

Calories: 131 kcal, Carbohydrates: 18 g, Protein: 4.4 g, Fat: 4.8 g

23. CHAHTA (CHOCTAW) TAMFULA

Cooking time: 1 hour Difficulty Level: Medium Servings: 4

Ingredients:

- 2 cups yellow cornmeal
- 1 teaspoon salt
- 1 teaspoon baking powder
- 1 tablespoon sugar
- 2 cups boiling water
- 2 tablespoons vegetable oil
- Honey or maple syrup (for serving, optional)

Directions:

- Preheat the oven to 350°F (175°C) and grease a baking dish.
- In a large bowl, combine the yellow cornmeal, salt, baking powder, and sugar.
- Gradually add the boiling water to the dry ingredients, stirring continuously to create a smooth batter.
- Stir in the vegetable oil until well incorporated.
- Pour the batter into the greased baking dish and spread it evenly.
- Bake in the preheated oven for 45 minutes to 1 hour, or until the tamfula is golden brown and cooked through.
- Remove from the oven and let it cool slightly before serving.
- Cut the tamfula into squares or slices and serve warm. Drizzle with honey or maple syrup, if desired.

Nutritional Information (per serving):

Calories: 235 kcal, Carbohydrates: 44 g, Protein: 4 g, Fat: 6 g, Fiber: 4 g, Sugar: 4 g, Sodium: 470 mg

24. CHEROKEE EGGS ALONGSIDE WILD ONIONS

Cooking time: 10-12 min, Difficulty Level: Easy, Servings: 4

Ingredients

- Wild Onions 2 dozen
- Eggs 6
- Water 2 tbsp
- Cooking Spray /Butter for frying 1-2tbsp
- Salt plus pepper to taste

Directions

- Gather or purchase 1 cup young delicate wild onions, scallions, or green onions.
- Roughly chop the onions.
- Place the onions and water in the cast iron fryer. Cook until they are limp, covered.
- Grease the pan with a pat of butter.
- Add the eggs to the mixture. Scramble the eggs and season with salt and pepper to taste. Avoid overcooking the dish.
- Serve right away..

Nutritional information

Calories: 149.2 kcal, Carbohydrates: 3.5 g, Protein: 9.8 g, Fat: 10.8 g

25. CHEROKEE GREEN ONIONS & EGGS HAVING A THAI FLAIR

Cooking time: 10-12 min, Difficulty Level: Easy, Servings: 2

Ingredients

- Egg whites 6
- Water 1-2 cups
- Wild green onions chopped 3 tbsp
- Thai chili paste. (option) ½ tsp
- Olive oil 2 tbsp
- Shredded cheese ½ cup
- Basil leaves 20
- Garnish with green onion, Thaipeppers cilantro

Directions

- Heat some oil in a skillet over medium heat.
- After adding the egg whites, chopped onion, and water, add the basil leaves and Thai chili paste.
- Toss the egg whites until they turn opaque white, then add the shredded cheese and toss it in with the eggs until it melts. Remove from the heat and garnish with green onion/cilantro.

Nutritional information

Calories: 225 kcal, Carbohydrates: 5.3 g, Protein: 18 g, Fat: 21.5 g

26. CHICKEN SOUP FOR THE SOUL

Preparation time: 15 minutes Cooking time: 1 hour and 30 minutes Difficulty Level: Easy Servings: 6

Ingredients:

- 1 whole chicken, about 4 pounds
- 8 cups chicken broth
- 2 carrots, peeled and diced
- 2 celery stalks, diced
- 1 onion, diced
- 3 cloves garlic, minced
- 1 bay leaf
- 1 teaspoon dried thyme
- 1 teaspoon dried rosemary
- Salt and pepper to taste
- Fresh parsley, chopped, for garnish

Directions:

- In a large pot, combine the chicken, chicken broth, carrots, celery, onion, garlic, bay leaf, thyme, and rosemary.
- Bring the mixture to a boil over medium-high heat. Reduce the heat to low and let it simmer for about 1 hour, or until the chicken is cooked through and tender.
- Remove the chicken from the pot and set it aside to cool.
- Once the chicken is cool enough to handle, shred the meat into bite-sized pieces and discard the bones and skin.
- Return the shredded chicken to the pot and season the soup with salt and pepper to taste. Simmer for an additional 30 minutes to allow the flavors to meld together.
- Remove the bay leaf from the soup before serving.
- Ladle the hot chicken soup into bowls and garnish with freshly chopped parsley.
- Serve the Chicken Soup for the Soul hot, comforting both the body and the spirit.

Nutritional Information (per serving): Calories: 250, Carbohydrates: 10g, Protein: 25g, Fat: 12g, Sodium: 800mg, Fiber: 2g

27. CLAM CHOWDER

Preparation time: 15 minutes Cooking time: 40 minutes Difficulty Level: Medium Servings: 4

Ingredients:

- 4 slices bacon, diced
- 1 onion, chopped
- 2 celery stalks, chopped
- 2 cloves garlic, minced
- 2 tablespoons all-purpose flour
- 2 cups clam juice
- 1 cup whole milk
- 1 cup heavy cream
- 1 bay leaf
- 1 pound potatoes, peeled and diced
- 2 cans chopped clams, drained
- Salt and pepper to taste
- Fresh parsley, chopped, for garnish

Directions:

- In a large pot, cook the diced bacon over medium heat until crispy. Remove the bacon from the pot and set it aside, leaving the bacon fat in the pot.
- Add the chopped onion and celery to the pot and sauté until they become tender, about 5 minutes. Add the minced garlic and cook for an additional 1 minute.
- Sprinkle the flour over the vegetables and stir well to coat. Cook for 1-2 minutes to cook off the raw flour taste.
- Gradually pour in the clam juice, whole milk, and heavy cream, stirring constantly to prevent lumps from forming.
- Add the bay leaf, diced potatoes, and drained chopped clams to the pot. Bring the mixture to a simmer and cook for about 20 minutes, or until the potatoes are tender.
- Season the clam chowder with salt and pepper to taste.
- Remove the bay leaf from the chowder before serving.

- Ladle the hot clam chowder into bowls, garnish with crispy bacon and freshly chopped parsley.
- Serve the Clam Chowder warm, savoring the creamy broth and tender clams.

Nutritional Information (per serving): Calories: 350, Carbohydrates: 22g, Protein: 12g, Fat: 24g, Sodium: 800mg, Fiber: 2g

28. CORNMEAL PORRIDGE

Cooking time: 0 min, Difficulty Level: Easy, Servings: 15

Ingredients

- Cornmeal 4 cups
- Boiling water 3 cups
- Wheat sprouts ½ cup
- One cup juniper ash in one cup boilingwater

Directions

- Pour water into cornmeal and carefully mix. Remove any lumps by vigorously swirling and combining.
- Sweeten the mixture by adding a few wheat sprouts at a time. When the porridge has thickened, add the juniper ash. The porridge is then allowed to cool outside overnight.
- Porridge is done when it turns into a frozen jello-like pudding.

Nutritional information

Calories: 142 kcal, Carbohydrates: 30 g, Protein: 3 g, Fats: 1 g

29. CUCUMBER AND TOMATO SALAD

Preparation time: 10 minutes Cooking time: 0 minutes Difficulty Level: Easy Servings: 4

Ingredients:

- 2 cucumbers, sliced
- 2 large tomatoes, diced
- 1/2 red onion, thinly sliced
- 1/4 cup fresh parsley, chopped
- 2 tablespoons olive oil
- 1 tablespoon lemon juice
- 1 teaspoon Dijon mustard
- Salt and pepper to taste

Directions:

- In a large bowl, combine the sliced cucumbers, diced tomatoes, thinly sliced red onion, and chopped parsley.
- In a small bowl, whisk together the olive oil, lemon juice, Dijon mustard, salt, and pepper until well combined.
- Pour the dressing over the cucumber and tomato mixture and toss gently to coat all the ingredients.
- Taste and adjust the seasoning with additional salt and pepper, if desired.
- Let the salad sit at room temperature for about 10 minutes to allow the flavors to meld together.
- Serve the Cucumber and Tomato Salad as a refreshing side dish, perfect for summer gatherings or as a light and healthy lunch.

Nutritional Information (per serving): Calories: 80, Carbohydrates: 8g, Protein: 2g, Fat: 6g, Sodium: 100mg, Fiber: 2g

30. FRIED PUMPKIN FLOWER

Cooking time: 10-11 min, Difficulty Level: Easy, Servings: 2

Ingredients

- Squash blossoms 16
- Red chili powder ¼ tsp
- Pinch of salt
- Canola sunflower /vegetable oil 2 cups
- Rice flour 2 tbsp

Directions

- Pour four teaspoons of water into one bowl. Combine the red chili powder, salt, and rice flour. To make a paste, properly combine all of the ingredients.
- Heat the oil in one pot. Test it with a pinch of flour paste to determine whether it's ready. If it rises, it's ready. Reduce the heat to medium-low until the pot is warm.
- Dip each flower in the paste, then carefully place it in the pan with a slotted spoon to fry.
- Fry each bloom for about 1 1/2 to 2 minutes, or until crispy brown.
- Transfer the blooms on a cloth to absorb any excess oil.

- Calories: 1,990 kcal, Carbohydrates: 14.2 g, Protein: 0.9 g, Fat: 216. 2 g

31. FRIED SQUASH BLOSSOMS ALONG WITH CORN & MOZZARELLA

Cooking time: 1 hr, Difficulty Level: Difficult, Servings: 4-6

Ingredients
- Fresh mozzarella ¼ pound
- Minced red onion 1 tbsp
- Kernels from corn 1
- Sea salt ¼ tsp
- Minced Garlic 1 tsp
- Butternut squash blossoms 18
- Pepper ¼ tsp
- Buttermilk ½ cup
- Canola oil (as required)
- Basil leaves (garnish)
- Rice flour ½ cup
- Lemon wedges (optional)

Directions
- Combine the corn, cheese, garlic, onion, salt, and pepper in a mixing bowl. Fill each blossom with about 1 1/2 teaspoons of filling and twist the petals closed.
- Heat the oil in one pot to 375 degrees Fahrenheit.
- Separate the buttermilk and rice flour into separate containers.
- Dip each packed bloom one at a time in buttermilk, allowing excess to drip off. Lightly but evenly coat with flour.
- Shake off extra flour before frying blooms in small batches for 45 seconds to 1 minute, or until golden brown.
- To cook the flower tops, gently submerge them in water using a slotted spoon. Absorb any excess liquid with paper towels.
- Season with salt, sprinkle with basil, and serve with lemon wedges.

Nutritional information
Calories: 98 kcal, Carbohydrates: 20.1g, Protein: 2.6 g, Fat: 0. 8 g

32. GOJI BERRY TADKA DAAL

Cooking time: 30 min, Difficulty Level: Medium, Servings: 4

Ingredients
- Toor dal 3/4 cup
- Water 3 cups
- Dried goji berries 1/4 cup
- Turmeric powder ½ tsp
- Red chili flakes 1 tsp
- Sal to tasteFor the tadka:
- Asafoetida a pinch
- Red onions 2
- Ghee 1 tbsp
- Green chili 1
- Cumin seeds 1 tsp

Directions
- Soak toor dal in two cups of water for around 30 minutes.
- Drain.
- In the pressure cooker, combine the soaked and drained toor dal, goji berries, 3 cups of water, turmeric powder, and chili flakes.
- Simmer until the pressure cooker whistles, then reduce to low and simmer for another two whistles.
- Allow the pressure to relax naturally before lifting the lid.
- Mash the boiling toor gently. Add a pinch of salt to taste.

Make the tadka
- Peel and thinly slice the onions. Slit any green chilis if using.
- In a heavy-bottomed pan, melt 1 tablespoon ghee.
- To the ghee, add one teaspoon cumin seeds.
- When the seeds begin to crackle, add one pinch of asafoetida powder. Finish with green chile and onion slices.
- Cook the onions in a skillet over medium heat, turning periodically.
- Cook the onions until they get golden brown around the edges.
- This work would take about 15 minutes to complete.

- When the onions are brown and aromatic, add your dal to the pan.
- Put the cover back on.
- Let the dal settle for about 4-5 minutes before serving.

Nutritional information

Calories: 127 kcal, Carbohydrates: 19 g,Protein: 3.6 g, Fat: 4.5 g

33. GOJI BERRY TEA

Cooking time: 5 min, Difficulty Level: Easy, Servings: 2

Ingredients

- Goji berries (dried) 1 tbsp
- Honey (if desired) 1 tsp
- Water 2 cups

Directions

- Place 1 tbsp dried goji berries in a teapot/infuser.
- Bring 2 cups of water to a boil on the stove.
- Place the dried berries in a dish of hot water.
- Steep the mixture for 3-4 minutes, then remove the goji berries and serve immediately.
- If desired, add honey to taste.

Nutritional information

Calories: 51 kcal, Carbohydrates: 11.5g, Protein: 0.4 g, Fat: 0.6 g

34. GOJI JUICE

Cooking time: 0 min, Difficulty Level: Easy, Servings: 4

Ingredients

- Soaked Goji berries 1/3 cup
- Filtered Water2 / Coconut water 2 cups

Directions

- Combine all ingredients in a standard/high-powered blender

Nutritional information

Calories: 50 kcal, Carbohydrates: 12.3g, Protein: 0.9 g, Fat: 0.5 g

35. GROUND CAKE

Cooking time: 8 hrs, Difficulty Level: Hard,

Servings: 30

Ingredients

- Yellow cornmeal (stone ground) 50 lb
- Whole wheat flour (stone ground) 50lb
- Sprouted wheat (coarsely ground) 12lb
- Simmering water 1 pail
- Brown sugar 10 lb
- Raisins 5 lb
- Corn husks 1 basket

Directions

- In a mixing dish, combine the cornmeal and wheat flour. The ideal method is to add the water in handfuls at a time, swirling regularly. Stir with sticks to remove any lumps.
- Remove any lumps by stirring with a wooden spoon. Add the sugar in little amounts until all of the cornmeal is used. In a mixing dish, combine the wheat sprouts and raisins.
- Soak the corn husks in water.
- Dig a 1-yard-long, 10-inch-deep trench in the ground.
- Light a fire in the pit. After the pit has achieved the desired temperature, remove the hot coals. The pit should be lined with multiple layers of pre-soaked corn husks. Cover the mush with the remaining corn husks and pour the soup into the rows. Before adding the coals, cover with damp dirt. Build a fire in the pit and cook for around 8 hours.

Nutritional information

Calories: 342 kcal, Carbohydrates: 30 g, Protein: 3 g, Fats: 1 g

36. GROUND CHERRY

Preparation time: 10 minutes Cooking time: 15 minutes Difficulty Level: Easy Servings: 4

Ingredients:

- 2 cups ground cherries
- 1 tablespoon olive oil
- 1 small onion, diced
- 2 cloves garlic, minced
- 1 teaspoon ground cumin

- 1 teaspoon paprika
- Salt and pepper to taste
- Fresh cilantro, for garnish (optional)

Directions:

- Rinse the ground cherries under running water to remove any dirt or debris. Pat them dry with a paper towel.
- In a skillet, heat the olive oil over medium heat.
- Add the diced onion and minced garlic to the skillet. Sauté until the onion becomes translucent and the garlic is fragrant.
- Add the ground cherries to the skillet and cook for about 5 minutes, stirring occasionally, until they start to soften.
- Sprinkle the ground cumin, paprika, salt, and pepper over the ground cherries. Stir well to coat them evenly with the spices.
- Continue cooking for another 3-4 minutes, or until the ground cherries are tender.
- Remove from heat and garnish with fresh cilantro, if desired.
- Serve the Ground Cherry as a side dish or use it as a topping for salads, tacos, or grilled meats.

Nutritional Information (per serving): Calories: 60 Carbohydrates: 9g Protein: 1g Fat: 3g Sodium: 80mg Fiber: 2g

37. GROUND CHERRY SALSA

Cooking time: 0 min, Difficulty Level: Easy, Servings: 2 cups

Ingredients

- Ground Cherries 1 cup
- Roasted tomatoes 1/3 cup
- Red onion 1/2 cup
- Chopped jalapeño seeds 1/4 cup
- Lime, juiced 1
- Sea Salt ¼ tsp
- Fresh cilantro leaves 1/4 cup

Directions

- Place all ingredients in a food processor and pulse to combine.
- Chill before serving to let flavors to blend. Place in the refrigerator for about a week.

Nutritional information
Calories: 71 kcal, Carbohydrates: 18 g,Protein: 1 g, Fat: 0.2 g

38. GROUND CHERRY COMPOTE

Cooking time: 20 min, Difficulty Level: Easy, Servings: 2 cups

Ingredients

- Husked ground cherries 1/2 pound
- Zest of lemon 1
- Granulated sugar 3/4 ounces
- Maple syrup 2-4 tbsp
- Water 2-4 tbsp

Directions

In a medium saucepan, combine the sugar, ground cherries, 2 tablespoons water, and addThe zest of a lemon. While the sugar dissolves and the fruit softens, stir occasionally.

- Cook the compote for another 10-15 minutes, turning regularly; if it begins to cling and burn, add the remaining water. The pulverized cherries should be mushy, but the majority of them should be whole and surrounded by a light fruit syrup. Remove from the heat and stir in the maple syrup, starting with two tablespoons and gradually increasing to taste.
- Allow to cool somewhat before serving, or transfer to a single heat-safe container, such as a mason jar; keep in the refrigerator for up to 1 week.

Nutritional information
Calories: 223 kcal, Carbohydrates: 56.1g, Protein: 0.5 g, Fat: 0.1 g

39. GROUND CHERRY SAUCE

Cooking time: 10 min, Difficulty Level: Easy, Servings: 32

Ingredients

- Water 1 cup
- Vanilla extract 1 tbsp
- White sugar 1 cup
- Ground nutmeg ¼ tsp
- Cinnamon 1 tsp

- Ground cherries, husked 4 cups
- Ground cloves ¼ tsp

Directions

- In a medium-sized saucepan, combine the sugar, water, vanilla extract, cinnamon, nutmeg, and cloves. Bring the mixture to a boil, then add the cherries. Reduce the heat to low and continue to simmer until the cherries are translucent. Fill resealable freezer bags with the mixture and pour into hot jars, leaving 1/4-inch headspace. Caps must be changed. Cook for approximately 15 minutes in a boiling water bath.

Nutritional information

Calories: 25 kcal, Carbohydrates: 8.5 g,Protein: 0.3 g, Fat: 0.1 g

40. GRILLED CORN, BASIL & GROUND CHERRY SALAD

Cooking time: 20 min, Difficulty Level: Easy, Servings: 4

Ingredients

- Olive oil 1/8 cup
- Zest of lime 1
- Pepper to taste
- Juice of lime 1
- Grilled corn 4 ears
- Salt to taste
- Cucumber 1 cup
- Ground cherries 1 cup
- Shallot 2 tbsp
- Basil 3 tbsp
- Jalapeno pepper 1 tsp

Directions

- Pinch the base of the husk away from the cherry, and it should easily come off.
- To make the vinaigrette, whisk together the lime zest, olive oil, salt, lime juice, and pepper. Place aside.
- In a mixing bowl, add the ground cherries, grilled corn, basil, jalapeño, cukes, and shallot; thoroughly incorporate the

Nutritional information

Calories: 679 kcal, Carbohydrates:124.7 g, Protein: 14.5 g, Fat: 21.6 g

ingredients.

- Toss in the vinaigrette, incorporate all of the ingredients, and set aside to chill.

Nutritional information

Calories: 71 kcal, Carbohydrates: 8.1 g,Protein: 0.9 g, Fat: 6.6 g

41. HERB PANZANELLA WITH HUSK CHERRIES & TOMATOES

Cooking time: 10 min, Difficulty Level: Easy, Servings: 4

Ingredients

- Tomatoes halved 16
- Small red onion 1/4
- Husk cherries 20
- Pepper to taste
- Olive oil 5 tbsp
- Salt to taste
- Italian bread 6 slices
- Garlic, crushed 4 cloves
- White balsamic vinegar 2 tbsp
- Fresh herbs like mint, tarragon, basil,chives, oregano 1 cup
- Vegetable stock 2/3 cup

Directions

- Preheat your oven to 300°F.
- Combine the husk cherries, tomatoes, and onion in a mixing dish; season with salt and pepper. Drizzle with 1 tablespoon olive oil, stir, and set aside.
- In a medium ovenproof skillet, heat three tablespoons olive oil. Cook, stirring occasionally, until the garlic is gently browned. Season with salt and pepper and toss in the bread. Place skillet in oven for about 12 minutes, or until bread is crisp.
- Combine the bread, tomatoes, tomato water, and vinegar in a mixing bowl. Allow 2–3 minutes for the liquid to absorb, tossing occasionally to achieve even saturation. Before serving, toss in the herbs and sprinkle with the remaining 1 tbsp olive oil.

42. HUARACHES DE NOPAL

Preparation time: 30 minutes Cooking time: 30

minutes Difficulty Level: Intermediate Servings: 4

Ingredients:

- 4 large nopal (cactus) paddles
- 1 tablespoon vegetable oil
- 1 onion, sliced
- 2 cloves garlic, minced
- 1 jalapeño pepper, seeded and diced
- 1 tomato, diced
- Salt, to taste
- Black pepper, to taste
- 1 cup cooked black beans
- 1 cup shredded lettuce
- 1 cup crumbled queso fresco
- Salsa, for serving
- Lime wedges, for serving

Directions:

- Carefully clean the nopal paddles, removing any thorns and tough edges. Slice them into long, thin strips.
- In a large skillet, heat the vegetable oil over medium heat.
- Add the sliced onion, minced garlic, and diced jalapeño pepper to the skillet. Sauté until the onion becomes translucent.
- Stir in the diced tomato and cook for a few minutes until the tomato softens.
- Add the nopal strips to the skillet and cook for about 15-20 minutes, or until they become tender and slightly browned, stirring occasionally.
- Season with salt and black pepper to taste.
- In a separate skillet, heat the cooked black beans over medium heat until warmed through.
- To assemble the huaraches, take a nopal strip and spread a layer of warm black beans on top.
- Top with shredded lettuce and crumbled queso fresco.
- Repeat with the remaining nopal strips and toppings.
- Serve the huaraches de nopal with salsa and lime wedges on the side.

Nutritional Information:

Calories: 210 Total Fat: 8g Saturated Fat: 4g

Cholesterol: 15mg Sodium: 420mg
Carbohydrates: 27g Fiber: 9g Sugar: 5g Protein: 11g

43. HULL CORN SOUP

Cooking time: 2-3 hrs, Difficulty Level: Medium, Servings: 12

Ingredients

- Dehydrated corn ½ lb
- Cooked salt pork ¾ lb
- Cooked beans 2 cups

Directions

- Soak the maize in enough water to cover it overnight. Drain.
- Place the corn in the water, cover, and cook for 1 hour.
- Stir in the beans and pork or. Cook for one to two hours.
- Add extra water as needed throughout the cooking process to keep the ingredients covered.

Nutritional information

Calories: 305 kcal, Carbohydrates: 21 g, Protein: 7 g, Fats: 23 g

44. KANUCHI

Cooking time: 2 hours Difficulty Level: Intermediate Servings: 6

Ingredients:

- 2 cups hickory nuts, shelled
- 2 cups water
- 2 cups cornmeal
- 1 cup maple syrup
- 1/2 cup butter
- 1 teaspoon salt

Directions:

- Preheat the oven to 350°F (175°C).
- Place the hickory nuts in a single layer on a baking sheet and roast them in the preheated oven for 10-12 minutes, or until they become fragrant. Remove from the oven and let them cool.
- Once the roasted hickory nuts have cooled, grind them into a fine powder using a food processor or a spice grinder.

- In a large saucepan, bring the water to a boil. Gradually whisk in the cornmeal, stirring constantly to prevent lumps from forming.
- Reduce the heat to low and continue cooking the cornmeal mixture, stirring frequently, for about 20 minutes or until it thickens and becomes creamy.
- Add the ground hickory nuts, maple syrup, butter, and salt to the cornmeal mixture. Stir well to combine all the ingredients.
- Continue cooking the mixture over low heat for another 30-40 minutes, stirring occasionally, until it reaches a thick and pudding-like consistency.
- Remove the Kanuchi from the heat and let it cool slightly before serving.
- Serve the Kanuchi warm in bowls or small dishes.

Nutritional Information (per serving):
Calories: 450 kcal, Carbohydrates: 47 g, Protein: 6 g, Fat: 29 g, Fiber: 5 g, Sugar: 20 g, Sodium: 400 mg

45. KNEEL DOWN BREAD

Cooking time: 1 hr, Difficulty Level: Medium, Servings: 12

Ingredients
- Fresh corn 12 ears
- Softened corn husks

Directions
- Fresh corn kernels should be scrapped.
- Mash the kernels until they form a mush. Wrap the mush in corn husks to form small bundles.
- Dig a one-yard-long, ten-inch-deep trench in the earth.
- Light a fire in the pit. Remove the hot coals from the pit and place the parcels in the ground, covering them with fresh leaves and damp earth before covering with coals. Build a fire and bake for at least an hour.

Nutritional information
Calories: 83 kcal, Carbohydrates: 19 g, Protein: 3 g, Fats: 1 g

46. LAMB WITH ROSEMARY

Preparation time: 15 minutes Marinating time: 2 hours Cooking time: 1 hour 30 minutes Difficulty Level: Medium Servings: 4

Ingredients:
- 2 pounds boneless lamb shoulder, cut into chunks
- 2 tablespoons olive oil
- 4 cloves garlic, minced
- 2 tablespoons fresh rosemary leaves, chopped
- 1 teaspoon salt
- 1/2 teaspoon black pepper
- 1/2 cup red wine
- 1 cup beef or vegetable broth

Directions:
- In a large bowl, combine the olive oil, minced garlic, chopped rosemary leaves, salt, and black pepper.
- Add the lamb chunks to the bowl and toss them until they are evenly coated with the marinade. Cover the bowl and refrigerate for at least 2 hours, or overnight for best flavor.
- Preheat the oven to 325°F (165°C).
- Heat a large oven-safe skillet or Dutch oven over medium-high heat. Add the marinated lamb chunks to the skillet and cook them until they are browned on all sides.
- Deglaze the skillet by pouring in the red wine. Stir well to scrape up any browned bits from the bottom of the skillet.
- Add the beef or vegetable broth to the skillet, then cover the skillet with a lid or aluminum foil.
- Transfer the skillet to the preheated oven and roast the lamb for 1 hour 30 minutes, or until it is tender and easily pulls apart with a fork.
- Remove the skillet from the oven and let the lamb rest for a few minutes before serving.
- Serve the Lamb with Rosemary with your favorite side dishes, such as roasted potatoes and steamed vegetables.

Nutritional Information (per serving):
Calories: 400 kcal, Carbohydrates: 2 g, Protein: 48 g, Fat: 20 g, Sodium: 600 mg

47. MARINATED CHERRY TOMATOES

Cooking time: 10 min, Difficulty Level: Easy, Servings: 4

Ingredients

- Cherry tomatoes 1/2 pound
- Garlic 1/2-1 clove
- Onion sliced thin 1/4 red
- Olive oil 1/4 cup
- Salt to taste
- Lemon juice 1
- Red wine vinegar 1 tbsp
- Optional fresh basil
- Pepper to taste

Directions

- Cherry tomatoes are quartered, and onions are thinly sliced.
- Using the flat end of your knife, crush peeled garlic to produce a paste. Season with salt and pepper and add to the bowl with the vegetables.
- Allow it to sit at room temperature for 1 to 2 hours, tossing occasionally, to coat the tomatoes. Serve at room temperature, seasoning with salt and pepper to taste.

Nutritional information

Calories: 141 kcal, Carbohydrates: 26.4g, Protein: 1 g, Fat: 14 g

48. MINTY MINT

Preparation time: 5 minutes Cooking time: None Difficulty Level: Easy Servings: 2

Ingredients:

- 2 cups fresh mint leaves
- 2 tablespoons fresh lime juice
- 2 tablespoons honey
- 1 cup crushed ice
- 1 cup sparkling water
- Lime slices, for garnish

Directions:

- In a blender, combine the fresh mint leaves, lime juice, honey, and crushed ice.
- Blend until the mixture becomes smooth and well combined.

- Divide the mint mixture between two glasses.
- Pour half a cup of sparkling water into each glass and stir gently.
- Garnish with lime slices.
- Serve immediately and enjoy the refreshing Minty Mint!

Nutritional Information (per serving):

Calories: 60 kcal, Carbohydrates: 16 g, Fiber: 2 g, Sugar: 12 g, Protein: 1 g, Fat: 0 g, Sodium: 5 mg

49. MOOSE MEAT CHILI

Cooking time: 2 hours Difficulty Level: Medium Servings: 6

Ingredients:

- 1 pound ground moose meat (substitute with beef if unavailable)
- 1 tablespoon vegetable oil
- 1 medium onion, chopped
- 2 cloves garlic, minced
- 1 bell pepper, diced
- 1 jalapeno pepper, seeded and minced
- 1 can (14 ounces) diced tomatoes
- 1 can (14 ounces) kidney beans, drained and rinsed
- 1 can (14 ounces) black beans, drained and rinsed
- 1 can (6 ounces) tomato paste
- 2 cups beef broth
- 2 tablespoons chili powder
- 1 teaspoon cumin
- 1 teaspoon paprika
- 1/2 teaspoon oregano
- Salt and pepper to taste
- Optional toppings: shredded cheese, sour cream, chopped cilantro

Directions:

- In a large pot, heat the vegetable oil over medium heat. Add the ground moose meat and cook until browned. If using beef, cook until browned and no longer pink. Drain any excess fat.
- Add the chopped onion, minced garlic, diced bell pepper, and minced jalapeno pepper to the pot. Sauté until the vegetables are tender.
- Stir in the diced tomatoes, kidney beans, black beans, tomato paste, beef broth, chili

powder, cumin, paprika, oregano, salt, and pepper. Mix well to combine.

- Bring the chili to a boil, then reduce the heat to low. Cover and simmer for approximately 1 1/2 to 2 hours, stirring occasionally, until the flavors meld together and the chili thickens to your desired consistency.
- Season with additional salt and pepper if needed.
- Serve the Moose Meat Chili hot, topped with shredded cheese, sour cream, and chopped cilantro if desired.

Nutritional Information (per serving):
Calories: 326 kcal, Carbohydrates: 32 g, Protein: 30 g, Fat: 8 g, Fiber: 9 g, Sugar: 6 g, Sodium: 750 mg

50. MORMAN TEA

Cooking time: 5-7 min, Difficulty Level: Easy, Servings: 1

Ingredients

- Morman stems 1 handful
- Water 1 cup
- Honey (for flavoring)

Directions

- Roast the stems over a fire. Bring 1 cup of water to a boil. Add a bunch of stems to the mix. Allow your tea to steep for at least 20 minutes after removing the kettle from the heat. It can be flavored with sugar, lemon, or honey.

Nutritional information
Calories: 16 kcal, Carbohydrates: 4.3 g, Protein: 0 g, Fat: 0 g

51. MUTTON LOAF

Cooking time: 1 hr, Difficulty Level: Medium, Servings: 6

Ingredients

- Diced mutton 2 cups
- Tomatoes ½ cup
- Bread 1 cup
- Onion ½ cup
- Salt ½ tsp
- Celery 1 tbsp

- Pepper ¼ tsp

Directions

- Grind the mutton in a meat grinder. Combine the tomatoes, bread, salt, onion, celery, and pepper in a mixing bowl. Mix thoroughly and shape into a loaf. In ashes, cook for 1 hour.

Nutritional information
Calories: 276 kcal, Carbohydrates: 29 g, Protein: 33 g, Fats: 2 g

52. NAVAJO CAKE

Cooking time: 4 hrs, Difficulty Level: Hard, Servings: 10

Ingredients

- Water 6 cups
- Raisins ½ cup
- Pre-cooked blue cornmeal 4 cups
- Wheat sprouts ½ cup
- Pre-cooked yellow cornmeal 2 cups
- Brown sugar ½ cup

Directions

- Mix the cornmeal and water together.
- Combine the wheat sprouts, raisins, and brown sugar in a mixing bowl. Blend until no lumps remain.
- Cook in ashes for 4 hours.

Nutritional information
Calories: 380 kcal, Carbohydrates: 84 g, Protein: 8 g, Fats: 1 g

53. NAVAJO TEA

Preparation time: 5 minutes Cooking time: 20 minutes Difficulty Level: Easy Servings: 1

Ingredients:

- 1 handful of Mormon stems
- 1 cup of water
- Honey (for flavoring)

Directions:

- Roast the Mormon stems over a fire.
- In a saucepan, bring 1 cup of water to a boil.
- Add the roasted Mormon stems to the boiling water.
- Reduce the heat to low and let the tea simmer for 20 minutes.

- Remove the saucepan from heat and allow the tea to steep for an additional 5 minutes.
- Strain the tea to remove the stems.
- Add honey, if desired, to flavor the tea.
- Serve hot and enjoy!

Nutritional Information:

Calories: 16 kcal Carbohydrates: 4.3 g Protein: 0 g Fat: 0 g

54. NAVAJO ROASTED CORN

Cooking time: 20 minutes Difficulty Level: Easy Servings: 4

Ingredients:
- 4 ears of corn
- 2 tablespoons melted butter
- 1 teaspoon chili powder
- 1/2 teaspoon salt
- 1/4 teaspoon black pepper
- Lime wedges, for serving
- Fresh cilantro, chopped (optional)

Directions:
- Preheat the grill to medium-high heat.
- Peel back the husks of the corn, but leave them attached at the base. Remove the corn silk and fold the husks back into place.
- In a small bowl, combine the melted butter, chili powder, salt, and black pepper.
- Brush the seasoned butter mixture evenly over the corn.
- Place the corn on the preheated grill and cook for approximately 15-20 minutes, turning occasionally, until the kernels are tender and lightly charred.
- Remove the corn from the grill and let it cool slightly.
- Once cooled, peel back the husks completely and serve the roasted corn with lime wedges.
- Optionally, garnish with fresh chopped cilantro for added flavor.

Nutritional Information (per serving):

Calories: 112 kcal, Carbohydrates: 19 g, Protein: 2 g, Fat: 4 g, Fiber: 2 g, Sugar: 5 g, Sodium: 308 mg

55. OJIBWE MENWAAGAMIG

Cooking time: 0 min, Difficulty Level: Easy, Servings: 4

Ingredients
- Water 4 cups
- Wild berries 1 cup
- Honey 4 tsp

Directions
- Crush and sieve the berries using a colander or a cheesecloth bag.
- Combine the strained berry juice, water, and honey in a mixing bowl.

Nutritional information

Calories: 33 kcal, Carbohydrates: 9 g, Protein: 1 g, Fats: 0 g

56. ONE SEED JUNIPER

Cooking time: 5-7 min, Difficulty Level: Easy, Servings: 1

Ingredients
- Juniper branches 1 handful
- Water 1 cup

Directions
- Boil a handful of juniper branches in a pan with water for about 5 minutes, or until the tea has achieved the appropriate strength.

Nutritional information

Calories: 41 kcal, Carbohydrates: 10 g, Protein: 0 g, Fat: 0 g

57. OSTRICH FERN (MATTEUCCIA STRUTBIOPTERIS)

Preparation time: 10 minutes Cooking time: 15 minutes Difficulty Level: Moderate Servings: 4

Ingredients:
- 1 pound Ostrich Fern fiddleheads
- 2 tablespoons butter
- 2 cloves garlic, minced
- Salt, to taste
- Black pepper, to taste
- Lemon wedges (optional, for serving)

Directions:
- Rinse the Ostrich Fern fiddleheads thoroughly under cold water to remove any dirt or debris.

- Bring a large pot of salted water to a boil.
- Add the fiddleheads to the boiling water and cook for about 10 minutes, or until they become tender.
- Drain the fiddleheads and rinse them with cold water to stop the cooking process.
- In a skillet, melt the butter over medium heat.
- Add the minced garlic to the skillet and sauté for about 1-2 minutes, until fragrant.
- Add the cooked fiddleheads to the skillet and sauté for an additional 3-4 minutes, stirring occasionally.
- Season with salt and black pepper to taste.
- Remove from heat and serve hot.
- Optionally, serve with lemon wedges for added flavor.

Nutritional Information:

Calories: 60 Total Fat: 4g Saturated Fat: 2g
Cholesterol: 10mg Sodium: 60mg ,
Carbohydrates: 6g Fiber: 3g Sugar: 0g Protein: 3g

58. PEACH GROUND CHERRY SALSA

Cooking time: 0 min, Difficulty Level: Easy, Servings: 2

Ingredients
- Canned black beans ½ cup
- Ground cherries husked ½ cup
- Fresh corn grilled 1 ear
- Jalapeno 1 tsp
- Peach diced 1
- Cilantro rough chopped 1 tbsp
- mint leaves 1 tbsp
- Juice of lime ½
- Red wine vinegar 1 tbsp
- Salt to taste

Directions
- Place all ingredients in a mixing bowl and toss well to combine flavors. Allow at least a half-hour at room temperature before re-seasoning if necessary. Allow to cool before serving.

Nutritional information

Calories: 285 kcal, Carbohydrates: 59.1g, Protein:

14 g, Fat: 1.9 g

59. PINON CAKES

Cooking time: 15 minutes Difficulty Level: Easy Servings: 10

Ingredients:
- 3 cups Pinon nuts
- 3 cups Water
- ½ tsp Salt
- 3 tbsp Oil

Directions:
- Finely chop or blend the pinon nuts until they reach a fine consistency.
- Season the nuts with salt and gradually add water while blending until a smooth mixture is obtained.
- Let the batter sit at room temperature for one hour.
- Heat the oil in a skillet.
- Drop the batter into the oil and shape each one into a small cake about 3 inches in diameter.
- Reduce the heat and continue to cook until both sides are golden.

Nutritional Information (per serving):

Calories: 252 kcal, Carbohydrates: 54 g, Protein: 2 g, Fat: 1 g

60. PORRIDGE HAVING FRESH FRUIT & GOJI BERRIES

Cooking time: 10-11 min, Difficulty Level: Easy, Servings: 1

Ingredients
- Rolled oats 45 g
- Vanilla extract ½ tsp
- Water (or milk) 115 ml
- Goji berries 1 tbsp
- Mixed nuts 1 tbsp
- Fruit

Directions
- In a small pot, combine the water or milk, rolled oats, and vanilla extract. Bring to a low heat and cook for 3-5 minutes, or until the porridge is creamy. If the mixture is too dry,

add more water or milk. Set it aside for now.

- Meanwhile, wash and cut fresh fruit into little pieces.
- Spoon the warm porridge into the serving bowl and delicately fold in the fruit. On top, goji berries and diced mixed nuts of your choice are sprinkled. Before serving, reheat the dish.

Nutritional information

Calories: 267 kcal, Carbohydrates: 32 g,Protein: 11 g, Fat: 11 g

61. POSOLE

Cooking time: 2.5 hrs, Difficulty Level: Hard, Servings: 8

Ingredients

- Dried red chiles 1.5 oz
- Chicken stock 8 cups
- Pork ribs 2 lb
- Salt and pepper as required
- Vegetable oil 3 tbsp
- White hominy 15 oz
- White onions (chopped) 2
- Garlic 5 cloves
- Fresh oregano 1 tbsp
- Lime juice 1 tbsp

Directions

- Season pork with salt andpepper on all sides.
- Cook for about 10 minutes, or until themeat is cooked. Place the cooked pork on a serving plate and leave aside.
- Sautee onion, chili, garlic before adding the stock.
- Add cooked pork, oregano, andpepper. Simmer for 90 minutes.
- Add hominy and continue to cook for 30 minutes. Finally, add the lime juice.

Nutritional information

Calories: 427 kcal, Carbohydrates:12 g,Protein: 33 g, Fats: 27 g

62. POYHA

Preparation time: 15 minutes Cooking time: 20 minutes Difficulty Level: Easy Servings: 4

Ingredients:

- 2 cups cornmeal
- 1 cup water
- 1 teaspoon salt
- 1 cup grated cheese (cheddar or mozzarella)
- 4 tablespoons butter
- 1 cup milk
- Fresh herbs (such as parsley or cilantro) for garnish

Directions:

- In a large mixing bowl, combine the cornmeal, water, and salt. Mix well until a thick batter forms.
- Heat a non-stick skillet or griddle over medium heat. Add a tablespoon of butter and let it melt.
- Take a small portion of the batter and flatten it in your hands to form a patty. Place it on the hot skillet.
- Cook the patty for about 2-3 minutes on each side until it turns golden brown. Repeat this process with the remaining batter, adding more butter as needed.
- Once all the patties are cooked, place them on a baking sheet. Sprinkle grated cheese on top of each patty.
- Preheat your oven's broiler.
- Place the baking sheet with the patties under the broiler for 2-3 minutes, or until the cheese melts and becomes bubbly.
- In a small saucepan, heat the milk and remaining butter over low heat until the butter melts.
- Serve the poyha patties hot, drizzled with the warm milk and butter mixture.
- Garnish with fresh herbs, such as parsley or cilantro, for added flavor and visual appeal.

Nutritional Information (per serving):

Calories: 380 kcal, Carbohydrates: 37 g, Protein: 12 g, Fat: 21 g, Fiber: 3 g, Sodium: 650 mg, Sugar: 2 g

63. PRICKLY PEAR

Preparation time: 15 minutes Cooking time: 10 minutes Difficulty Level: Easy Servings: 4

Ingredients:

- 4 prickly pears
- 1 tablespoon honey
- Juice of 1 lime
- Mint leaves (for garnish)

Directions:
- Using a sharp knife, carefully slice off the ends of each prickly pear.
- Make a lengthwise slit along the skin of each prickly pear.
- Use your fingers or a spoon to peel off the skin, revealing the flesh inside.
- Cut the peeled prickly pears into small cubes or slices.
- In a small saucepan, combine the prickly pear cubes, honey, and lime juice.
- Cook over medium heat for about 10 minutes, stirring occasionally, until the prickly pear softens and the flavors combine.
- Remove from heat and let the mixture cool.
- Once cooled, transfer the mixture to a blender or food processor and blend until smooth.
- Strain the mixture to remove any remaining seeds or pulp.
- Transfer the strained prickly pear mixture to a serving dish.
- Garnish with fresh mint leaves.
- Serve chilled and enjoy!

Nutritional Information:
Calories: 85 Total Fat: 0g Saturated Fat: 0g Cholesterol: 0mg Sodium: 2mg Carbohydrates: 22g Fiber: 5g Sugar: 15g Protein: 1g

64. PUMPKIN VEGAN BLOSSOM FRITTERS

Cooking time: 10-11 min, Difficulty Level: Easy, Servings: 2

Ingredients
- Pumpkin blossoms 4
- Garlic 1 pods
- Wild rice soaked 2 tbsp
- Cumin seeds ¼ tsp
- Thai green pepper 1
- Salt to taste
- Turmeric ¼ tsp

- Oil 1 tsp

Directions
- Soak two to three teaspoons of wild rice in a water cup.
- Drain the soaking rice and combine it with a blender.
- Stir in one garlic pod, one green pepper, and 1/4 teaspoon cumin seeds.
- Add the salt and blend until the purée is smooth.
- Stir in the turmeric thoroughly.
- Before utilizing your pumpkin blossoms, wash and dry them.
- Remove the stem and discard the sepals and stigma.
- Prepare the Fritters
- Add a few drops of oil to a heated griddle.
- A skillet could also be used.
- After dipping the flowers in the batter, cook them on a greased griddle / Tawa.
- Flip the fritters when the bottoms start to crisp. Gently press down on the fritters with your spatula to flatten them.
- Cook for five minutes more after spraying with oil.
- Each fritter would take around 10-15 minutes to cook thoroughly over low heat.
- As a side dish, serve with chutney, dressing, or cauliflower rice and lentils.

Nutritional information
Calories: 54.8 kcal, Carbohydrates: 7.4g, Protein: 1.5 g, Fat: 2. 5 g

65. ROASTED SQUASH STUFFED BLOSSOMS

Cooking time: 20 min, Difficulty Level: Easy, Servings: 4

Ingredients
- Olive oil divided 3 tbsp
- Rainbow chard 1 bunch
- Cloves Garlic, minced 3
- Salt to taste
- Chopped fresh basil 3 tbsp
- Pepper to taste
- Zucchini blossoms 8

- Chevre (goat cheese) 3 ounces

Directions

- Preheat your oven to 400°F.
- Heat 1 tablespoon olive oil in a pan over medium heat; add garlic and sauté for 1 minute. Cook, stirring occasionally, until the chard is soft, about 10 minutes. Add the salt, basil, and pepper and cook for 2 minutes, or until the basil is soft. Set aside for about 15 minutes to totally cool. Press the cooled chard mixture between two towels to remove excess moisture.
- Combine the chevre and chard in a mixing dish. Fill zucchini blooms 3/4 full with goat chevre mixture and crimp the ends shut. • Place full flowers in a roasting pan; spritz with 2 tablespoons olive oil; season with salt and pepper.
- Roast for 10 minutes in a preheated oven until the blossoms become hot.

Nutritional information

Calories: 244 kcal, Carbohydrates: 16.6g, Protein: 10.6 g, Fat: 17. 3 g

66. ROASTED TURNIP WITH AGAVE GLAZE

Cooking time: 35 minutes Difficulty Level: Easy Servings: 4

Ingredients:

- 4 medium-sized turnips, peeled and cut into wedges
- 2 tablespoons olive oil
- 2 tablespoons agave nectar
- 1 tablespoon balsamic vinegar
- Salt and pepper to taste
- Fresh parsley for garnish

Directions:

- Preheat the oven to 400°F.
- In a mixing bowl, combine the olive oil, agave nectar, balsamic vinegar, salt, and pepper. Whisk until well blended.
- Add the turnip wedges to the bowl and toss them in the glaze until evenly coated.
- Arrange the turnip wedges in a single layer on a baking sheet lined with parchment paper.
- Roast in the preheated oven for 30-35 minutes, or until the turnips are tender and caramelized, flipping them halfway through the cooking time for even browning.
- Remove from the oven and let the roasted turnips cool for a few minutes.
- Transfer the roasted turnips to a serving dish and garnish with fresh parsley.
- Serve the Roasted Turnip with Agave Glaze as a side dish alongside your favorite main course.

Nutritional Information (per serving):

Calories: 110 kcal, Carbohydrates: 17 g, Protein: 1 g, Fat: 5 g, Fiber: 3 g, Sugar: 10 g, Sodium: 80 mg

67. ROSEMARY AND GARLIC ROASTED POTATOES

Preparation time: 10 minutes Cooking time: 40 minutes Difficulty Level: Easy Servings: 4

Ingredients:

- 1.5 pounds baby potatoes
- 2 tablespoons olive oil
- 2 cloves garlic, minced
- 1 tablespoon fresh rosemary leaves, chopped
- Salt, to taste
- Black pepper, to taste

Directions:

- Preheat the oven to 425°F (220°C).
- Rinse the baby potatoes and pat them dry with a paper towel. Cut any larger potatoes in half for more even cooking.
- In a large bowl, combine the olive oil, minced garlic, chopped rosemary leaves, salt, and black pepper. Mix well.
- Add the potatoes to the bowl and toss them until they are evenly coated with the oil and herb mixture.
- Transfer the potatoes to a baking sheet, spreading them out in a single layer.
- Place the baking sheet in the preheated oven and roast the potatoes for 35-40 minutes, or until they are golden brown and crispy on the outside, and tender on the inside. Stir the potatoes once or twice during cooking for

even browning.

- Remove the roasted potatoes from the oven and let them cool for a few minutes.
- Serve the Rosemary and Garlic Roasted Potatoes as a delicious side dish to accompany your favorite main course.

Nutritional Information (per serving):

Calories: 180 kcal, Carbohydrates: 28 g, Fiber: 3 g, Sugar: 1 g, Protein: 3 g, Fat: 6 g, Sodium: 150 mg

68. ROSEMARY BREAD

Cooking time: 5 min, Difficulty Level: Easy, Servings: 6

Ingredients

- Whole-wheat flour (organic) 4 cups
- Baking powder 2 tbsp
- Salt 1 tsp
- Rosemary 50 g
- Warm water 1 ½ cups

Directions

- Combine all the ingredients and knead intoa dough.
- Divide the dough into tiny balls and rollout the dough to diameter of 8 to 10 inches.
- Cook for around 2 to 3 minutes per side.

Nutritional information

Calories: 169 kcal, Carbohydrates:31 g, Protein: 5 g, Fats: 4 g

69. SEGO-LILY

Preparation time: 10 minutes Cooking time: 20 minutes Difficulty Level: Moderate Servings: 4

Ingredients:

- 1 pound Sego-Lily bulbs
- 2 tablespoons vegetable oil
- 1 onion, chopped
- 2 cloves garlic, minced
- 1 teaspoon ground cumin
- 1 teaspoon chili powder
- Salt, to taste
- Black pepper, to taste
- 1 cup vegetable broth
- 1 can (14 ounces) diced tomatoes
- 1 can (14 ounces) black beans, drained and

rinsed

- 1 cup frozen corn kernels
- Fresh cilantro, for garnish
- Lime wedges, for serving

Directions:

- Peel and trim the Sego-Lily bulbs, discarding any tough outer layers. Cut them into bite-sized pieces.
- In a large skillet, heat the vegetable oil over medium heat.
- Add the chopped onion and minced garlic to the skillet. Sauté until the onion becomes translucent and the garlic is fragrant.
- Stir in the ground cumin, chili powder, salt, and black pepper. Cook for another minute to toast the spices.
- Add the Sego-Lily bulbs to the skillet and cook for 5 minutes, stirring occasionally.
- Pour in the vegetable broth and diced tomatoes. Bring the mixture to a simmer.
- Cover the skillet and let it cook for about 10 minutes, or until the Sego-Lily bulbs become tender.
- Stir in the black beans and frozen corn kernels. Cook for an additional 5 minutes, until the beans and corn are heated through.
- Taste and adjust the seasoning as needed.
- Serve the Sego-Lily stew hot, garnished with fresh cilantro. Provide lime wedges for squeezing over the stew for added flavor.

Nutritional Information:

Calories: 245 Total Fat: 7g Saturated Fat: 1g Cholesterol: 0mg Sodium: 786mg Carbohydrates: 42g Fiber: 10g Sugar: 7g Protein: 9g

70. SISTERS BEAN STEW

Cooking time: 5-7 min, Difficulty Level: Easy, Servings: 4-6

Ingredients

- Canola oil 2 tbsp
- Garlic 2 cloves
- Small onion 1
- Bay leaf 1
- Fresh thyme 2 sprig

- Stalk celery diced 1/2
- Carrot diced ½
- Cooked kidney beans 177 g
- Salt plus black pepper
- Cooked black beans 185 g
- Cooked cannellini beans 155 g
- Chicken / vegetable stock 600 ml
- Diced tomatoes 90 g

Directions

- Heat some oil in a large, heavy-bottomed pot over medium heat. To the heated oil, add the garlic, onion, bay leaf, thyme, and carrot.
- Season with salt and pepper and cook, turning occasionally, for about 5 minutes, or until the onion is soft and translucent.
- Combine the chopped tomatoes, boiled beans, and stock; bring to a boil, then reduce to a low heat and continue to cook for several minutes, or until the stock thickens.
- Adjust the seasoning as needed, remove the bay leaf and thyme sprigs, and serve immediately.

Nutritional information

Calories: 353 kcal, Carbohydrates: 57.2g, Protein: 20.3 g, Fat: 5.8 g

71. SQUASH BLOSSOMS

Cooking time: 5-7 min, Difficulty Level: Easy, Servings: 4

Ingredients

- Blossoms 30
- Water 1 cup
- Salt 1/4 tsp

Directions

- Blossoms are cooked for about 10 minutes in mildly salted water; they should not be overcooked or boiled dry. The final texture is similar to cooked spinach.

Nutritional information

Calories: 38 kcal, Carbohydrates: 7.5 g, Protein: 0 g, Fat: 0 g

72. SQUASH BLOSSOMSOUP

Preparation time: 15 minutes Cooking time: 25 minutes Difficulty Level: Easy Servings: 4

Ingredients:

- 1 tablespoon olive oil
- 1 small onion, diced
- 2 cloves garlic, minced
- 4 cups vegetable broth
- 2 cups squash blossoms, stems removed and roughly chopped
- 2 cups zucchini, diced
- 1 cup corn kernels
- 1 teaspoon ground cumin
- 1 teaspoon dried oregano
- Salt and pepper to taste
- Fresh cilantro, chopped (for garnish)

Directions:

- Heat olive oil in a large pot over medium heat. Add the diced onion and minced garlic. Sauté for about 5 minutes until the onion becomes translucent.
- Add the vegetable broth, squash blossoms, diced zucchini, and corn kernels to the pot. Stir well to combine.
- Sprinkle ground cumin, dried oregano, salt, and pepper into the soup. Stir again.
- Bring the soup to a boil, then reduce the heat and simmer for 15 minutes until the vegetables are tender.
- Using an immersion blender or a regular blender, puree the soup until smooth and creamy.
- Return the soup to the pot and heat it for an additional 5 minutes.
- Ladle the Squash Blossom Soup into bowls, garnish with fresh cilantro, and serve hot.

Nutritional Information (per serving):

Calories: 130 kcal, Carbohydrates: 20 g, Protein: 4 g, Fat: 5 g, Fiber: 4 g, Sodium: 600 mg, Sugar: 6 g

73. SQUASH FRIED BLOSSOMS SNACK

Cooking time: 30 min, Difficulty Level: Easy, Servings: 1 dozen

Ingredients

- All-purpose flour 1/2 cup
- Garlic salt ¼ tsp
- Baking powder ½ tsp
- Large egg 1

- Ground cumin ¼ tsp
- Canola oil 1 tbsp
- 2% milk 1/2 cup
- Squash blossoms 12

Directions

- In a mixing bowl, combine flour, garlic salt, baking powder, and cumin. In a separate bowl, whisk together the egg, milk, and oil; add to the dry ingredients and stir until smooth. Preheat a skillet with 2 inches of oil to 375°. Dip the blooms in the batter, then cook them in batches in heated oil until golden brown. Absorb any excess liquid with paper towels. Continue to heat until ready to serve.

Nutritional information

Calories: 45 kcal, Carbohydrates: 5.7 g,Protein: 1.3 g, Fat: 1.8 g

74. SPICED CARROT SALAD

Preparation time: 10 minutes Cooking time: 10 minutes Difficulty Level: Easy Servings: 4

Ingredients:

- 4 large carrots, peeled and grated
- 1/4 cup raisins
- 1/4 cup chopped almonds
- 2 tablespoons olive oil
- 1 tablespoon lemon juice
- 1 teaspoon ground cumin
- 1/2 teaspoon ground coriander
- 1/4 teaspoon ground cinnamon
- Salt, to taste
- Fresh parsley, for garnish

Directions:

- In a large bowl, combine the grated carrots, raisins, and chopped almonds.
- In a small bowl, whisk together the olive oil, lemon juice, ground cumin, ground coriander, ground cinnamon, and salt.
- Pour the dressing over the carrot mixture and toss well to coat all the ingredients.
- Let the spiced carrot salad sit for at least 10 minutes to allow the flavors to meld together.
- Garnish with fresh parsley before serving.

Nutritional Information:

Calories: 150 Total Fat: 9g Saturated Fat: 1g Cholesterol: 0mg Sodium: 70mg Carbohydrates: 16g Fiber: 4g Sugar: 9g Protein: 3g

75. SPICED OOLONG EGGS ALONG WITH BEAN CURD & WOLFBERRIES

Preparation time: 15 minutes Cooking time: 30 minutes Difficulty Level: Intermediate Servings: 4

Ingredients:

- 4 large eggs
- 2 cups water
- 2 tablespoons soy sauce
- 2 tablespoons oolong tea leaves
- 1 cinnamon stick
- 2 star anise
- 1 teaspoon Sichuan peppercorns
- 1 block bean curd, diced
- 1/4 cup dried wolfberries (goji berries)
- 1 tablespoon sesame oil
- 2 green onions, chopped
- Salt, to taste

Directions:

- Place the eggs in a medium saucepan and add enough water to cover them. Bring the water to a boil over medium heat and cook the eggs for 6 minutes for a soft-boiled consistency. Remove the eggs from the saucepan and place them in a bowl of cold water to cool. Once cooled, peel the eggs and set them aside.
- In the same saucepan, add 2 cups of water, soy sauce, oolong tea leaves, cinnamon stick, star anise, and Sichuan peppercorns. Bring the mixture to a boil, then reduce the heat and simmer for 10 minutes to infuse the flavors.
- Add the diced bean curd and dried wolfberries to the saucepan and simmer for another 10 minutes to allow the flavors to meld. Season with salt to taste.
- Remove the saucepan from the heat and carefully add the peeled eggs back into the liquid. Allow the eggs to marinate in the

spiced tea mixture for at least 4 hours or overnight in the refrigerator for the best flavor.

- When ready to serve, gently remove the eggs from the marinade and slice them in half lengthwise.
- In a separate pan, heat the sesame oil over medium heat. Add the chopped green onions and sauté for 1-2 minutes until fragrant.
- Arrange the spiced oolong eggs on a serving plate along with the diced bean curd and wolfberries. Drizzle the sautéed green onions and sesame oil over the dish.
- Serve the Spiced Oolong Eggs along with Bean Curd & Wolfberries as an appetizer or side dish.

Nutritional Information: Calories: 180 Total Fat: 10g Saturated Fat: 2g Cholesterol: 186mg Sodium: 660mg Carbohydrates: 11g Fiber: 3g Sugar: 5g Protein: 14g

76. STEWED CHICKEN WITH GOLDEN TOMATOES

Cooking time: 1 hour 30 minutes Difficulty Level: Intermediate Servings: 4

Ingredients:

- 4 chicken thighs, bone-in and skin-on
- Salt and pepper to taste
- 2 tablespoons olive oil
- 1 onion, diced
- 2 cloves garlic, minced
- 1 red bell pepper, diced
- 1 yellow bell pepper, diced
- 1 can (14 ounces) golden tomatoes, diced
- 1 cup chicken broth
- 1 teaspoon dried thyme
- 1 bay leaf
- Chopped fresh parsley for garnish

Directions:

- Season the chicken thighs with salt and pepper on both sides.
- In a large Dutch oven or pot, heat the olive oil over medium heat.
- Add the chicken thighs, skin-side down, and sear them until golden brown, about 5

minutes per side. Remove the chicken from the pot and set it aside.

- In the same pot, add the diced onion, minced garlic, and diced bell peppers. Sauté for about 5 minutes until the vegetables are softened.
- Return the chicken thighs to the pot, along with any accumulated juices. Add the diced golden tomatoes, chicken broth, dried thyme, and bay leaf. Stir to combine.
- Bring the mixture to a boil, then reduce the heat to low. Cover the pot and let it simmer for 1 hour, or until the chicken is cooked through and tender.
- Remove the bay leaf from the pot. Taste and adjust the seasoning with salt and pepper if needed.
- Serve the Stewed Chicken with Golden Tomatoes hot, garnished with chopped fresh parsley.
- This dish pairs well with steamed rice or crusty bread.

Nutritional Information (per serving): Calories: 320 kcal, Carbohydrates: 10 g, Protein: 24 g, Fat: 20 g, Fiber: 2 g, Sugar: 5 g, Sodium: 600 mg

77. STUFFED ONION SQUASH BLOSSOM

Cooking time: 20 min, Difficulty Level: Easy, Servings: 4

Ingredients

- Oil for frying
- Fresh Squash blossoms 10-15Batter mix
- Rice flour 1 cup
- Oregano seeds 1/4 tsp
- Pancake mix 1/4 cup
- Salt to tasteFilling
- Onion julienned 1
- Thin flattened rice 3-4 tsp
- Salt to taste
- Green chilies (optional) 1-2
- Coriander to taste
- Chaat masala 1 tsp

Directions

Filling with blossoms for the squad
- Combine sliced onions, poha, and green chilis in a mixing bowl. Chaat masala, chili powder, and salt should be added as well.
- Toss in the ginger and coriander leaves and put aside. Make the batter.

Batter
- In a separate skillet, combine the pancake mix, rice flour, salt, and oregano seeds, and stir thoroughly.
- Add water as needed and fully blend. It must be thick enough to coat the blooms but also have a lovely flowing consistency.
- Pour oil into the pan.
- Thoroughly stuff the washed and dried squash blossoms with the filling.
- Check that the filling isn't too thick and that it stays in place.Remove it from the oil when it has turned golden brown. Serve with a spicy sauce on the side.

Nutritional information
Calories: 177 kcal, Carbohydrates: 38.6g, Protein: 2.8 g, Fat: 0. 7 g

78. SUCCOTASH
Cooking time: 20 minutes Difficulty Level: Easy Servings: 4

Ingredients:
- 2 cups fresh or frozen lima beans
- 2 cups fresh or frozen corn kernels
- 1 red bell pepper, diced
- 1 small onion, diced
- 2 tablespoons butter
- 1 tablespoon olive oil
- 2 cloves garlic, minced
- 1 teaspoon dried thyme
- Salt and pepper to taste
- Optional toppings: chopped fresh parsley, crumbled bacon

Directions:
- In a large pot of boiling salted water, cook the lima beans for about 5 minutes until tender. Drain and set aside.
- In a large skillet, melt the butter and olive oil over medium heat. Add the diced onion,

diced bell pepper, minced garlic, and dried thyme. Sauté until the vegetables are softened and fragrant.
- Add the corn kernels and cooked lima beans to the skillet. Stir well to combine.
- Cook the succotash for an additional 10 minutes, stirring occasionally, until the flavors meld together and the vegetables are cooked through.
- Season with salt and pepper to taste.
- Remove from heat and garnish with chopped fresh parsley and crumbled bacon, if desired.
- Serve the Succotash as a side dish or as a main course with bread or rice.

Nutritional Information (per serving):
Calories: 210 kcal, Carbohydrates: 29 g, Protein: 6 g, Fat: 9 g, Fiber: 6 g, Sugar: 7 g, Sodium: 220 mg

79. SUMAC NAVAJO LAMB LEG WITH ONION SAUCE
Cooking time: 1 hour 30 min, Difficulty Level: Difficult, Servings: 6-8

Ingredients
For the lamb
- Leg of lamb 3-pound
- Cracked black pepper 1 tsp
- Fine salt 1 tsp
- Canola oil 3 tbsp
- Ground sumac 1/3 cupFor onion sauce
- Canola oil 2 tbsp
- Fresh thyme 2 sprigs
- Onion 1
- Dried juniper berries 5
- Fresh rosemary 1 sprig
- Black pepper 1 tsp
- Chicken stock 2 cups
- Salt 1 tsp
- Water, as needed

Directions
- Preheat your oven to 375°F. Insert a rack into it. Season the lamb on all sides with salt and pepper, then coat it with sumac.
- Heat the oil in a skillet. Add the meat and sear on all sides for about 8 minutes, or until evenly browned.

- The roast took about 40 minutes to cook.
- To make the onion sauce, heat the oil in a saute pan over medium heat while the lamb roasts. Place the rosemary, pepper, onion, juniper berries, thyme, and salt in a mixing bowl. Reduce the heat to medium-low and cook, stirring regularly, for almost 20 minutes, or until the onions are soft and golden.
- To make the onion sauce, heat the oil in a saute pan over medium heat while the lamb roasts. Place the onion, thyme, rosemary, juniper berries, salt, and pepper in a mixing bowl. Reduce the heat to medium-low and cook, stirring regularly, for almost 20 minutes, or until the onions are soft and golden. Stir with a little water if the onions start to cling or discolor in any spots. After the bacon has browned, add the stock and cook for about 10 minutes, or until the liquid has been reduced by half. Remove and discard the herb stems and juniper berries from the container.
- Serve immediately with an onion sauce on the side.

Nutritional information

Calories: 509 kcal, Carbohydrates: 1.7 g, Protein: 34.2 g, Fat: 39.4 g

80. SWEET TAMALES

Cooking time: 1 hour 30 minutes Difficulty Level: Medium Servings: 12

Ingredients:
- 2 cups masa harina (corn flour)
- 1 teaspoon baking powder
- 1/2 teaspoon salt
- 1/2 cup unsalted butter, softened
- 1/2 cup granulated sugar
- 1 cup water
- 1 teaspoon vanilla extract
- 1 cup sweetened shredded coconut
- 1/2 cup raisins
- 12 dried corn husks, soaked in water until pliable

Directions:
- In a mixing bowl, combine the masa harina, baking powder, and salt.
- In a separate bowl, cream together the softened butter and granulated sugar until light and fluffy.
- Gradually add the butter and sugar mixture to the dry ingredients, mixing well.
- Slowly add water and vanilla extract to the mixture, stirring until a smooth dough forms.
- Stir in the shredded coconut and raisins, ensuring they are evenly distributed throughout the dough.
- Drain the soaked corn husks and pat them dry with a clean towel.
- Take a soaked corn husk and spread about 1/4 cup of the dough mixture onto the center of the husk.
- Roll the husk tightly around the dough, folding in the sides to enclose it completely.
- Repeat the process with the remaining dough and corn husks.
- Prepare a steamer by filling the bottom with water and placing a steamer insert or rack over it.
- Arrange the wrapped tamales upright in the steamer, ensuring they are tightly packed but not crushed.
- Cover the steamer and steam the tamales over medium heat for approximately 1 hour and 30 minutes, or until the dough is firm and cooked through.
- Carefully remove the tamales from the steamer and let them cool slightly before serving.

Nutritional Information (per serving):

Calories: 250 kcal, Carbohydrates: 33 g, Protein: 3 g, Fat: 12 g, Fiber: 3 g, Sugar: 12 g, Sodium: 170 mg

81. TABOULEH WITH MINT, CUCUMBER & GOJI BERRIES

Preparation time: 15 minutes Cooking time: No cooking required Difficulty Level: Easy Servings: 4

Ingredients:

- 1 cup bulgur wheat
- 1 1/2 cups boiling water
- 1 cucumber, finely diced
- 1/2 cup fresh mint leaves, chopped
- 1/4 cup fresh parsley, chopped
- 1/4 cup goji berries
- 2 tablespoons olive oil
- Juice of 1 lemon
- Salt, to taste
- Black pepper, to taste

Directions:

- Place the bulgur wheat in a large bowl and pour the boiling water over it. Cover the bowl and let it sit for about 15 minutes, or until the bulgur is tender and has absorbed the water.
- Once the bulgur is ready, fluff it with a fork and let it cool for a few minutes.
- Add the finely diced cucumber, chopped mint leaves, chopped parsley, and goji berries to the bowl with the bulgur.
- Drizzle the olive oil and lemon juice over the mixture. Season with salt and black pepper to taste.
- Toss all the ingredients together until well combined.
- Let the tabouleh sit at room temperature for about 15-20 minutes to allow the flavors to meld together.
- Serve the Tabouleh with Mint, Cucumber & Goji Berries as a refreshing salad or as a side dish.

Nutritional Information:

Calories: 180 Total Fat: 7g Saturated Fat: 1g Cholesterol: 0mg Sodium: 150mg Carbohydrates: 27g Fiber: 6g Sugar: 3g Protein: 5g

82. TANGY ORANGE SALAD

Preparation time: 15 minutes Cooking time: 0 minutes Difficulty Level: Easy Servings: 4

Ingredients:

- 4 oranges, peeled and segmented
- 1 small red onion, thinly sliced
- 1/4 cup fresh mint leaves, chopped
- 1/4 cup pitted black olives, halved
- 2 tablespoons olive oil

- 1 tablespoon white wine vinegar
- 1 teaspoon honey
- Salt and pepper to taste

Directions:

- In a large bowl, combine the orange segments, thinly sliced red onion, chopped mint leaves, and halved black olives.
- In a small bowl, whisk together the olive oil, white wine vinegar, honey, salt, and pepper until well combined.
- Pour the dressing over the orange salad and toss gently to coat all the ingredients.
- Taste and adjust the seasoning with additional salt and pepper, if desired.
- Let the salad sit at room temperature for about 10 minutes to allow the flavors to meld together.
- Serve the Tangy Orange Salad as a refreshing side dish or as a light and vibrant appetizer.

Nutritional Information (per serving): Calories: 120, Carbohydrates: 16g, Protein: 2g, Fat: 7g, Sodium: 150mg, Fiber: 4g

83. THREE SISTERS HOMINY HARVEST STEW

Preparation time: 15 minutes Cooking time: 45 minutes Difficulty Level: Medium Servings: 6

Ingredients:

- 2 tablespoons olive oil
- 1 large onion, diced
- 2 cloves garlic, minced
- 2 bell peppers, diced (any color)
- 2 medium zucchini, diced
- 2 cups fresh or frozen corn kernels
- 1 can (15 ounces) black beans, rinsed and drained
- 1 can (15 ounces) diced tomatoes
- 1 can (15 ounces) hominy, drained
- 4 cups vegetable broth
- 2 teaspoons chili powder
- 1 teaspoon ground cumin
- 1/2 teaspoon smoked paprika
- Salt and pepper to taste
- Fresh cilantro for garnish

Directions:

- Heat the olive oil in a large pot or Dutch oven over medium heat. Add the diced onion and minced garlic, and sauté until the onion becomes translucent and fragrant.
- Add the diced bell peppers and zucchini to the pot, and cook for 5 minutes until they start to soften.
- Stir in the corn kernels, black beans, diced tomatoes (with their juice), and drained hominy.
- Pour in the vegetable broth and add the chili powder, cumin, smoked paprika, salt, and pepper. Stir well to combine all the ingredients.
- Bring the stew to a boil, then reduce the heat to low. Cover the pot and simmer for 30 minutes to allow the flavors to meld together.
- After 30 minutes, remove the lid and give the stew a taste. Adjust the seasoning if needed.
- Serve the Three Sisters Hominy Harvest Stew hot, garnished with fresh cilantro.

Nutritional Information (per serving):
Calories: 235 kcal, Carbohydrates: 42 g, Protein: 9 g, Fat: 5 g, Fiber: 8 g, Sodium: 680 mg, Sugar: 9 g

84. TOMATO WITH ROSEMARY AND CORIANDER

Preparation time: 10 minutes Cooking time: 20 minutes Difficulty Level: Easy Servings: 4

Ingredients:

- 4 large tomatoes
- 2 tablespoons olive oil
- 2 cloves garlic, minced
- 1 tablespoon fresh rosemary leaves, chopped
- 1 tablespoon fresh coriander leaves, chopped
- Salt and pepper to taste

Directions:

- Preheat the oven to 400°F (200°C).
- Cut the tomatoes in half horizontally and remove the seeds.
- Place the tomato halves in a baking dish, cut side up.
- In a small bowl, mix together the olive oil,

minced garlic, chopped rosemary leaves, chopped coriander leaves, salt, and pepper.

- Drizzle the olive oil mixture over the tomato halves, making sure they are well coated.
- Place the baking dish in the preheated oven and roast the tomatoes for 20 minutes, or until they are tender and slightly caramelized.
- Remove the baking dish from the oven and let the tomatoes cool slightly before serving.

Nutritional Information (per serving):
Calories: 80 kcal, Carbohydrates: 6 g, Protein: 1 g, Fat: 6 g, Sodium: 50 mg

85. TUMBLEWEED (SALSOLA KALI)

Cooking time: 5-7 min, Difficulty Level: Easy, Servings: 4

Ingredients

- Sprouts a bundle
- Water 1 cup

Directions

- The sprouts are boiled in moderately salted water for around 10 minutes.
- They should not be overcooked or dried out. It's also buttered or topped with a small amount of mutton grease. If the sprouts are still young, they can be chopped raw and used in salads.

Nutritional information
Calories: 53 kcal, Carbohydrates: 11.5 g, Protein: 2 g, Fat: 0.3 g

86. TURMERIC ROASTED WILD CARROTS WITH SEEDS

Preparation time: 10 minutes Cooking time: 25 minutes Difficulty Level: Easy Servings: 4

Ingredients:

- 1 pound wild carrots, peeled and trimmed
- 2 tablespoons olive oil
- 1 teaspoon ground turmeric
- 1 teaspoon cumin seeds
- 1 teaspoon sesame seeds

- Salt, to taste
- Black pepper, to taste
- Fresh cilantro, for garnish

Directions:
- Preheat your oven to 425°F (220°C).
- In a large bowl, toss the wild carrots with olive oil, ground turmeric, cumin seeds, sesame seeds, salt, and black pepper. Make sure the carrots are well coated with the spices.
- Arrange the carrots in a single layer on a baking sheet.
- Roast in the preheated oven for about 20-25 minutes, or until the carrots are tender and slightly caramelized, stirring once halfway through.
- Remove from the oven and let the carrots cool slightly.
- Garnish with fresh cilantro before serving.

Nutritional Information:
Calories: 110 kcal Total Fat: 7g Saturated Fat: 1g Cholesterol: 0mg Sodium: 110mg Carbohydrates: 12g Fiber: 4g Sugar: 6g Protein: 2g

87. VANILLA GOJI BERRY BALLS

Preparation time: 15 minutes Cooking time: No cooking required Difficulty Level: Easy Servings: 12

Ingredients:
- 1 cup Medjool dates, pitted
- 1 cup almonds
- 1/2 cup goji berries
- 1/4 cup unsweetened shredded coconut
- 1 teaspoon vanilla extract
- Pinch of salt

Directions:
- Place the pitted dates, almonds, goji berries, shredded coconut, vanilla extract, and salt in a food processor.
- Pulse the ingredients until they are well combined and form a sticky mixture.
- Transfer the mixture to a bowl.
- Using your hands, roll small portions of the mixture into bite-sized balls.
- Place the balls on a parchment-lined baking sheet or plate.
- Once all the mixture has been rolled into balls, refrigerate them for at least 30 minutes to firm up.
- After chilling, the Vanilla Goji Berry Balls are ready to be enjoyed!

Nutritional Information:
Calories: 100 Total Fat: 4g Saturated Fat: 0.5g Cholesterol: 0mg Sodium: 0mg Carbohydrates: 15g Fiber: 3g Sugar: 11g Protein: 2g

88. WATERMELON, CUCUMBER & HUSKCHERRY SALSA

Cooking time: 0 min, Difficulty Level: Easy, Servings: 2

Ingredients
- Seeded watermelon 2 cups
- Husk cherries 1 pint
- Cucumber 1
- Minced fresh cilantro 2 tbsp
- Jalapeno 1
- Squeezed lime juice 2 tbsp
- Honey 2 tsp

Directions
- Combine all of the ingredients in a mixing dish. Allow 15 minutes for it to rest. Serve.

Nutritional information
Calories: 157 kcal, Carbohydrates: 39.4g, Protein: 2.9 g, Fat: 0.7 g

89. WILD GITIGAN SALAD

Preparation time: 15 minutes Cooking time: None Difficulty Level: Easy Servings: 4

Ingredients:
- 6 cups mixed salad greens
- 1 cup fresh wild berries (such as raspberries, blackberries, or blueberries)
- 1 cup cherry tomatoes, halved
- 1/2 cup sliced almonds
- 1/4 cup crumbled feta cheese
- 1/4 cup balsamic vinaigrette dressing
- Salt and pepper to taste

Directions:
- In a large salad bowl, combine the mixed

salad greens, fresh wild berries, cherry tomatoes, sliced almonds, and crumbled feta cheese.

- Drizzle the balsamic vinaigrette dressing over the salad.
- Season with salt and pepper to taste.
- Gently toss all the ingredients together until well coated with the dressing.
- Serve the Wild Gitigan Salad immediately as a refreshing and nutritious side dish.

Nutritional Information (per serving):
Calories: 150 kcal, Carbohydrates: 10 g, Protein: 5 g, Fat: 11 g, Fiber: 4 g, Sodium: 220 mg, Sugar: 4 g

90. WILD MUSHROOMSAUTEE

Cooking time: 20 minutes Difficulty Level: Easy Servings: 4

Ingredients:

- 1 pound mixed wild mushrooms (such as cremini, shiitake, and oyster), sliced
- 2 tablespoons butter
- 2 cloves garlic, minced
- 1 teaspoon fresh thyme leaves
- Salt and pepper to taste
- 1 tablespoon chopped fresh parsley for garnish

Directions:

- In a large skillet, melt the butter over medium heat.
- Add the minced garlic and sauté for about 1 minute until fragrant.
- Add the sliced mushrooms to the skillet. Cook for 8-10 minutes, stirring occasionally, until the mushrooms are tender and lightly browned.
- Stir in the fresh thyme leaves and season with salt and pepper to taste. Cook for an additional 2 minutes to allow the flavors to meld together.
- Remove from heat and garnish with chopped fresh parsley.
- Serve the Wild Mushroom Saute as a side dish or as a topping for grilled meats or toasted bread.

Nutritional Information (per serving):
Calories: 80 kcal, Carbohydrates: 6 g, Protein: 3 g,

Fat: 5 g, Fiber: 2 g, Sugar: 2 g, Sodium: 80 mg

91. WILD RICE AND CARROTS

Preparation time: 10 minutes Cooking time: 45 minutes Difficulty Level: Easy Servings: 4

Ingredients:

- 1 cup wild rice
- 2 cups vegetable broth
- 2 cups water
- 2 large carrots, diced
- 1 small onion, finely chopped
- 2 cloves garlic, minced
- 2 tablespoons olive oil
- 1/2 teaspoon dried thyme
- Salt, to taste
- Black pepper, to taste
- Fresh parsley, for garnish

Directions:

- Rinse the wild rice under cold water and drain.
- In a large saucepan, heat the olive oil over medium heat. Add the diced carrots, chopped onion, and minced garlic. Cook for about 5 minutes, or until the vegetables start to soften.
- Add the wild rice to the saucepan and stir to coat the grains with the vegetable mixture.
- Pour in the vegetable broth and water. Season with dried thyme, salt, and black pepper.
- Bring the mixture to a boil, then reduce the heat to low. Cover the saucepan and simmer for about 45 minutes, or until the wild rice is tender and the liquid is absorbed.
- Remove the saucepan from heat and let it sit, covered, for about 5 minutes.
- Fluff the wild rice with a fork and garnish with fresh parsley before serving.

Nutritional Information:
Calories: 210 kcal Total Fat: 7g Saturated Fat: 1g Cholesterol: 0mg Sodium: 450mg Carbohydrates: 32g Fiber: 4g Sugar: 4g Protein: 5g

92. WILD RICE AND MUSHROOM

Cooking time: 50 minutes Difficulty Level: Medium Servings: 4

Ingredients:

- 1 cup wild rice
- 2 cups vegetable broth
- 2 tablespoons butter
- 1 small onion, diced
- 8 ounces mushrooms, sliced
- 2 cloves garlic, minced
- 1 teaspoon dried thyme
- Salt and pepper to taste
- Chopped fresh parsley for garnish

Directions:

- Rinse the wild rice thoroughly under cold water.
- In a saucepan, combine the wild rice and vegetable broth. Bring to a boil, then reduce the heat, cover, and simmer for 40-45 minutes until the rice is tender and the liquid is absorbed. Remove from heat and let it rest for 5 minutes.
- In a large skillet, melt the butter over medium heat. Add the diced onion and sliced mushrooms. Sauté until the mushrooms are golden brown and the onions are translucent.
- Add the minced garlic and dried thyme to the skillet. Cook for an additional 2 minutes until fragrant.
- Stir in the cooked wild rice and season with salt and pepper to taste. Cook for 5 minutes, allowing the flavors to blend together.
- Remove from heat and garnish with chopped fresh parsley.
- Serve the Wild Rice and Mushroom as a side dish or as a main course with roasted vegetables or grilled chicken.

Nutritional Information (per serving):
Calories: 220 kcal, Carbohydrates: 38 g, Protein: 7 g, Fat: 6 g, Fiber: 4 g, Sugar: 3 g, Sodium: 470 mg

93. WILD RICE SALAD

Cooking time: 45 min, Difficulty Level: Easy, Servings: 4

Ingredients

- Dijon mustard 1 ½ tsp
- Dried cranberries 40-45 g
- orange juice 1(orange)
- Apple cider vinegar 1 ½ tsp
- Chicken stock 4 cups
- Olive oil ¼ cup
- Chopped chives 1 ½ tbsp
- Spring onions 3
- Pumpkin seeds ¼ cup
- Maple syrup 1 tbsp
- Wild rice 1 cup

Directions

- Drain and put the rice out to let it cool.
- Bring the rice and chicken stock to a boil together. Reduce to a low heat and cover for 45 minutes. Drain the rice and set it aside to cool.
- Roast pine nuts and pumpkin seeds together for 5-10 minutes.
- To make the vinaigrette, combine the olive oil, orange juice, apple cider vinegar, maple syrup, and mustard in a mixing bowl.
- In a serving dish, combine the wild rice, pumpkin seeds, spring onions, chives, pine nuts, cranberries, and vinaigrette.

Nutritional information
Calories: 244 kcal, Carbohydrates: 30 g, Protein: 7 g, Fats: 12 g

94. WILD RICE SAUTÉ ALONG WITH SWEETPOTATO

Preparation time: 10 minutes Cooking time: 40 minutes Difficulty Level: Easy Servings: 4

Ingredients:

- 1 cup wild rice
- 2 cups vegetable broth
- 2 tablespoons olive oil
- 1 large sweet potato, peeled and diced
- 1 onion, chopped
- 2 cloves garlic, minced
- 1 teaspoon dried thyme
- Salt, to taste
- Black pepper, to taste
- Fresh parsley, for garnish

Directions:

- Rinse the wild rice under cold water and

drain.

- In a medium saucepan, bring the vegetable broth to a boil. Add the wild rice, reduce the heat to low, cover, and simmer for about 40 minutes, or until the rice is tender and cooked through. Drain any excess liquid.
- In a large skillet, heat the olive oil over medium heat.
- Add the diced sweet potato to the skillet and sauté for about 10 minutes, or until the sweet potato becomes slightly tender.
- Add the chopped onion, minced garlic, dried thyme, salt, and black pepper to the skillet. Continue sautéing for another 5 minutes, until the onions are translucent and the sweet potato is fully cooked.
- Stir in the cooked wild rice and cook for an additional 2-3 minutes to combine the flavors.Remove from heat and garnish with fresh parsley.
- Serve the wild rice sauté along with sweet potato as a side dish or a main course.

Nutritional Information:

Calories: 250 Total Fat: 7g Saturated Fat: 1g Cholesterol: 0mg Sodium: 450mg Carbohydrates: 42g Fiber: 5g Sugar: 5g Protein: 5g

95. WOJAPI

Cooking time: 5-10 min, Difficulty Level: Easy, Servings: 12

Ingredients

- Berries 3 cups
- Sugar ¾ cups
- Water 2 ¼ cups
- Corn starch 3 tbsp

Directions

- Crush the berries completely.
- In a mixing basin, combine the berries and 1 1/2 cups water. Bring to a boil, stirring occasionally. Reduce the heat and leave it alone.
- Stir in the sugar thoroughly. In a mixing dish, combine the corn starch and 3/4 cup water.Mix with the berry sauce. Cook for 4 to 5 minutes, or until the sauce thickens.

Nutritional information

Calories: 76 kcal, Carbohydrates: 19 g, Protein: 0 g, Fats: 0 g

96. WOLFBERRY LEAVES PLUS SEEDS SOUP

Cooking time: 17-18 min, Difficulty Level: Easy, Servings: 4

Ingredients

- Wolfberry leaves 1 bundle
- Ginger 5 slices
- Wolfberry seeds one tbsp.
- Pork liver slices
- Egg 1
- Salt to taste

Directions

- Soak the wolfberry leaves in salted water for about 15 minutes. Then, thoroughly clean. Bring 10 cups of water to a boil, then add the ginger and heat for 5 minutes before adding the liver and wolfberries.
- Cook the liver until it is half done, then add the leaves. Instead of overcooking your leaves, season them with salt, whisk in the egg, and slowly pour it over them. Cook, covered, for several minutes before removing.

Nutritional information

Calories: 224 kcal, Carbohydrates: 28.2g, Protein: 14.5 g, Fat: 7.4 g

97. ZUCCHINI BLOSSOM PAKORA

Cooking time: 15 min, Difficulty Level: Easy, Servings: 10

Ingredients

- Zucchini blossoms 10
- Cumin seeds ½ tsp
- Besan (chickpea flour) ¾ cup
- Cayenne ½ tsp
- Salt to taste
- Ajwain seeds ½ tsp
- Baking soda ¼ tsp
- Turmeric ½ tsp

Directions

- Cumin and ajwain seeds are coarsely

ground.Combine everything except the flowers in one bowl. Add just enough water to make a thick paste.

- Heat two inches of oil in a skillet to 350-375 degrees.
- Drop each zucchini blossom into the heated oil after uniformly coating it with batter. Deep-frying three or four at a time is acceptable, but do not overcrowd the skillet.
- Fry until golden brown and puffy on both sides, then serve immediately.

Nutritional information

Calories: 37 kcal, Carbohydrates: 6 g,Protein: 2 g, Fat: 1 g

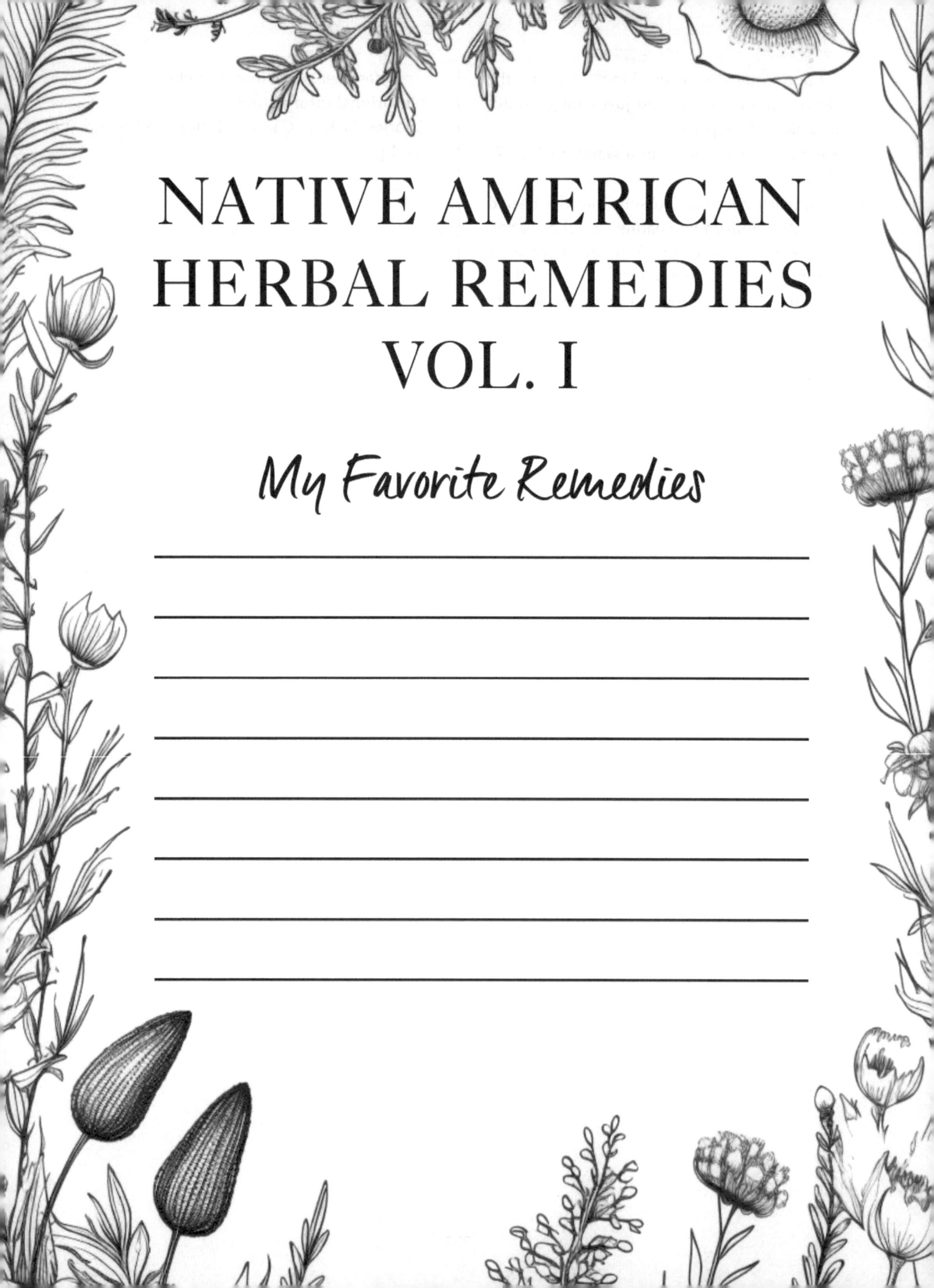

NATIVE AMERICAN HERBAL REMEDIES VOL. I

My Favorite Remedies

_____

_____

_____

_____

_____

_____

_____

INTRODUCTION

The Native Americans' traditional food preparation skills and medical herb list were widespread; numerous plants were employed for therapeutic purposes, such as the cowberry (Vaccinium arboreum), whose berries are used to make blue-black color.

The wood is also utilized for a variety of purposes. Smudging, firestarter, and dyeing are examples of these. This will focus on a plant that is extensively used in herbal medicine and has a role in the Thanksgiving holiday: chicory coffee!

Chicory coffee is a popular ingredient in the wintertime drink "chicory" or "Kaffee." During wartime or when money was short, mixing chicory root with coffee was a means to stretch the coffee supply. The Native Americans combined their chicory root with coffee but never drank it. To assist in curing other disorders, they drank a whole different beverage.

This plant was utilized for medical purposes by Native Americans, as were many other Native American herbs described by ethnobotanists. The herb was also utilized in cooking and was described by the first Europeans to explore the New World. Native Americans taught European settlers how to use this herb as a coffee substitute and a medicinal herb for green tea. I'll concentrate on the therapeutic uses of chicory for this.

Chicory was utilized for various purposes, the most prominent of which was as a coffee replacement. It was necessary during times of war when money was scarce, and coffee supplies were few. Chicory may be easily cultivated and gathered yearly because it grows on the roots. This suggests that Native Americans have access to these plants at all times to manufacture coffee replacements.

"Chicory root has long been one of Canada's premier native wild plants, farmed for millennia by Caughnawaga Indians and used as a coffee replacement and natural dye" - Wabanaki Medicinal Plants' Alex Colville.

The roots were really bitter. The place where the roots were collected also yielded the most bitter flavor. As a result, "chicory tea" was created by boiling dark-colored roots in wood ashes and roasting them in hot ashes." It's known as "black tea."

"Both this drug and black tea contain caffeine as a component of their alkaloids, making them more stimulating for persons who require that stimulant in their everyday routine tasks." - Wabanaki Medicinal Plants' Alex Colville

Chicory plant leaves have been utilized as greens. "Chicory is a useful plant to eat if eaten as greens, because it contains nausea (a bitter substance), a property many other plants lack." The arrangement of the leaves in the stalk is supposed to mimic the letters X and Z or an 'X' and a 'Y'; this letter-like shape is said to represent a symbol for a star.'" "The root also has medicinal properties." – Alex Colville, Wabanaki Medicinal Plants

"The root also has medicinal properties." – Alex Colville, Wabanaki Medicinal Plants

"For example, chicory was used as an ointment in places like Montreal [in Canada], where ringworm was prevalent." "The roots were roasted in ashes before being pounded and mixed with lard oil." - Wabanaki Medicinal Plants' Alex Colville

The entire plant was utilized. "The root is harvested when it is green or ripe. The root is cut into strips and boiled in water until the bitterness is removed. While the water is still boiling, it is squeezed out of the strips. The plant milk is then strained through a napkin or cloth to remove any garbage, and a little water may be added to make it more liquid and drinkable. The remaining root milk is cooked down to a thicker, syrupy consistency. This paste is then placed in a tightly sealed container and stored in a cool place. This paste can be stored for several weeks to months. It can be smeared on round or flatbread like bannock before cooking, and possibly also after cooking in hot ashes." -Wabanaki Medicinal Plants' Alex Colville

NATURAL HERBS' HEALTH BENEFITS

Many people are looking for natural solutions to stay healthy.

There is a growing demand for herbs with multiple health advantages as more people become more careful of their food.

Natural herbs have grown in popularity in recent years because they can effectively treat various diseases while having no side effects.

Natural herbs include parsley, ginger, garlic, and peppermint leaves, to name a few. Humans have utilized these plants to treat various illnesses and disorders for ages because we were formed with an intrinsic understanding of how our bodies work and what they require to stay healthy and whole.

Some of these natural herbs are also frequently used to produce food and beverages, such as teas, cosmetics, soaps, and spices.

Natural herbs have several advantages

Blood Pressure Regulation (Lowering High Blood Pressure) - Regular consumption of ginger or raw garlic has been demonstrated to lower blood pressure. Ginger can be consumed as a tea or in pill form. This herb helps to stabilize blood pressure by lowering artery enlargement caused by elevated salt levels in the body.

Reducing Menstrual Cramps - Taking ginger as a tea daily may help ease regular menstrual cramps by encouraging ovulation, lowering uterine contractions, and preventing uterine spasms. Ginger also lowers uterine inflammation, prevents pre-eclampsia, and relieves pregnancy sickness. Ginger's activities are related to its capacity to raise prostaglandin levels in the body, which is responsible for many of these health advantages.

Thinning Blood - Garlic is an excellent plant for thinning the blood, and it lowers excessive clotting, which can lead to dangerous conditions in people with this condition. People with atrial fibrillation, for example, are recommended to consume a lot of garlic since it reduces blood clotting and prevents strokes.

Gastric Ulcers - Ginger is a good plant for treating gastric ulcers because it encourages the creation of mucus in the stomach, the activity of digestive fluids, and the protection of the stomach mucous membrane. Ginger also eliminates harmful microorganisms in the stomach and is employed in treating intestinal infections, indigestion, and diarrhea.

Garlic's antioxidants battle free radicals, which cause cellular damage, aging, and disease. Garlic is also a fantastic natural detox herb since it helps cleanse the body of toxins and heavy metals like lead, mercury, and cadmium.

Heart Protection - There is much evidence that garlic can help prevent heart disease by lowering cholesterol levels in the bloodstream, improving blood pressure, and strengthening blood vessels to increase circulation.

Hair Growth - Ginger is used to promote hair development. Of course, it may be more useful to some than others, but many claim it has helped them with their hair. Ginger promotes hair development by increasing the activity of enzymes in the body, which are necessary for maintaining healthy hair follicles. It also softens and heals the scalp, reducing itching and irritation on the skin.

Hydration (Lubrication) - It lubricates the inside walls of the body and aids in the relief of joint and muscle pain, particularly in situations of arthritis. Ginger is also particularly effective in cases of persistent skin dryness. This herb is beneficial in improving the body's absorption of key nutrients that are required to maintain strong and healthy hair follicles.

Immunity - Ginger contains antiviral, antibacterial, and antifungal characteristics that aid in preventing and treating ailments such as cold sores, sinus infections, bronchitis, and sore throats. As a result, it can be used to alleviate the symptoms of lower respiratory tract diseases such as bronchitis.

Liver Support - Ginger includes curcumin, an antioxidant, anti-inflammatory, and antiviral plant that can help reduce the risk of liver damage.

Nausea - Taking ginger as a tea or supplement can help many people who suffer from nausea. Ginger relieves nausea by increasing the formation of gastrin, which increases the flow of digestive juices from the pancreas and duodenum into the stomach. These juices aid in nutrient absorption and assimilation, especially iron absorption. Furthermore, ginger promotes bile synthesis from the liver, which aids with fat digestion and food absorption. Nausea is typically a result of a shortage of nutrients being expelled from the body, and this herb can aid with that. Ginger also modulates digestive fluid secretions and increases peristalsis, which is food movement through the intestines.

Pain Relief - Taking cloves as a tea or supplement might help relieve pain caused by arthritis, bursitis, gout, and other joint issues. Its capacity to enhance circulation in the joints and encourage blood flow to these places reduces swelling and pain levels associated with these illnesses.

TRADITIONAL CURE FOR COMMON ALIMENTS

ABSCESS AND GINGIVITIS

1. Make the Mullein poultice in three sections and the Lobelia poultice in one piece. Apply it to the affected area.
2. Make one onion poultice with five garlic cloves. Use it on the abscess.
3. Take half a cup of basil leaves and half a cup of crushed Vetiver roots. Soak them in a jug of boiling water overnight.
4. Collect an equal amount of Vetiver and Sandalwood scraps. Grind them together. Mix one teaspoon of powder into Rosewater and add it once a day, or mix any leftover Vetiver and Sandalwood. Dip for 2 hours in a mud pot filled with water. Frequently Consume it. Combine Sandalwood, Vetiver, and Turmeric powder in similar amounts.
5. Combine equal parts Sandalwood, Vetiver, and Turmeric powder.
6. Take Woodfordia Fruticosa (Dhawan) blossoms. Blend of Camel Thorn (Java) oil. Hold it for 10 to 15 minutes on a medium flame. Apply the affected area warmly.
7. Combine 1 teaspoon Bush Grape (Amalbel) root powder and 1/4 teaspoon black pepper. Make a paste with a small amount of water. Apply twice a day for 20 minutes on the affected area
8. Drink it on an empty stomach. This helps boils that are packed with blood.

ACNE

Acne can appear at any age and can be caused by allergies, high-sugar or high-fat diets, inheritance, the use of oral contraceptives and other medicines (such as cortisone), hormone fluctuations, or stress.

Toner for the Skin

If you're having trouble getting rid of acne, use this toner twice or thrice a day, rinsing softly with water first and not scrubbing too hard or using harsh soaps.

1. Facial Steam

Yields 2 cups of dried herb mix (for 4 to 8 steams)

- ½ cup dried chamomile flower
- ½ cup dried sage leaf
- ½ cup dried thyme leaf
- ½ cup dried yarrow leaf and flower
- ½ gallon water

1. Combine the chamomile, sage, thyme, and yarrow in a mixing bowl.
2. Keep it in an airtight container.

Making and Using Herbal Steam

In a medium pot over high heat, bring water to a boil. Remove the pot from the fire and place it on a heat-proof surface next to which you can sit, creating a tent with a towel or blanket.

Add 14 to 12 cups of the herb mixture to the hot water. Place your face above the steam and hold it there for 5 to 20 minutes (Keep tissues handy because the smoke also clears your sinuses!). Apply raw or herb-infused honey to specified locations after that.

2. Acne Wash Tea

- 1 cup horsetail tea
- 30 drops Gotu kola tincture

Use when in need to wash the skin three times daily.

3. Acne-Fighting Tea

- 1 cup Oregon grape root tea
- 50 drops yellow dock tincture

Stir together the Ingredients. Use one-third of the mixture three times daily.

AGING

Free radicals are unstable chemicals that damage the DNA of cells and impair their capacity to operate. Several herbs function as antioxidants, efficiently removing free radicals.

1. Anti-Aging Tea 1

- 5 drops cayenne tincture
- 30 drops burdock tincture
- 15 drops goldenseal tincture
- 10 drops ginger root tincture
- ½ cup slippery elm tea,

ANEMIA

Anemia is a blood condition characterized by either too few red blood cells or too few red blood cells in the blood (Hemoglobin is a protein found in red blood cells that transports oxygen).

Alcoholism, heavy bleeding, sickness, infections, poor bone marrow function, poor food, and pregnancy are all potential causes of anemia..

1. Anemia Tea
- 2 teaspoons barberry root
- 2 teaspoons Oregon grape root
- 4 tablespoons nettle leaves
- 2 cups cold water

1. Stir together the herbs in a glass container.
2. Cover with the water.
3. Allow to soak overnight.
4. Strain.
5. Take up to one-half cup three times each day.

ARTHRITIS

Rheumatoid arthritis and osteoarthritis are the two kinds of arthritis. Antibodies produced by the immune system assault the joints and soft tissues, producing inflammation, discomfort, and slow degeneration of the joint. RA can be a devastating disorder, especially in young children.

In addition to the herbs listed below, other useful herbs for arthritis include bilberry, black currant, nettle, and vervain.

The medications listed below are beneficial for both osteoarthritis and rheumatoid arthritis.

1. Nightly Arthritis Tea

- 1 teaspoon black cohosh root
- 1 teaspoon chamomile flowers
- 1 teaspoon cascara sagrada bark
- 2 cups of water

1. Steep 1-1/2 tablespoons of the mixture in one cup hot water for 10 minutes before straining..
2. Take one cup in the evening, right before bed.

2. Quick Analgesic Arthritis Tea

- 25 drops black cohosh tincture
- 90 drops wild cherry bark tincture
- 90 drops mullein tincture
- 1 cup warm water

1. Take a third of the mixture three times each day.

3. Arthritis Milding Tea

- 2 teaspoons devil's claw tuber
- 3 teaspoons white willow bark
- 1 teaspoon feverfew herb
- 2 teaspoons yucca root
- 2 teaspoons sarsaparilla root
- 3 cups cold water

1. Stir Together the spices in a container of glass and cover them with water.
2. Allow to Soak overnight.
3. Drain.
4. Take one-half cup three times each day.

4. Arthritis Ointment

- 1 pound petroleum jelly
- 1 tablespoon Canada balsam
- 2 tablespoons cayenne
- 2 tablespoons chamomile

1. In a double boiler, melt one pound of petroleum jelly.
2. Stir in the herbs and cook for 2 hours.
3. Remove from heat and strain through a cheesecloth, pressing the cloth to extract all of the liquid.
4. While the ointment is still warm, pour it into glass containers to chill.
5. As needed for arthritis pain, apply topically and massage until completely absorbed.

ASTHMA

If you've ever heard a child with asthma struggle for air, you'll never forget the wheezing sound or the dread you feel as their skin turns blue from a lack of oxygen.

The trachea and bronchial tubes become irritated with this condition. An asthma episode can last anywhere from a few minutes to a few days and, if severe, can be fatal.

For many people, there is no known cause of asthma; nevertheless, allergies to molds, pollen, or other allergens, as well as certain foods and medicines, can trigger asthma episodes. Cold, moist weather, inhaling dust, smoke, various irritants, and even illnesses can all exacerbate asthma. Unfortunately, asthma is on the rise in the country, maybe due to the problems caused by filthy air.

1. Quick-Acting Asthma Tea

- 1 teaspoon elecampane root
- 2 teaspoons horehound herb

- 1 teaspoon blue vervain leaves
- 2 cups water

1. Stir together the spices in a pan, then cover the mixture with water.
2. **Soothing Tea**

- 2 teaspoons powdered Indian root
- 2 teaspoons coarse echinacea root
- 2 teaspoons elecampane root

1. Allow to soak for several hours, then strain.
2. Take one-half cup two times each day.

BACK PAIN

Back pain is sometimes accompanied by pain that spreads down your leg. This is known as sciatica, and it indicates that pressure is being applied to the spinal cord's nerves. Back discomfort is frequently relieved by relaxing the back muscles.

1. Warming Compress
- 16 fluids ounces water
- ½ cup dried ginger
- ¼ cup Epsom salts

1. Mix together all of the ingredients. Bring to a boil, covered. Fill a hot water bottle in the meantime.
2. Soak a towel in hot tea, then place it in a dry place to cool until it is still hot but may be touched without getting burned.
3. Lie down and drape the moist cloth across your back. Cover the affected area with a dry cloth and place the hot water bottle on top. Make yourself at ease and leave it for 10 to 20 minutes. You should experience relaxation, warmth, and pain relief.
4. Repeat as many times as required.
   Tip: Have you have pain but no dried ginger? You can also use fresh ginger from the grocery store—sliced, diced, or grated.

2. Spine's Fine Tincture

These analgesic herbs soothe and relax the spasms that cause most back pain, whether acute or chronic, muscular or connective, and so on. If you have fresh goldenrod or ginger oil on hand, use it as a massage oil after using this solution topically.

Take 1 to 4 drops of wild lettuce tincture by mouth to help you sleep: this will also relieve pain.

- 1 fluid ounce tincture of Solomon's seal

- 1 fluid ounce tincture of ginger
- ½ fluid ounce mixture of goldenrod
- ½ fluid ounce remedy of meadowsweet
- ½ fluid ounce tincture of mullein root
- ½ fluid ounce tincture of St. John's wort

1. Str together the tinctures in a small bottle, then Seal and label it.
2. Take 1 to 4 drops by mouth 3 to 5 times daily.
3. Also, place 1 to 4 drops in your palm and rub them into your back muscles.

Tip: Increase the amount of mullein root to 1 fluid ounce if your spinal discs are painful or worn away. It strongly supports these issues. If you have sciatica or other radiating nerve pain, you should also take St. John's wort. It regenerates nerve tissue that has been injured.

3. Analgesic Daily Tea For Back Pain
- 1 teaspoon coltsfoot leaf
- 2 teaspoons St. John's wort leaves
- 2 cups boiling water

1. Mix together the herbs in a glass container and cover with boiling water.
2. Allow to steep for 15 to30 minutes, then strain.
3. Take daily, twice: one-half cup in the morning and one-half cup at night.

4. Sciatic Pain Tea
- 2 teaspoons crampbark
- 2 teaspoons kava gout root

2. Cook for 30 minutes on low heat.
3. Allow to cool and strain.
4. Take up to one cup daily.

BITES AND STINGS

Although we call it a "bite," most insects and other critters pierce the skin rather than bite. The substance left in the wound by the animal, rather than the injury itself, frequently causes the damage.

Native Americans have been utilizing plants to treat snakebites for thousands of years. Echinacea and Seneca snakeroot are two of the most effective medicines for this illness.

Most bug bites, whether from mosquitos, fire ants, or black flies, are straightforward: the goal is to reduce inflammation.

Bee and wasp stings are more painful: in this situation, we must first extract the venom, if possible, to minimize inflammation and assist the immune system in dealing with the poison injected into the body. Keep an eye out for anaphylaxis! If someone has been stung or bitten and is having trouble breathing, get aid right once.

You could be allergic to the sting and require immediate medical assistance. Needless to say, if you are stung by a rattlesnake or any dangerous snake, get medical attention immediately.

1. Bug Bite Relief Spray

Makes eight fluid ounces

If you frequently travel through clouds of mosquitoes or black flies or live in a chigger-infested area, keep this cooling, itch-relieving spray on hand for when you come inside.

a. 4 fluids ounces nonalcoholic witch hazel extract or apple cider vinegar
b. 2 fluids ounces' tincture of rose
c. 1 fluid ounce tincture of self-heal
d. 1 fluid ounce tincture of yarrow

1. Mix all the Ingredients in a bottle with a fine-mist sprayer top. Cap and label the bottle.
2. Spray wherever you've been bitten.

2. Cooling Compresses

The menthol in peppermint provides a soothing sensation to the skin while also boosting blood circulation and dispersing irritants from the bite or sting location..

- 16 fluid ounces of water
- ½ cup dried peppermint leaf
- ¼ cup Epsom salts

1. Mix all the **Ingredients**. Cover and bring to a boil., then emove from the heat.
2. Apply the cloth to the bite or sting.

3. Bites and Stings Topical Wash

1 cup boiling water, 2 teaspoons comfrey leaves, 2 tablespoons marshmallow leaves, 1 tablespoon dried yarrow

BREATH

According to the EPA, humans take between 17,280 and 23,040 breaths daily. We want each of them to smell good.

Common Causes of Bad Breath:

- Gingivitis: This main source of stinky breath occurs due to plaque collection and tooth decay between the teeth.
- When your halitosis is accompanied by deep purple gums, inflammation, bleeding, and painful brushing, you need specialized dental treatment and natural medicines.
- Cavities: Anaerobic bacteria can colonize a cavity over time. These microorganisms emit a bad odor in the mouth. This frequently involves a doctor, and if ignored, it can develop into a potentially fatal infection.
- Dry Mouth: Stinky breath can arise from a variety of causes, including dry mouth. Your mouth will dry out if you snore, breathe with an open mouth, speak a lot, and so on.

Lemon Balm

Make a leaf decoction and swish it around.

Ginger Mango

Prepare the decoction rhizomes. Gargle with it twice a day.

Dill

Chew half a tablespoon of the seeds of Dill. Or:

Make a tea with Dill leaves and drink twice.

Cubeb

Take a somewhat wet glass of water. Pour in five drops of Cubeb oil. Swish it around two or three times per day. Make the Cubeb infusion instead. Swish it around.

Guava (Amrood)

Have a leaf decoction prepared, then swish with it.

Further Recipes

1. Chop the parsley leaves. You're putting four cloves in water. Simmer. Use it as a mouthwash.
2. Combine one teaspoon Carom (Ajwain) and four teaspoons Laung. In a cup, bring the water to a boil. Cool. Swish this water twice a day.
3. In the morning, gargle with 1 teaspoon of Dalchini powder.
4. As a combination, use Solanum Xanthocarpum and some Vinegar.
5. Combine 1-2 tbsp. Vinegar in 1/4 cup Solanum Xanthocarpum juice. Use as a mouthwash twice a day. Combine a few Asafoetida pieces with 2-3 cloves in half a water bowl. We are only leaving it overnight. Gargle with this water to avoid foul breath.

BRONCHITIS

A fever, strong coughing, thick sputum, trouble breathing, chills, and a sore throat may accompany bronchitis. Bronchitis is typically caused by an infection, although it can also occur due to inhaling dust, smoke, or other irritants.

Don't conceal your cough if you have a lung infection—it's a necessary bodily response!

We aim to cough productively so that all infectious or irritating material is removed as you cough up all the phlegm and to prevent unproductive coughing. If you can't cough out the phlegm, a simple cough may become pneumonia due to mucus buildup (Seek medical attention if you have true pneumonia. Meanwhile, take garlic and elecampane - these are your most powerful buddies against this problem.)

1. Fire Cider

It makes about 1 quart

Traditional fire cider recipes are concoctions of spicy and aromatic stimulating expectorants that will warm you and aid in removing junk. We slip in several immunity boosters and a rich source of vitamin C in this version. If you are currently on pharmaceutical blood thinners, do not take this.

- 1 whole head garlic, cloves peeled and chopped
- 1 (2-inch) piece fresh ginger, chopped
- ¼ cup dried pine needles
- ¼ cup dried sage leaf
- ¼ cup dried thyme leaf
- ¼ cup dried elderberry
- ¼ cup dried rose hips
- 2 tablespoons dried elecampane root
- 2 tablespoons dried angelica root
- 1-quart apple cider vinegar
- Honey or water, for sweetening or diluting

1. Combine the garlic, ginger, and other herbs in a mixing bowl.
2. Pour the vinegar into the pot. Before screwing down the ring, place a wax paper sheet under the jar cover (When exposed to vinegar, the coating on the bottom of the metal mason jar lids corrodes).
3. Allow the herbs to macerate in the vinegar for at least two weeks.
4. Strain the final fire cider, bottle and label it. If the vinegar is excessively powerful and troubles your stomach, dilute it with honey (up to one-fourth of the entire volume) or water.
5. Give yourself a shot (approximately 12 fluid ounces) at the first sign of mucus buildup in the lungs, and then every couple of hours until the symptoms disappear.

2. Bronchitis Tea #3
- 1 teaspoon elecampane root
- 2 tablespoons nettle leaves
- 1 cup boiling water
1. Mix the above herbs.
2. Strain.
3. Sweeten with honey, if you like.
4. Take up to two cups daily.

3. Sweet Soothing Tea
- 1 teaspoon marshmallow leaves or flowers
- 1 teaspoon coltsfoot leaves
- 1 teaspoon mullein leaves and flowers
- ½ cup boiling water, Honey

Mix all the herbs listed above; steep one teaspoon of the mixture in the boiling water and strain.Sweeten with honey. Take one-half hot cup, three or four times daily.

4. Bronchitis Tea #4
- 1 to 2 slices of fresh ginger root
- 1 teaspoon pearly everlasting flowers or leaves
- 1 teaspoon redroot
- 1 cup boiling water

Stir together all the herbs; steep in the boiling water for 30 thirty minutes, then strain. Take one-half cup of tea three times each day.

BURNS AND SUNBURNS

A burn is a tissue or skin injury caused by fire (or another form of heat), electricity, chemicals, or radiation. A first-degree burn causes the skin to get red and swell, but it does not blister. Complete healing without scars occurs in a matter of days.

A second-degree burn causes substantially more severe damage. The skin turns bright red and blisters, yet it cures without leaving scars.

The third-degree burn penetrates the skin, killing both the epidermis and the dermis. Scar tissue can occur as a result of a third-degree burn. Burn tissue can become necrotic and cause a severe infection. Skin suppleness can be lost. Internal burns can also develop from swallowing scalding liquids or inhaling hot air. A severe burn can result in potentially fatal systemic damage such as respiratory tract injury, infection, and shock. Anyone suffering from a serious burn should seek medical assistance immediately to avoid these possibly fatal consequences. On the other hand, herbs can help ease the discomfort of a mild burn and promote faster recovery.

Run cold water over the affected area immediately after a burn—the skin holds heat for far longer than you might believe (If blisters form in the burned region, be very gentle with them and avoid breaking them before they naturally peel off, if possible.) Then, gently clean your wound, eliminating any dirt or pollutant. Apply the herbs, combining antiseptics to prevent infection with cooling, wound-healing herbs to induce tissue regeneration.

Use any herbal composts as a wash, compress, poultice, or infused honey on burns; avoid using oily solutions because they trap heat in the tissue.

Never underestimate the therapeutic properties of a marshmallow root poultice! Soak a handful of marshmallow root in cold water until it becomes a gloopy mass and apply it to the burn. Repeat as needed.

1. Burn Poultice
- 1 tablespoon dried coneflower flower
- 1 tablespoon dried hyssop flowers
- 1 tablespoon dried goldenrod flowers
- 1 tablespoon dried sunflower petals

1. Stir together all the **Ingredients**, moisten with boiling water, and place between two cheesecloth layers; let cool and then apply the mixture to the affected area.
2. Remoisten once dry. Use when in need.

2. Immunity Strengthener
- 30 drops echinacea tincture
- 20 drops wild indigo root tincture
- 1 cup warm water

1. Mix all the above herbs in warm water.
2. Take up to five times daily.

A burn can weaken your body, making you more susceptible to sickness and infection. Use this tea to boost your immune system.

3. Burn-Healing Honey

It yields about 1 pint

Honey is by far the most effective burn-healing agent. Even if all you have is raw honey, you're still in good hands. It's even better if you infuse it with these medicinal herbs beforehand.

- ½ cup fresh calendula flower
- ½ cup fresh rose petals
- 1-pint honey, gently warmed

1. Fill a pint-size mason jar halfway with calendula and rose petals.

2. Fill the pot halfway with heated honey, set it aside in a warm location, and leave it to infuse for one month.

3. Gently reheat the lidded pot in a double boiler until the honey is liquefied. Press the marc against the sieve to extract as much honey as possible from the infused honey.

4. Apply a layer of the infused honey to a burn site after heating the honey and washing it. Cover lightly with a gauze bandage. Apply the solution at least twice a day.

4. Sunburn Cream

A few spritzes will start to cool the skin and relieve inflammation.

- 1 tablespoon dried peppermint leaf
- 1 tablespoon dried self-heal leaf and flower
- 1 tablespoon dried plantain leaf
- 1 tablespoon dried linden leaf and flower
- 4 fluid ounces rose water
- 1-quart boiling water.

1. Make a hot infusion by combining peppermint, self-heal, plantain, and linden in a mason jar.

2. Place the container in the refrigerator to cool.

3. Strain four fluid ounces of the infusion into an 8-ounce bottle fitted with a fine-mist sprayer tip. Use the remainder of the input to make compresses or a cooling drink. It will keep in the fridge for three days.

4. Fill the spray bottle halfway with rose water. Close and label the bottle.

5. Use liberally and frequently. When finished, store the spray in the refrigerator.

CANKER SORES

Canker sores are small sores that commonly appear on the lining of the mouth, but they can also appear on the lips, tongue, or neck. Aphthous ulcers, which can be white or yellow, are bordered by red, inflamed tissue. These tiny ulcers, which are accompanied by fever and enlarged lymph glands, can be excruciating for several days. Canker sores can also be caused by injuries (such as particular dental procedures).

SORES FROM THE COLD

The herpes simplex virus causes cold sores, which are tiny, painful, fluid-filled blisters on the lips. Tingling, tingling, and burning sensations may indicate that a cold sore is going to emerge. Blisters may occur hours or days after the first warning symptoms. They ultimately dry and create a crust after a few days. They normally heal entirely in a week or two.

1. Cold Sore Tea
- 1 teaspoon burdock root
- 1 teaspoon dried and powdered goldenseal root
- 1 cup boiling water
- Honey, to taste

1. Mix all the ingredients in a glass container
2. Steep for 30 minutes, calm and then strain.

3. Sweeten with honey, if you like.
4. Take up to one cup daily.

2. Cold Sore Mouthwash
- 1 teaspoon echinacea root
- 1 teaspoon yerba mansa root
- 1 tablespoon white oak bark
- 1 cup boiling water

1. Stir together the above herbs in a glass container.
2. Steep 30 minutes, calm and strain. Use the solution as a wash to treat cold sores.

3. Cold Sore Compress

Makes 5 cups dried herb mixture

- 1 cup dried calendula flower
- 1 cup dried plantain leaf
- 1 cup dried chamomile flower, dried self-heal leaf, and flower
- ½ cup dried St. John's wort leaf and flower

1. Combine all the herbs.
2. Store in an airtight container.
3. Apply the moist towel over the affected area. Place a dry cloth on top and place the hot water bottle on top. Allow it to soak in for 10 to 20 minutes.
4. Repeat 2 to 3 times daily.

4. Cold Sore Balm

Makes 5 ounces

- 1 fluid ounce calendula-infused oil
- 1 fluid ounce plantain-infused oil
- ½ fluid ounce self-heal–infused oil
- ½ fluid ounce chamomile-infused oil
- ½ fluid ounce St. John's wort–infused oil
- ½ fluid ounce thyme-infused oil
- 1-ounce beeswax, plus more as needed

1. As usual, make a salve. If you're going to store it in little jars, make it soft; if you're going to use lip balm tubes, make it slightly harder.

CONSTIPATION

Constipation, formerly known as "costiveness," refers to any irregularity or absence of bowel movements. Most people have one action each day, however some people can go two days or more without constipation. However, the longer waste products remain in the colon, the more water is absorbed, and the waste becomes drier and more compact.

Constipation can be caused by a variety of conditions, including thyroid issues, circulatory difficulties, and intestinal problems.

1. Infusion for Bowel Hydration

Makes 2½ cups dried herb mix

- 1 cup dried linden leaf and flower
- ¼ cup dried cinnamon bark
- 1 cup dried marshmallow root
- ¼ cup dried licorice root
1. Combine all herbs. Keep it in an airtight container.
2. Prepare a cold infusion. Pour in cold or room temperature water and set aside for 4 to 8 hours before straining.

2. Bowel-Stimulating Tincture

Bitters and carminatives stimulate bile flow and intestinal peristalsis, causing the bowels to move.

- 1-½ fluid ounces tincture of dandelion root
- 1-½ fluid ounces tincture of St. John's wort
- ½ fluid ounce mixture of angelica root
- ½ fluid ounce medicine of ginger
1. Combine the tinctures in a small bottle. Cap and label the bottle.
2. Take 2 to 4 drops every 20 minutes until you feel better.

3. Purifying Digestive Tea

- 2 teaspoons cascara sagrada

- 3 to 4 slices ginger root
- 1 teaspoon cayenne
- 1 teaspoon Oregon grape root

- 2 cups boiling water

Take up to two cups each day, one tablespoon at a time.

COUGH AND COLD

Watery eyes, a runny or stuffy nose (rhinitis), head congestion (with a mild, moderate, or severe headache), lethargy, sneezing, and coughing are all common cold symptoms. Malaise is a broad throbbing feeling of discomfort and listlessness. As the cold progresses, you may get mild to severe sore throat. Any or all of these symptoms could exist.

To use herbs effectively, we must first distinguish between a hot, dry, and unpleasant cough and a wet, cold, and ineffective one. When your lungs are dry, you will have a frustrating, never-ending cough; we employ moistening herbs to help with this. Wet lungs are most usually a reaction to infection.

1. Cough Syrup
- 2 teaspoons coltsfoot leaves
- 1 tablespoon wild plum root
- 2 teaspoons mullein leaves
- 2 cups boiling water
- 1 pound honey
1. Combine the above herbs in a pot of boiling water, soak them for 30 minutes, and filter them into nonmetallic containers.
2. Heat and stir in one pound of honey until it is dissolved; cool and store in a glass container.

2. Lung-Lubricating Tea

Yields 2¾ cups dried herb mix

- 1 cup dried marshmallow root
- ½ cup fennel seed
- 1 cup dried mullein leaf
- Honey (optional)
- ¼ cup dried licorice root, or to taste

1. Combine all of the herbs in an airtight jar.

2. Make a cold infusion by adding cold or room temperature water and leaving it to steep for 4 to 8 hours.

3. Strain the liquid and serve immediately, or warm if preferred.

4. If used, add honey for added soothing.

3. Soothing Cough And Cold Formula
- 30 drops echinacea tincture
- 20 drops wild indigo root tincture
- 2 cups white cedar leaf tips tea
1. Combine the above-mentioned ingredients and take half a cup at a time, hot.
2. Use up to three times per day.

4. Lakota Cough And Cold Formula
- 1 teaspoon goldenseal root
- 1 teaspoon mullein leaves
- 1 teaspoon osha root
- 1 teaspoon pleurisy root
- 1 teaspoon yerba mansa root
- 2 teaspoons yerba sante leaves
- 2 cups boiling water
1. Combine the above herbs and cover with boiling water; soak for 30 minutes, then cool and drain.
2. As needed, take two teaspoons at a time, up to two cups each day.

5. Antitussive Oxymel

It yields approximately 1 quart (20 to 60 doses).

An oxymel is a vinegar and honey mixture that combines honey's moistening and soothing properties with the astringent and stimulating properties of vinegar. The addition of lung-specific herbs makes this popular for all types of coughs.

- 1/3 cup dried sage leaf
- 1/3 cup dried pine needles
- 1/3 cup dried thyme leaf
- ¼ cup dried ginger
- 1-quart apple cider vinegar
- Honey, as needed for topping off the jar

1. Fill the jar four-fifths of the way with vinegar; top with honey.
2. Cover the saucepan and set aside for four weeks to macerate.
3. Strain and store the oxymel in a bottle. Cap and label the bottle.
4. As needed, take 1 to 3 tablespoons.

6. Lumbee Cough And Cold Formula

- 3 teaspoons goldenrod leaves
- 4 teaspoons horehound leaves
- 2 teaspoons white pine inner bark
- 4 cups boiling water

1. Wrap the herbs in cheesecloth and tie them with a string.
2. Place the bag in the boiling water for 15 minutes and cool before removing the bundle.
3. As needed, take half a cup of the heated mixture at a time, up to two cups each day.

7. Quick-Acting Cough And Cold Formula

- 4 teaspoons agrimony leaves
- 2 teaspoons mullein leaves
- 2 teaspoons blue vervain leaves
- 1 teaspoon oxeye daisy
- 3 teaspoons horehound leaves
- 2 teaspoons speedwell
- 2 cups boiling water

8. Decongestant Tea

- 2 slices fresh ginger
- 2 teaspoons pleurisy root
- 1 cup boiling water

1. Place the herbs in a glass container and steep for 30 minutes before calming and straining.
2. Start with a tablespoon and work up to two cups daily. This tea is beneficial for bronchial congestion.

9. Quick-Acting Mullein Cough Syrup

- 1 cup of mullein tea
- 1 pound honey

1. Heat the honey until it is liquid.
2. Remove from the fire, allow to cool, and pour into a glass container. As needed, take a spoonful at a time.

10. Expectorating Cough And Cold Tea

- 2 teaspoons boneset herb
- 2 teaspoons licorice root
- 2 to 3 slices ginger root
- 2 teaspoons wild cherry bark
- 2 cups boiling water

11. Horehound Lozenges

- 1-½ cups horehound leaves
- 1-½ cups water
- 3 cups sugar three tablespoons corn syrup.

Fill a pan halfway with water and add the horehound leaves.

FATIGUE

Fatigue is more than just tiredness. Instead, weariness is defined as a protracted or extreme decline in one's ability to operate, over and beyond what would be caused by regular activity. Fatigue is familiar to those who push themselves to the brink of physical weariness. Fatigue, on the other hand, can be a symptom of more than just overexertion. It can be a symptom of anemia, circulatory problems (such as angina pectoris, atherosclerosis, and high blood pressure), chronic fatigue syndrome, diabetes, hepatitis, inflammatory bowel disease, multiple sclerosis, and respiratory conditions such as pneumonia and pleurisy.

Fatigue is an indication that something is interfering with healing. Most of the time, it's only a result of a lack of sleep (it has been scientifically shown that healthy adults require 8 to 10 hours of sleep every night — and most Americans only get six during the week and eight during the weekend!). Even if a good night's sleep does not immediately cure your exhaustion, it is still crucial to prioritize your sleep, a factor - with other ones as malnutrition, chronic sickness, stress, pharmaceutical side effects, and so on - that is vital.

In contrast to tiredness, we should not underestimate the value of movement in generating energy. If you cultivate it carefully and persistently, a little motion can expand into more tremendous dynamic energy, and Tai chi and qigong are good methods for accomplishing this.

1. Up-And-About Morsels

It takes about 24 pieces

These tasty, refreshing treats are an excellent way to get a substantial dose of beneficial herbs. This format is handy because it provides the full complement of plant compounds instead of just water-soluble or alcohol soluble, as happens with a tea or tincture.

- ¼ cup powdered ashwagandha root
- ¼ cup powdered tulsi leaf
- ¼ cup crushed milk thistle seed
- ¼ cup powdered nettle leaf
- 3 tablespoons powdered licorice root
- ¾ cup nut butter
- ½ cup honey

For coating, use unsweetened shredded coconut, cocoa powder, powdered cinnamon, powdered ginger, cayenne pepper, or whatever tastes good to you.

1. Combine the powders.
2. Stir in the nut butter and honey. Stir together to make a thick "dough."
3. Roll the balls in your preferred coating.
4. Consume 1 to 4 per day.

2. Shake-It-Off Formula

Makes three fluid ounces (45 to 90 doses)

- 1 fluid ounce tincture of licorice
- 1 fluid ounce tincture of ashwagandha
- 1 fluid ounce tincture of tulsi

1. Combine the tinctures in a small bottle. Cap and label the bottle.

2. Feel free to take extra doses whenever you need a pick-me-up.

3. Invigorating Tea
- 1 teaspoon blackberry leaf
- 1 teaspoon strawberry leaves
- 1 teaspoon raspberry leaves
- 2 cups boiling water, Honey
a. Cover with boiling water and steep for 10 minutes before straining.
b. 2. If desired, sweeten with honey. Drink only as needed.

4. Pick-Me-Up Tea

One teaspoon Ginkgo biloba leaves, one teaspoon dried mirabilis root, one teaspoon dried ginseng root, one teaspoon pulsatilla herb, one teaspoon gotu kola leaves, one teaspoon of St. John's wort leaves.

FEVER

Fever is your ally: It's a critical immunological reaction, and herbalists aren't the only ones who believe it! Please don't succumb to fever phobia; instead, assist your body in doing its job.

Keep hydrated! Almost all serious complications connected with fever are caused by dehydration rather than the fever itself. Sitting in a warm bath is a wonderful rehydration technique if someone cannot keep water down.

1. Fever Relief Tea

- One teaspoon angelica root
- 1 teaspoon ground ivy leaves
- 1 teaspoon barberry berries
- 2 teaspoons peppermint leaves
- 2 teaspoons blue vervain leaves
- 1 tablespoon dried yarrow
- 1 teaspoon catnip leaves
- 1 cup boiling water

1. Combine the herbs listed above.

2. Put one tablespoon of the mixture in a cup and soak for 30 minutes before straining.

2. Fever-Inducing Tea

Makes 3 cups dried herb mix (enough for 18 to 24 quarts of tea)

- 1 cup dried tulsi leaf
- ½ cup dried sage leaf
- ½ cup dried thyme leaf
- ½ cup dried yarrow leaf and flower
- ¼ cup dried angelica root
- ¼ cup dried ginger, one garlic clove, sliced, for a real kick (optional)

1. Combine all of the herbs. Keep it in an airtight container.

2. Stir in the garlic (if using).

3. For the greatest results, reheat before drinking and consume very hot.

3. Fever-Breaking Tea

Makes 1¾ cups dried herb mix (enough for 14 to 24 pints of tea)

- ½ cup dried catnip leaf and flower
- ½ cup dried elderflower
- ½ cup dried peppermint leaf
- ¼ cup dried wild lettuce leaf and stalk
- 1 pint boiling water

1. Combine all of the herbs. Keep it in an airtight container.

2. Make a hot infusion by putting 1 to 2 tablespoons of herbs in a pint-size mason jar. Drink this tea with a little more ease than normal.

3. Drink a mugful when you're feeling under the weather.

FOOD INTOLERANCES

Food allergies are common and range from moderate to life-threateningly severe. They cause various gastrointestinal issues, including heartburn, IBS, bloating, and others, and contribute to systemic inflammation, neurological issues, and autoimmune.

Gluten, dairy, soy, maize, eggs, and nightshades (potatoes, tomatoes, peppers, eggplant, and so on) are all major culprits that we believe everyone should test for regularly.

1. Gut-Heal Tea

This digestive herb mix contains all the functions required to restore a healthy stomach, intestines, and liver function. It is the single most frequently prescribed formula in our business and is highly customizable individually.

- ½ cup dried calendula flower
- ½ cup dried plantain leaf
- ½ cup dried chamomile flower
- ½ cup dried tulsi leaf
- ½ cup dried marshmallow leaf
- ¼ cup dried ginger
- ¼ cup dried licorice root
- ¼ cup dried yarrow leaf and flower
- ¼ cup dried St. John's wort leaf and flower

1. Combine all of the herbs. Keep it in an airtight container.

2. Quick-Acting Flatulence Tea

- 1 teaspoon catnip leaf
- 1 teaspoon grated ginger root
- 2 teaspoons dandelion leaves
- 2 cups boiling water

1. Cover the herbs with boiling water and steep for 20 to 30 minutes before straining.

2. Take just as needed.

3. Build-Up Broth

It takes about 3 quarts

The amino acids in these components aid in restoring intestinal integrity, which has been compromised by the food allergy reaction. The addition of herbs boosts these anti-inflammatory and healing properties. If your intestines are very disturbed, skip solid food for a day and consume only broth!

Another incentive to start drinking bone broth: broth derived from bones that still have collagenous tissue attached is high in chondroitin and glucosamine. The body uses these nutrients to construct connective tissues and maintain healthy joints. You can buy glucosamine and chondroitin pills, but bone broth is a far cheaper option with many more benefits!

- 1 cup dried calendula flower
- ¼ cup dried dandelion root
- ¼ cup fennel seed
- ¼ cup dried ginger
- ¼ cup dried kelp
- Bones (such as from 1 rotisserie chicken; 6 pork chop bones; 1 lamb or beef shank; orthe bones, head, and tail from 2 medium fish—really, any bones will do)
- 3 quarts water, plus more as needed
- 1 tablespoon apple cider vinegar
- Oyster, shiitake, or maitake mushrooms, for their nutritional and healing properties
- Salt
- Freshly ground black pepper

1. Combine the bones, water, herbs, vinegar, and mushrooms (optional) in a large pot over high heat and season with salt and pepper. Bring the water to a boil, and continue to boil for 4 to 8 hours. Check frequently and refill any water that has burnt away.

2. Reserve the liquid after straining it. If desired, compost the bones and herb marc.

3. Drink a cup of heated broth two to three times per day

4. Colon-Soothing Tea

- 2 teaspoons bee balm leaves
- 2 teaspoons peppermint leaves
- 2 teaspoons chamomile flowers

- 1 cup boiling water

1. In a container, combine the herbs.

HANGOVER

Milk thistle capsules are the most effective and simple hangover treatment.

You might not have a hangover at all if you do this!

1. Take-It-Easy Next Day Infusion

Yields about 3¼ cups dried herb mix (enough for 20 to 28 quarts of tea)

This mild tea relieves fundamental hangover symptoms and aids in rehydrating the body. It's best to make it ahead of time so it's ready when you need it. Drink a quart or more throughout the day, slowly.

- ½ cup dried chamomile flower
- Self-heal leaf and flower
- 1 tablespoon dried licorice root
- 1 tablespoon dried ginger
- ¼ cup dried St. John's wort leaf and flower

1. Combine all of the herbs. Keep it in an airtight container.

2. No-Fuss Hangover Tea
- 1 teaspoon ripe barberry berry
- 2 cups boiling water
- 1 teaspoon Oregon grape root
1. In a nonmetallic jar, combine the herbs and cover with boiling water; soak for 30 minutes, then cool and filter.

2. Take up to one cup daily, diluted with plenty of lukewarm water

3. Quick-Acting Hangover Tea
- 1 teaspoon bayberry root
- 1 teaspoon dried goldenseal root
- 2 cups boiling water
- 1 teaspoon Oregon grape root
1. In a nonmetallic jar, combine the herbs and cover with boiling water; steep for 30 minutes; strain.
2. Throughout the day, drink several glasses of water

4. Spicy Hangover Tea
- 1 teaspoon catnip leaf
- 1 teaspoon peppermint leaves
- 2 cups boiling water
- 1 teaspoon dried chaparral leaves
1. In a nonmetallic pot, combine the herbs and cover with boiling water; soak for 20 to 30 minutes before rinsing.
2. Drink up to two cups daily, half a cup at a time

HEADACHE

Headaches are common and can range from dull and steady to stabbing, gnawing, or throbbing. There are numerous types of headaches, each with its own set of causes. A headache can be caused by tension, weariness, or stress. Allergies, traumas, infections, tumors, and numerous disorders can cause headaches in the eyes, ears, nose, throat, or teeth. Headaches are another major business; most people use NSAIDs like aspirin, ibuprofen, or indomethacin, or even stronger medications. However, these medications have unfavorable and often severe side effects, such as ulcers and an increased tendency to bleed. Herbs may provide a safer alternative.

Headaches are caused by a variety of imbalances. Some are one-time events, such as dehydration, sleep deprivation, dietary excesses, alcohol, caffeine, and pharmaceuticals. For individuals who require immediate pain relief while supplying what is lacking or just waiting for the body to heal.

Long-term treatment requires identifying your triggers as well as the underlying patterns that contribute to your pain; this requires some trial and error. The herbal medicines listed below are intended to treat the most common forms of headaches we experience, but experiment with different combinations of herbs to refine the prescription and make it as personalized as possible. If you experience recurring headaches and discover that this helps, drink a quart or more daily as a preventive measure.

1. Peppery Headache Tea

- 1 teaspoon feverfew leaf
- 1 teaspoon peppermint leaves
- 1 cup boiling water
- Honey
1. In a nonmetallic jar, combine the above herbs, then cover with boiling water and soak for 30 minutes before straining.
2. To taste, add honey. Take one tablespoon to one cup every day.

2. Soothing Headache Tea

- 1 teaspoon catnip leaf
- 2 teaspoons feverfew leaves
- 1 to 2 cups boiling water
1. In a glass jar, combine the catnip and feverfew.
2. Steep for 30 minutes before straining.
3. A tablespoon at a time, up to one cup daily.

3. Cooling Headache Tea

This is the ideal cure for you if your headache pain is acute, hot, and very sensitive to touch. Tension, nasal congestion, stress or anxiety, or direct nerve pain are all common causes of this type of headache. These herbs can soothe, relax, and drain you (be cautious that the wild lettuce may make you asleep).

- 1 cup dried betony leaf and flower
- ½ cup dried linden leaf and flower
- 1 cup dried meadowsweet flower
- ¼ cup dried wild lettuce leaf and stalk
- ½ cup dried marshmallow leaf

1. Combine all of the herbs. Keep it in an airtight container. Drink hot or cold. A cup of this tea should provide some relief.

4. Warming Headache Tea

If you experience headaches, a pale complexion, and the pain feels chilly, dull, and broad, you should try this blend. These herbs warm, astringe gently, and enhance circulation; if caffeine is normally your go-to headache remedy, try this. If you get frequent headaches and find this helps, drink a quart or more daily as a preventive.

- 1 cup dried betony leaf and flower
- ½ cup dried chamomile flower
- 1 cup dried tulsi leaf
- ¼ cup dried ginger
- ½ cup dried sage leaf

1. Combine all of the herbs. Keep it in an airtight container. Warm to hot to drink, and a cup of this tea should provide some relief.

HYPERTENSION

High blood pressure is normal on sometimes; it is a natural response to stressful events. High blood pressure, however, can induce or worsen other cardiovascular diseases over time. Herbs have many effects that can help reduce high blood pressure, generally by addressing the underlying causes rather than just treating the symptoms.

It's worth noting that high blood pressure isn't always insufficient: new research suggests that hypertension developed in the elderly may assist in lessening the incidence of dementia.

1. Anti-Congestive Tea

- 2 teaspoons black cohosh root
- 2 cups boiling water
- 4 teaspoons ginkgo Biloba leaves
1. In a nonmetallic vessel, combine the herbs above, then pour the boiling water over them. Immerse for 30 minutes, then calmly strain.
2. Take two to three teaspoons at a time up to six times per day

2. Arteriosclerosis Preventive Tea

- 2 to 3 ginger slices
- 2 teaspoons Ginkgo biloba leaves
- 4 teaspoon ginseng leaves Take up to half a cup daily.

3. Softhearted Tea

Makes 2 cups dried herb mix (enough for 12 to 16 quarts of tea)

Stress reduction makes a significant difference in your life, thus herbs that can both calm the heart and rest the mind are perfect. If you have an extremely dry constitution, prepare this as a cold infusion instead. Every day, drink a quart or more of water.

- 1 cup dried linden leaf and flower
- ½ cup dried rose petals
- ½ cup dried marshmallow leaf.
1. Combine all of the herbs. Keep it in an airtight containe.

4. Free-Flowing Circulation Tea

- 1 teaspoon burdock root
- 1 teaspoon goldenseal root
- 1 teaspoon cayenne
- 2 teaspoons slippery elm bark
- 3 cups boiling water
- 2 slices of ginger root
1. In a nonmetallic bowl, combine the above herbs and filter.
2. Take 2 tablespoons at a time, up to 1 cup
3. daily.

INDIGESTION/DYSPEPSIA

Indigestion is defined as any gastrointestinal problem, such as a stomachache. Indigestion can occur if you eat too quickly, overeat, eat while emotionally agitated, or eat the wrong meals. Caffeine, high-fiber foods, alcohol, and carbonated drinks are frequently blamed for indigestion. Allergies can sometimes cause dyspepsia. Indigestion can be a synptom of various disorders, including pancreatitis, ulcers, gastritis, and cholecystitis. However, dyspepsia is frequently undiagnosed.

Whether you have chronic digestive problems, evaluate your diet to discover whether you are allergic to any foods. However, herbs provide a quick cure for indigestion—read on for two simple, portable alternatives.

1. Digestive Tea
- 1 teaspoon blue cohosh root
- 1 cup boiling water
- 1 teaspoon coneflower root
1. In a glass jar, combine the herbs.
2. Steep for 30 minutes before cooling and straining.
3. Consume up to one cup every day as needed.

2. Strong Digestive Tea
- 1 teaspoon angelica root
- 1 teaspoon grated ginger root
- 2 teaspoons chamomile flowers
- 2 teaspoons peppermint leaves
- 1 cup boiling water
1. In a vessel, combine the ingredients listed above.
2. Place one tablespoon of the herb mixture in a cup of boiling water; steep for 30 minutes; cool and drain.
3. Take up to two cups each day as needed.

3. Pre-Emptive Bitter Tincture

Indigestion is frequently caused by inadequate digestion. This solution stimulates all of your digestive fluids—saliva, stomach acid, bile, and pancreatic enzymes—to ensure proper digestion.

- 1 fluid ounce tincture of dandelion root

- 1 fluid ounce tincture of catnip
- 1 fluid ounce tincture of sage
- 1 fluid ounce tincture of chamomile
1. Combine the tinctures in a small vial. Seal and label the bottle.
2. 10 minutes before meals, take 1 to 2 drops.

4. Carminative Tincture
This solution heats the center of your body, boosting your digestive organs and keeping you warm.

To keep your bowels from becoming sluggish, try angelica instead of peppermint.

- 1-½ fluid ounces tincture of ginger
- 1 fluid ounce tincture of peppermint
- 1 fluid ounce tincture of fennel
- ½ fluid ounce tincture of licorice
1. Combine the tinctures in a small vial. Seal and label the bottle.
2. 1 to 2 drops after each meal or whenever your stomach and intestines feel clogged

5. Quick-Acting Digestive Tea
- 1 teaspoon licorice root
- 2 cups boiling water
- 1 teaspoon peppermint leaves
1. In a nonmetallic jar, combine the herbs and cover with boiling water; steep for 15 to 20 minutes, then sieve.
2. Drink up to one cup every day as needed.

INSOMNIA

Insomnia is defined as any trouble sleeping. Nearly one-fourth of all Americans experience intermittent sleep problems, however certain people (up to 10% of the American population) have chronic insomnia. Insomnia can be caused by various factors, including stress and nervous tension, excessive caffeinated beverages, and inconsistent sleeping habits.

1. **Insomnia Relief Tea**
- One teaspoon chamomile flower
- one teaspoon hops, one teaspoon valerian root, 1 cup boiling water

1. Combine the herbs listed above.

2. Warm half a cup at a time as needed.

2. **Sweet Dreams Tea**
- 2 teaspoons catnip leaves
- 1 teaspoon hops
- 2 teaspoons chamomile flower
- 2 teaspoons passionflower

1. Take one hour before going to bed.

3. **End-Of-The-Day Elixir**
This combination of moderate sedatives and relaxants relieves the tension, anxiety, and distraction that make falling asleep difficult. This combination works best when taken in "pulse doses," which are far more effective than taking the entire amount shortly before bedtime. It allows the herbs to begin functioning in your system and signals the body that it is time to sleep.

- 1 fluid ounce tincture of chamomile
- 1 fluid ounce tincture of betony
- ½ fluid ounce tincture of catnip

- ¾ fluid ounce tincture of ashwagandha
- ¼ fluid ounce honey
- ½ fluid ounce tincture of linden
1. Combine the tinctures and honey in a small vial. Seal and label the bottle.
2. Take 1 or 2 drops one hour before going to bed.
3. Take 1 or 2 more drops 30 minutes before bedtime.
4. Take the final 1 - 2 drops before going to bed.

4. **Sleep Formula**

For this mixture, we use wild lettuce, one of the strongest hypnotic (sleep-inducing) herb. This is especially useful if physical pain keeps you awake at night, as wild lettuce has a pain-relieving effect. Like End-of-the-Day Elixir, this formula is best taken in "pulse doses".

- 2 fluid ounces tincture of wild lettuce
- 1 fluid ounce tincture of betony
- ½ fluid ounce tincture of linden
- ½ fluid ounce tincture of chamomile
1. Combine the tinctures in a small vial. Seal and label the bottle.
2. Take 1 or 2 drops one hour before going to bed.
3. Take 1 or 2 more drops 30 minutes before bedtime.
4. Take the final 1 - 2 drops before going to bed.

SINUSITIS/STUFFY NOSE

Sinusitis is a sinus infection characterized by sinus congestion, headache, and pain around the eyes or cheekbones. Sinus discharge, weariness, cough, fever, earache, and increased susceptibility to sinus infections are all possible symptoms.

Sinusitis can also be caused by nasal injury, a deviated septum (the separator between the two nasal passageways), a large conchae nasal polyp, or restricted sinuses, as well as cigarette smoke, dusty or dry air, or infected tonsils or teeth.

A runny nose is a necessary response to a cold or flu! Mucus, believe it or not, contains antibodies. Using prescription decongestants to dry it out makes the tissue more prone to infection. Maintaining a comfortable medium for mucous membranes—not too dry or drippy—helps shorten the sickness and prevent complications.

If the symptoms are not caused by a full respiratory infection or are chronic or recurring, they are most likely caused by a mix of bacterial, fungal, and viral components (this is why illness can persist even after numerous rounds of antibiotics). Antimicrobial herbs are less specific than antibiotic medications, which is a plus in this case because they can combat multiple diseases and weakened states at the same time.

It is beneficial to clear the sinuses by grating fresh horseradish and inhaling its fumes, or by eating prepared horseradish or wasabi.

1. Sinus-Clearing Steam Bath

Makes 2 cups dried herb mix (enough for 4 to 8 steams)

Steaming is a universal remedy throughout cultures for all respiratory system problems, including sinus problems. Combining heated steam and evaporating volatile oils from herbs makes pathogen survival extremely difficult and triggers an immune response in the mucous membranes.

- 1 cup dried pine needles
- ½ cup dried sage leaf
- ½ cup dried thyme leaf
- ½ gallon water

Five garlic cloves, chopped, per steam (optional)

1. Combine the pine, sage, and thyme in a bowl. Keep it in an airtight container.
2. To make and use herbal steam, boil the water in a medium pot over high heat.
3. Place the pot on a heat-resistant surface near where you can sit and construct a tent with a blanket or towel.
4. Add 14 to 12 cups of the herb mixture, along with the garlic (if using), to the water.
5. Bring a tissue since your nose will run as your sinuses clean!
6. Repeat two to three times per day.

Tip: Working with aromatic herbs such as incense or a smudge stick (a tightly wrapped bundle of leaves ignited on one end to produce medicinal smoke) can provide similar microbe-clearing advantages. A study published in the Journal of Ethnopharmacology by Nautiyal et al. discovered that "[when] using medicinal smoke [,] it is possible to eliminate different plant and human pathogenic bacteria of the air within confined space." Conifer trees, such as pine, are especially suited for this.

2. Mucus-Freeing Tea

- 1 teaspoon bayberry root
- 1 teaspoon white willow bark
- 2 cups boiling water
1. Combine the herbs listed above.

SPRAINS AND STRAINS

A sprain occurs when a ligament is excessively twisted, whereas a strain is caused by muscle fiber tearing and overstretching. The same injuries that create a sprain might also cause a piece. The distinction is that a sprain affects ligaments and tendons, whereas a strain affects muscles. Because of the discomfort and swelling make movement in the affected area is frequently restricted.

1. Soft Tissue Injury Liniment

It makes about eight fluid ounces

- 3 fluid ounces ginger-infused oil
- 2 fluid ounces Solomon's seal-infused oil or tincture of Solomon's seal
- 1 fluid ounce tincture of St. John's wort
- 1 fluid ounce tincture of self-heal
- 1 fluid ounce tincture of meadowsweet

- 40 drops peppermint essential oil
- 40 drops cinnamon essential oil
1. Combine the infused oils, tinctures, and essential oils in a small bottle. Cap and label the bottle, including shaking well before each use.
2. Place your palm over the lip of the bottle and tilt to deposit a small bit in your palm. Warm the therapy between your palms before applying it to the hurting joints.
3. Massage the oil into your joints until your hands are no longer greasy. Incorporate the cream into the tissue.

4. Apply the solution 3 to 5 times per day. More is more!

2. Sweet Relief Tea
- 1 tablespoon raspberry leaf
- 1 teaspoon white willow bark
- 2 cups boiling water
1. Cover the herbs with boiling water and soak for 30 minutes before straining.
2. Take just as needed

STRESS

Stress manifests as increased heart rate, blood pressure, muscle tension, irritability, depression, stomachache, and indigestion. Many people associate stress with emotional distress, because both stimulate the body's production of adrenaline.

A well-balanced diet and lifestyle are the most effective tools for combating the effects of stress.

Everyone is stressed, and everyone has a different priority. Whatever is causing you to stress, herbs can assist both in the short term to provide quick relief and in the long term to build more "nerve reserve" and poise in the face of adversity.

1. Calm Down Tea
- 1 teaspoon powdered ginger
- 1 teaspoon powdered valerian root
- 1 teaspoon powdered pleurisy root
- 2 cups boiling water
Combine the above ingredients.

2. Rescue Elixir

Makes five fluid ounces

- 1 fluid ounce tincture of tulsi

- 1 fluid ounce tincture of betony
- ½ fluid ounce tincture of catnip
- ½ fluid ounce tincture of chamomile
- ½ fluid ounce tincture of elderflower
- ½ fluid ounce tincture of rose
- ¼ fluid ounce tincture of goldenrod
- ¼ fluid ounce tincture of sage
- ½ fluid ounce honey
1. Combine the tinctures and honey in a small vial. Cap and label the bottle.
2. Take 2 to 4 drops as needed

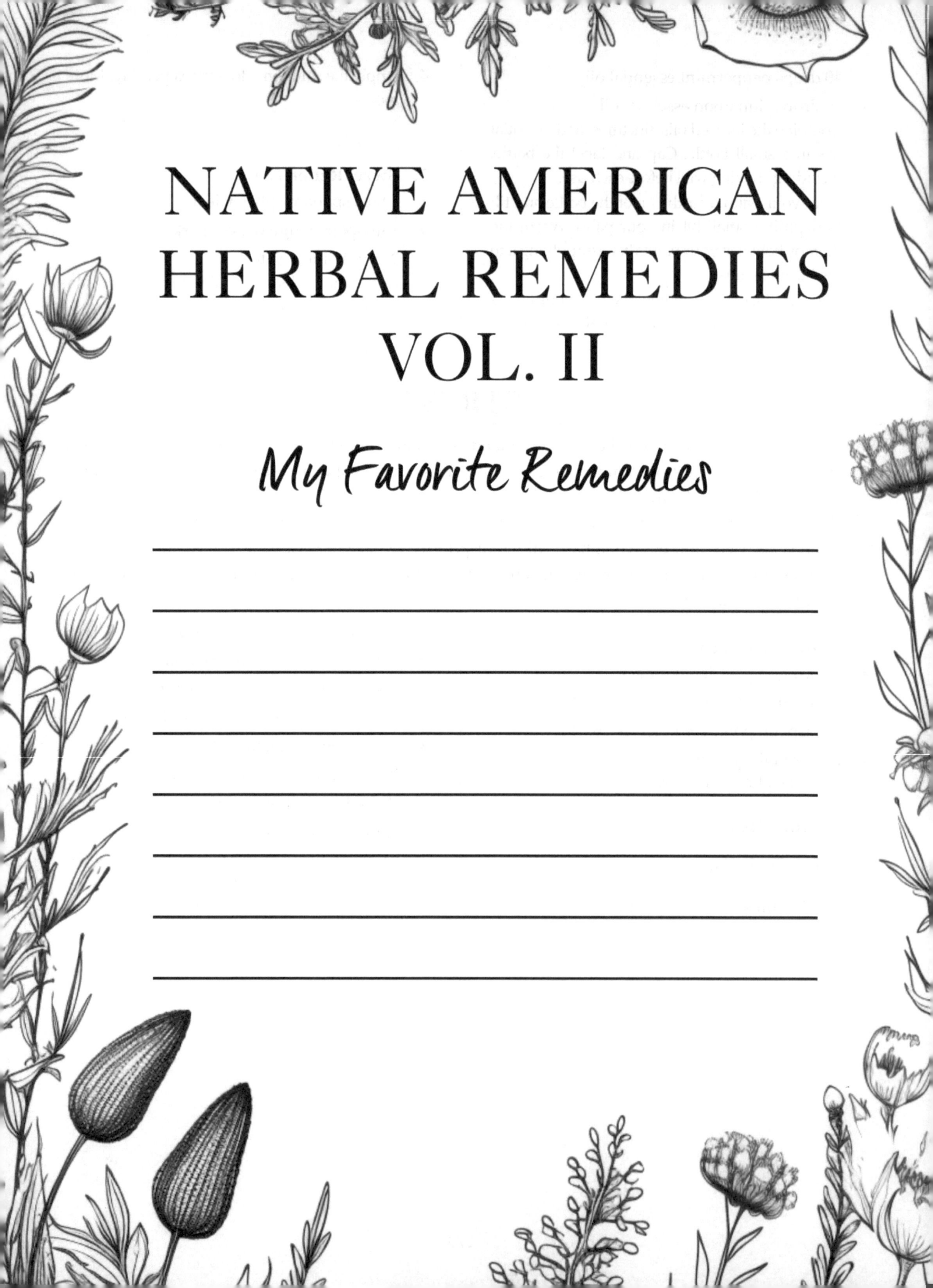

NATIVE AMERICAN HERBAL REMEDIES VOL. II

My Favorite Remedies

_____

_____

_____

_____

_____

_____

_____

1. ROSE TEA

Ingredients
- Black tea (loose-leaf) like Ceylon, Darjeeling, or Assam 1 cup
- Green cardamom seeds, powdered/chopped fine 2 tsp
- Wild rose petals ¼ cup

Directions
1. With scissors, chop the rose petals into little pieces. This meal is worth trying if you can obtain entire green cardamom pods. They have a much stronger flavor and scent than powdered cardamom.
2. Remove the dark seeds from the green pods using your fingernail. They may appear to be nothing more than mouse droppings at first glance, but after you eat one, you'll understand why they've influenced chefs for hundreds of years.
3. Finely chop the seeds.
4. Combine everything and keep it in an airtight jar.

2. WILD ROSE TONER

Rose is thought to be the most skin-balancing herb. This traditional formula can compete with today's high-priced face care products. Witch hazel tree bark is both astringent and soothing. It is extracted using water, with around 15% alcohol added as a preservative. It's available in various herb shops, natural food stores, and pharmacies.

Ingredients
- Wild rose ½ cup
- Witch hazel extract 1 jar

Directions
1. Fill a glass jar halfway with dried wilted/wild rose petals.
2. Cover the entire surface with witch hazel essence.
3. Cover the rose and witch hazel container and leave it aside for at least two weeks. Shake the fluid every couple of days to ensure the medicine is equally dispersed.
4. Strain and cover with a muslin cloth inside one glass jar/spray bottle. Label. As a mild astringent, spray or apply this liquid on the face to tighten pores and balance skin. Adding 25% rose water to this extract provides more rose scent and medicament.

3. LICORICE TEA

Native Americans used American Licorice extensively throughout the country. This plant's peeled, dried roots were used to make a medicinal tea to treat digestive disorders or diarrhea. The Montana Indians, Cheyenne, and Northwestern Tribes ate the tender spring shoots raw. The Lakotas used the plant's root as a flu remedy, while the Dakotas boiled licorice leaves in boiling hot water to make a topical earache remedy. The Blackfeet prepared a tea from the root to alleviate coughs, chest discomfort, and sore throats.

Ingredients
- 1 tablespoon dried licorice root
- 1/4 cup water

Directions
1. You can make licorice root tea by boiling the dried root in water for 15 minutes before filtering it and drinking it like tea.

4. SORE THROAT COUGH SYRUP

Thyme is the key ingredient in this cough syrup. Thyme has various medicinal properties, including enhancing your immune system due to its high vitamin C level. This cough remedy works especially well if the cough is accompanied by a cold. It also has thymol, an antibiotic that might help with a sore throat. Coughing is not necessarily a bad thing. It's the body's way of clearing the airways, so you'd only have to stop it if it hurts you or causes sleep loss.

Ingredients
- 1 cup of honey
- 1/2 cup water
- Sprig of fresh thyme (or some dried thyme)

- 1/4 cup water.

Directions
1. Bring the water to a boil in a saucepan.
2. Warm the honey in a separate pan.
3. Combine the two to make the basis.
4. Remove the thyme sprigs leaves and set them in a pestle and mortar.
5. Lightly bruise the thyme to release the active components.
6. Soak the thyme in boiling water for about 15 minutes.
7. Pour or pour the water into the honey mixture.

5. SOOTHING COUGH SYRUP

Wild Ginger was also used to treat colic, garnering it the moniker "Colic Root" among many others. Native Americans utilized wild ginger to treat open wounds. The roots contain antibiotic chemicals that, when sliced up and applied on a plantain leaf, could be used to treat skin inflammations as a poultice.

Wild ginger should never be eaten whole.

This dish is ideal for relaxing at night and can be used with anyone over the age of two. It alleviates coughing.

Ingredients
- 1 cup of honey
- 1/2 cup water
- Lemon zest – from 2 lemons
- Several teaspoons lemon juice (to your taste)
- ¼ cup peeled and sliced ginger or ¼ teaspoon ground ginger.

Directions
1. A honey mixture combines boiling water and wild honey.
2. Boil the lemon zest and ginger in a small amount of water for a few minutes. Strain the shards from the mixture to remove them.
3. Combine the honey mixture, filtered water, and lemon juice.

6. BLACKBERRY LEAF TEA

The Cherokee Indians have always used blackberry as medicine, among other things, to settle an unsettled stomach. Blackberry tea helps relieve joint swelling, while eating blackberry leaves can relieve painful gums. All-natural cough syrup are prepared from blackberry root and maple syrup or honey. It is also good for the immune system as a whole.

Ingredients
- 1 teaspoon blackberry leaf
- 1 cup water.

Directions
1. Fill a cup halfway with boiling water.
2. Add the leaves.
3. After covering the cup, soak it for around 5 minutes.

7. THE EXPECTORANT COUGH SYRUP

This is for your persistent phlegmy cough. Licorice root is an expectorant that aids in the breakdown of mucus. Licorice contains the chemical glycyrrhizin. Glycyrrhizin, which gives licorice its sweetness, and that is also an anti-inflammatory that can help with inflammatory respiratory diseases.

Ingredients
- 1 cup honey
- 1/2 cup water
- 1 tablespoon dried licorice root
- 1/4 cup water

Directions
1. Heat the water to a boil.
2. Warm the honey in a separate saucepan.
3. Combine the two to make the basis. You are free to experiment with the doses. You'll add extra liquid while making the cough mixtures, so make sure it's smooth.
4. Bring the licorice root and water to a boil and

set it aside for about 15 minutes.

5. Take the licorice water out of the filter.
6. Combine with honey mixture and whisk well.

8. BLACKBERRY TEA

Blackberries include antioxidants, minerals, and vitamins that have a variety of health benefits. Anthocyanins, for example, are anti-inflammatory and antibacterial antioxidants, and they may also be useful in treating diabetes and some malignancies.

Blackberries contain a high concentration of insoluble fiber. Fiber improves digestion by increasing the number of stools and making them pass more quickly. A fiber-rich diet can help ease constipation.

Ingredients
- Blackberries 3-4
- Water 1 cup

Directions
1. Place blackberries in a pan.
2. Pour in water and bring to a boil for about 5 minutes.
3. Strain the solids through a small hole sieve or a colander lined with cheesecloth.

9. COFFEE & TURMERIC FACE MASK

The two main benefits of this mask are caffeine and antioxidants: caffeine helps to reduce inflammation, such as puffy eyes, while antioxidants brighten the complexion.

Curcumin, turmeric's most active ingredient, has many scientifically verified health advantages, including improving heart health and protecting against Alzheimer's and cancer; it is also anti-inflammatory, antioxidant and may help with depression and rheumatic disorders.

Ingredients
- Instant/ Ground Coffee 1 tbsp
- Greek Yogurt 1 tbsp
- Powdered Turmeric 1tbsp

Directions
1. Combine all of the ingredients.
2. Apply to the entire face, paying special attention to the area around the eyes.
3. Allow for a 20-minute break.
4. Remove it with a warm, moist cloth.

10. PAPAYA LEAF TEA

The papaya leaf, which is usually consumed as a tea, extract, or juice, has been shown to lessen dengue fever symptoms. Other common applications include reducing inflammation, improving blood sugar management, enhancing skin and hair health, and avoiding cancer.

Papaya leaf extract helps also improing the function of your liver. The fluids' therapeutic qualities can cure chronic liver illnesses such as jaundice and liver cirrhosis. It naturally cleanses the liver of toxins while detoxifying it.

Ingredients
- Small leaf papaya 1
- Small piece ginger 1
- Glass water 2
- Honey as desired

Directions
1. Combine water, papaya leaf, and ginger slice in a saucepan. Boil until the color changes and the water content drops. This would take approximately 8-10 minutes.
2. Remove the leaf and then add the tea dust. Bring to a boil for about 2-3 minutes, then pour into serving glasses. To taste, add honey and a few drops of lemon juice.
3. Warm through before serving.

11. YARROW TEA

Because yarrow is a diuretic, it is an excellent "carrier" herb to use alongside urinary antibacterial medications to guarantee that the herbs reach the urinary tract. It can be used to clean cuts and scrapes.

The Cherokee, Iroquois, Gosiute, and Mohegan peoples have traditionally used yarrow for digestive aid, which makes sense given that bitter plants aid digestion by stimulating the production of pancreatic and bile secretions. Because of her astringent characteristics, yarrow is a good cure for diarrhea. The bitter components of yarrow stimulate the liver and aid in bile flow, while the antispasmodic properties (a chemical that reduces spasms or cramps) help with cramps induced by stress, colic, wind, or nervous digestion. Yarrow has been shown to aid with menstrual cramps.

Face steams using yarrow leaves can help with clogged pores. Yarrow tea can also be used as a hair rinse to soothe irritated or dry scalps. To obtain the above-mentioned therapeutic health benefits, drink some of the tea before washing, or soak a cloth in it and place it over your closed eyes for a headache.

Ingredients
- 1 teaspoon dried yarrow flower
- 1 cup water.

Directions
1. Add 1 cup of boiling water to 1 cup of dried yarrow flower.
2. Cover and set aside for 30 minutes before filtering and serving.

12. YARROW TINCTURE

Yarrow is an anti-flu and fever remedy!

Anti-inflammatory and antibacterial effects are found in yarrow. It soothes pain, serves as an anti-catarrhal, increases circulation, and has soothing properties. Yarrow is used to treat a range of unpleasant conditions. Salicylate-like substances found in yarrow teas and tinctures, such as beta-sitosterol and stigmasterol, aid in the reduction of inflammation and accelerate healing. These compounds block the formation of enzymes, which are essential for a series of chemical reactions that cause inflammation and discomfort.

The anti-inflammatory properties of yarrow are believed to be effective for dull, pounding headaches or migraines that seem to continue forever.

Ingredients
- 1 oz dried yarrow
- 5 oz alcohol (80 or more proof)

Directions
1. Dissolve dried yarrow in alcohol. Allow it to infuse for 6 to 8 weeks.
2. Strain it and store it in a dark glass bottle.

13. YARROW POLICE OR COMPRESS

Yarrow is widely used to tone veins, so can be used in treating varicose veins and hemorrhoids. Because of their ability to flow blood (vasodilation) and their cytoprotectant and antioxidant properties, yarrow leaves and blossoms are good for overall heart health. The cytoprotective and antioxidant properties of yarrow leaves and blossoms may also aid in wound healing. As wound healer, Yarrow includes anti-inflammatory and antibacterial oils, as well as astringent tannins and resins. It also contains silica, which helps to regenerate wounded tissue.

Ingredients
- Yarrow leaves
- Water

Directions
1. To prepare the police, produce a paste with just enough hot water and ground yarrow, then apply it to the affected area. If you're using dried herbs that aren't powdered, mash them up a little to make a paste.
2. Soak a cloth or towel in a strong brewed tea or tincture before applying it to the affected area to create a compress.

14. MINT TEA

The Cherokee produced mint tea to help with digestive difficulties and upset stomachs. They also made a salve from the leaves to cure itching skin and rashes. This plant has been used by healers to treat inflammation and respiratory disorders.

Wild Mint is a popular plant used by various Native American tribes to treat various ailments; a leaf infusion is used by California Indians to cure renal disease; Cherokee, Okanagan, and Navajo Ramah tribes use a leaf infusion to cure fever and colds. The plant is used as a ceremonial plant in the Sun Dance Ceremony. The leaves are eaten and applied to the body to improve one's personal love life, and infusions of the leaves are consumed to activate important organs. The Flathead used a leaf infusion to treat colds and fevers. Leaves were also used to treat infected teeth.

Ingredients
- 6-7 mint leaves
- ½ tsp grated ginger
- ½ cup water

Directions
1. In a pan, combine all of the ingredients.
2. Allow it to heat until it reaches a boil. Reduce the heat to low and continue to cook for 3-7 minutes, depending on your preference.

15. WILD ROSE TEA

Rosehip tea is an herbal tea made from the pseudo-fruits of the rose plant. It has a delicate, floral flavor that is slightly sweet with a tart finish. Rose hips are tiny, spherical fruits that are generally crimson or orange in color and are found right beneath the rose petals. Rose hips were used in a variety of ways by Native Americans. They can be consumed raw, dried, cooked, or roasted. To hasten labor, women nibbled on rose hips. Children's necklaces and bracelets were made from hard hips that served as beads.

Ingredients
- 2 cups wild rose with rose hips
- 1 lemon
- 41/2 cups boiling water
- ½ cup raw sugar cane
- A handful of wild rose petals

Directions
1. Simmer for two minutes until sugar dissolves. Remove the flowers and place them on a cooling rack to cool. The simple rose syrup is finished. Refrigerate in an airtight container.
2. To cover the wild roses, fill a big glass jar halfway with boiling water (about 4 cups). Soak for approximately 12 hours, covered.
3. Using a strainer, scoop out the flowers. Taste. If the finished tea is too strong or bitter, add more water.
4. Fill the cup halfway with tea, then add 1/2 teaspoon rose syrup and 1/2 teaspoon lemon.
5. After stirring, serve chilled.

16. CABBAGE CINNAMON APPLE JUICE

Cabbage juice is a formidable force in treating stomach ulcers. It's also abundant in antioxidants including Vitamins A, C, and K and Folate. The cabbage, on the other hand, is the principal source of ulcer-healing nutrients.

Drink no more than 4 oz of cabbage juice at a time to avoid overstimulating the gastric secretions, which can produce bowel cramping and gassiness when the sulfur in the juice reacts with the bacteria in the gut. By combining cabbage juice and carrot juice, sulfur can be reduced and intestinal walls toned. In addition to its ability to heal stomach ulcers, cabbage is also a helpful treatment for various other health issues such as constipation and colitis.

Ingredients
- Cabbage, tough stem sliced out ¼ head
- Small organic apple of a variety 1
- Large carrot peeled 1
- Cinnamon for additional heart health ¼ tsp

Directions
1. Place an eight-ounce glass beneath the spout

of a professional juicer and add ingredients one at a time until the juicer has expelled all of the juice.

2. Toss everything together and serve immediately.

17.GINGER HOPPER JUICE

Ginger aids in the elimination of intestinal gas, motion sickness and the treatment of pregnancy-related vomiting and diarrhea; it also contains anti-inflammatory properties. Carrots contain beta-carotene, which after digestion, is transformed into vitamin A: it enhances vision and treats skin problems such as acne and rough, dry skin. It reduces blood pressure, boosts the immune system, and fights cancer.

Apples are high in vitamins A and B and folic acid. They reduce cholesterol and aid in weight loss. It is beneficial to the skin, hair, and fingernails. They are also strong in quercetin and antioxidants and benefit the heart and lungs.

Ingredients

- Piece of ginger 1/4 inch
- Carrots 4
- Apple, peeled, cut into wedges 1

Directions

1. Juice the ingredients in a juicer and enjoy

18.HONEY FACE MASK

This face mask does wonders for scars and dark spots. It's also quite easy to make. This recipe depicts the use of honey as a face mask by Native Americans.

Its anti-inflammatory characteristics aid in removing excess oil from the skin's surface; when applied daily, it helps to balance your skin's microflora. It can be used as a spot treatment for stubborn breakouts and even autoimmune skin conditions such as eczema and psoriasis.

Ingredients

- Lemon Juice ½ tsp
- Raw Honey 2 tsp

Directions

1. In a mixing bowl, combine the lemon juice and honey.
2. Allow this mixture to sit on your face for a few minutes.
3. Allow around 20-30 minutes for relaxing.
4. Rinse. Because lemon juice is so potent, you should only use it 1-2 times a week

19.ALOE VERA & ALMOND OIL FACE MASK

Almond oil , high in enzymes, antioxidants, and vitamins A and C, has long been used to treat dry skin conditions such as eczema, psoriasis and acne. Fatty acids in the oil may aid in the breakdown of excess oil on the skin, whereas retinoids in the oil may aid in reducing acne and enhancing cell turnover. It Assist in the repair of solar damage.

With all of these benefits, Aloe Vera is undeniably good for the skin.

Ingredients

- Aloe Vera Gel 1 tsp
- Banana 1 tsp
- Almond Oil ½ tsp

Directions

1. This mask is great for moisturizing and moisturizing the skin and treating dry, flaky skin.
2. In one mixing dish, mash a banana with a fork.
3. Add 2 tbsp aloe vera gel to the mixture.
4. Stir until all of the ingredients are properly combined.
5. Add 3 tablespoons of almond oil to the mixture.
6. Mix everything thoroughly.
7. Use on a clean surface.
8. Allow for about 15 minutes of relaxation time.
9. Rinse

20.SUMAC TEA

Although this plant is utilized for various medical applications, it is one of the few herbs recommended by healers to treat eye diseases. Sumac decoctions have been used as a gargle to relieve sore throats and to treat diarrhea. The berries and berries were used to produce a fever-reducing tea or a poison ivy treatment. Sumac contains antioxidants that have been demonstrated to help decrease inflammation. Antioxidants shield human cells from damage and help to reduce oxidative stress in the body, helping also to prevent inflammatory disorders.

Ingredients
- Sumac 1 teaspoon
- Water 1/2 cup

Directions
1. Begin by bringing the water to a boil.
2. Fill a mug halfway with Sumac.
3. Half-fill the mug with boiling water.
4. Allow the sumac to soak for 4 minutes.

21. CRANBERRY ROSEMARY COCKTAIL

Native American tribes regarded the Rosemary plant as sacred. It was primarily used as an analgesic to alleviate joint discomfort. This plant improves the circulatory and neurological systems, improves memory, and relieves muscle pain and spasms. It alleviates indigestion and boosts immunity.

Ingredients
- 12 oz fresh cranberry
- ½ cup fresh rosemary
- 1 cup water.

Directions
1. Bring cranberries, water, and rosemary needles to a boil in a saucepan. After that, reduce the heat to low and cover for 45 minutes.
2. Strain through a fine-mesh sieve, scraping the sides as you go, and it will transform the mixture into a smooth purée.

22. GREEN NOURISHING SMOOTHIE FOR DIGESTIVE, SKIN & IMMUNE HEALTH

Dodecenal, an antibacterial component present in cilantro, may aid in the prevention of infections and ailments caused by contaminated food. Salmonella, a germ that can cause fatal food poisoning, is resistant to the chemical.

Lutein, which is found in spinach, aids in cholesterol reduction: it helps in maintaining good vision, energy levels, heart, and bone health.

Ingredients
- Fresh/frozen spinach 2 cups
- Cilantro 1/2 cup
- Fresh/ frozen kale 2 cups
- Coconut water 1 cup
- Fresh/ frozen pineapple chopped 1 cup
- Chia seeds 1 tbsp
- Hemp seeds 2 tbsp
- Ground turmeric/ half inch fresh turmeric knob 1/2 tsp
- Black pepper 1 pinch
- One inch fresh ginger knob/ ground ginger 1 tsp
- Lime peeled 1/2
- Green apple 1/2
- Medium-sized cucumber 1/2

Directions
1. Combine all of the ingredients in a blender.
2. Blend until the mixture is absolutely smooth.

23. YUCCA SHAMPOO

Yucca is the common name for the genus Yucca, which includes more than 40 plant species. The root of this non-flowering plant is used to make medicine.

Yucca treats osteoarthritis, migraine headaches, high blood pressure, high cholesterol, intestinal inflammation (colitis), diabetes, stomach problems, gallbladder illnesses, and liver disease. Some people apply yucca directly to their skin to treat wounds, sprains, skin disorders, joint soreness, bleeding, dandruff, and baldness.

Yucca extract is a foaming and flavoring ingredient in carbonated beverages. Many yucca compounds have been used in the creation of new drugs.

Chemicals contained in yucca may help reduce high blood pressure and cholesterol and aslo also aid in the relief of arthritic symptoms such as pain, swelling, and stiffness.

Yucca was an important plant for the Ancestor Pueblo people because of its many uses. The plant's roots were peeled and mashed to create a frothy pulp; the pulp was then blended with water and used to manufacture soap or shampoo.

Ingredients

- Tap water/ distilled water 4 cups
- Yucca root 1/2 cup/ medium size roots 2

Directions

1. Please wash your hands.
2. Cut the roots into big pieces.
3. Cut the dice into little pieces. Because the pulp is stringy, combining it into small pieces is recommended.
4. Half-fill the blender with water.
5. Add the yucca root.
6. Blend everything thoroughly to obtain as much soap as possible.
7. Drain the liquid and sift out the particles with a sieve.
8. Use the pulp to fertilize your plants or to make paper.
9. Using a funnel, fill the bottle with liquid soap.

24. WILD ROSE

Rose has a mythical air about her. It is associated with saints and gods and represents love, beauty, protection, and elegance. Rose tales are deeply rooted throughout history, from China to the Middle East, Europe to the native Americas. After all, it appears to be an elderly soul who has lived for 35 million years and seen various civilizations grow and fall. Her enormous presence has reigned in poetry, art, singing, and religious ceremony since ancient times, and her influence continues to reign today.

Ingredients

- Honey 1 jar
- Wild rose ½ cup

Directions

1. Gather aromatic petals and allow them to wilt for a day or two until half-dry. Fill a glass jar halfway with petals and a tight-fitting lid.
2. Warm the honey slowly on the burner until it is extremely liquid but not hot.
3. Fill the container with enough honey to completely encircle the blooms. Cap.
4. Place in a warm spot in the garden or on the vent.
5. Stir it well and wipe the moisture from underneath the lid. This will be advantageous.
6. Remove any excess water from your honey.Strain using a muslin cloth after around 2-3 weeks. Tea can be made from crushed petals and drunk or soaked in for a soothing "rose honey" bath.
7. Honey should be stored in a glass jar in a cool, dark place. Some people prefer to keep their honey in the refrigerator, although this is only necessary if it contains a little water.

REMEDY PREPARATION PLANNER

Embarking on the path of creating your herbal remedies is an exciting and rewarding adventure. To assist you in this journey, we introduce the Remedy Preparation Planner, a tool meticulously designed to facilitate a seamless and organized approach to remedy creation. This planner will be your companion, helping you to note down all the essential details, from ingredients and quantities to the preparation methods and storage instructions.

Beyond merely being a tool for recording details, this planner aims to instill a structured approach to remedy preparation, allowing you to plan and strategize your creations with utmost precision. It serves as a canvas where you can jot down your thoughts, ideas, and experiences, fostering an enriching learning experience.

Furthermore, by scanning the provided QR code, you unlock access to an additional 100 pages, granting you an expansive space to refine your craft and experiment with new recipes!

REMEDY PREPARATION PLANNER

DATE

PREPARATION TIME

DIFFICULTY ● ● ● ● ●

REMEDY NAME:

INGREDIENTS	QTY	NOTES

PREPARATION STEPS

USAGE INSTRUCTIONS

REMEDY PREPARATION PLANNER

DATE _____

PREPARATION TIME _____

DIFFICULTY ⬤ ⬤ ⬤ ⬤ ⬤

REMEDY NAME:

INGREDIENTS	QTY	NOTES

PREPARATION STEPS

_____

_____

_____

_____

_____

_____

USAGE INSTRUCTIONS

_____

_____

_____

_____

_____

_____

REMEDY PREPARATION PLANNER

DATE _____

PREPARATION TIME _____   DIFFICULTY ⚫ ⚫ ⚫ ⚫ ⚫

REMEDY NAME:

INGREDIENTS	QTY	NOTES

PREPARATION STEPS

_____

_____

_____

_____

_____

USAGE INSTRUCTIONS

_____

_____

_____

_____

_____

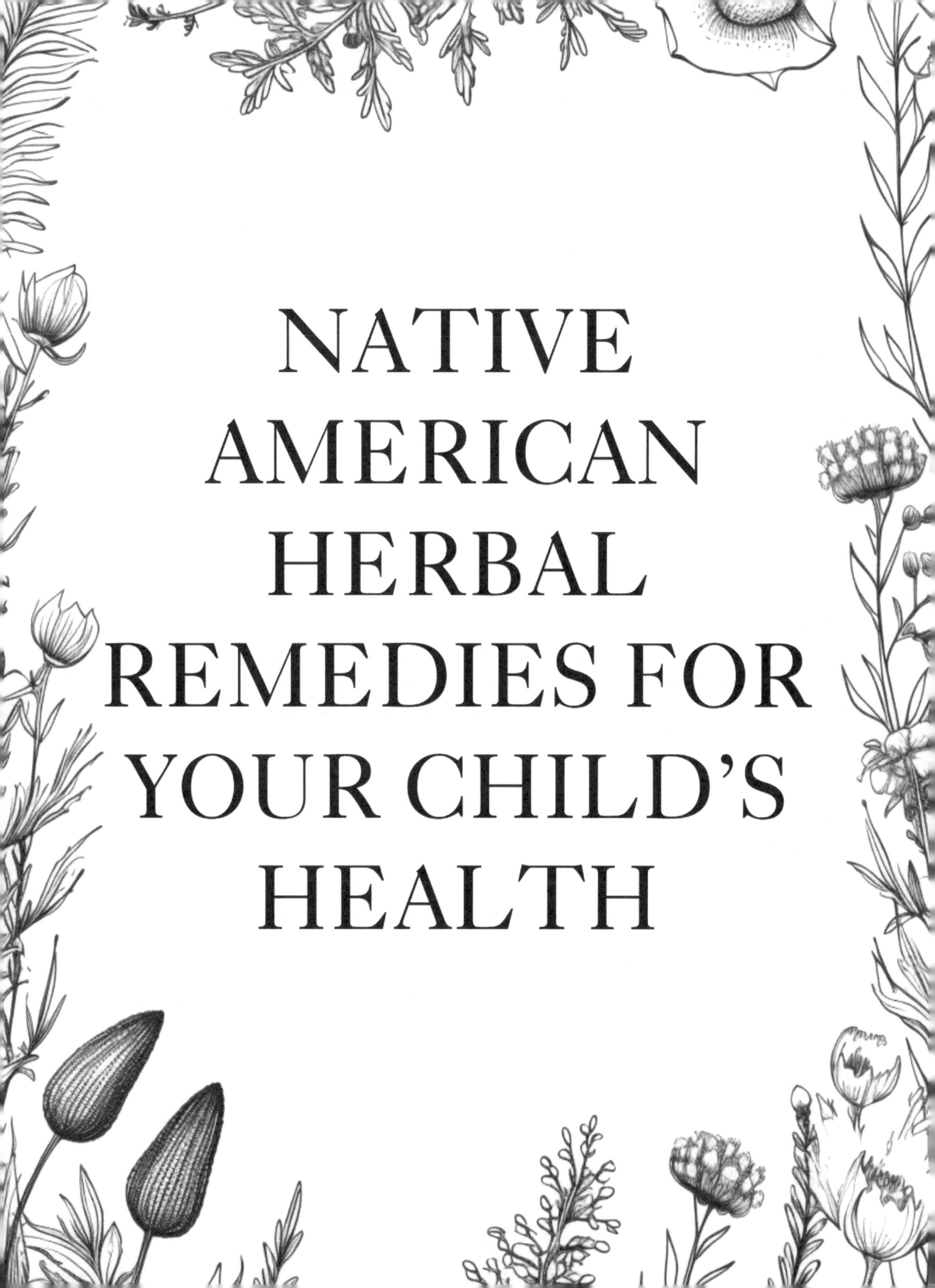

NATIVE AMERICAN HERBAL REMEDIES FOR YOUR CHILD'S HEALTH

HERBAL RECIPE FOR CHILDREN'S ILLNESS

Herbal treatments can be an excellent method to manage common difficulties that your child may be experiencing. We've collected a list of cures to try on your 0-12-month-old child.

For Children aged 2 to 12 months

1. DIAPER RASH WITH THYME AND COMFREY SALVE

Ingredients:
- 1 ounce of beeswax
- 1 ounce of dried thyme herb
- 1 cup olive oil (mild)
- 1 ounce dried comfrey herb

Directions:
1. Combine all ingredients except the beeswax in a saucepan, mix well, and heat for at least six to twelve hours. The oil will properly combine with the herbs, and the herbal extracts will permeate into the oil, offering therapeutic effects.
2. Melt the beeswax over low heat in a double boiler, then strain the oil through a cheesecloth before putting it in. It should be twisted and pressed firmly enough to allow every drop of oil to enter the bowl.
3. Remove and discard any residual debris from the cheesecloth. Turn off the boiler after thoroughly mixing the wax and oil to obtain a well-consistent mixture.
4. To treat a diaper rash, apply one teaspoon of this ointment to the affected area and gently rub it in.
5. Store in a cool, dry place.

2. NIGHT-NIGHT TEA

In a tea ball, combine 1/4 cup chamomile, 1/4 cup elderberry, 2 teaspoons valerian root, and 2 teaspoons lemon balm. Allow your child to drink this before bedtime to help them fall asleep faster.

3. BANANA BABY FOOD RECIPE

Give your infant mashed banana with 2 teaspoons of honey. The honey will provide a lot of energy. Before modifying your baby's food, always consult with your doctor.

4. FRUIT SMOOTHIE RECIPE

Combine 1 banana, 1/2 cup mixed berries, and 1 tablespoon of honey. Before modifying your baby's food, always consult with your doctor.

5. ELDERBERRY SYRUP

Blend 1/2 teaspoon dried elderberries with 1 cup water or apple juice in a blender. Place in the refrigerator for about 3 hours, or until cooled. Mix with 1 tablespoon of raw honey and drink 2-3 tablespoons per day to help relieve cold and flu symptoms like fever and congestion.

6.OATMEAL BATH

Soak for 20-30 minutes in a full bath with 1/4 cup oatmeal. This can aid in the relief of painful, dry skin, and rashes.

7.COLIC TREATMENT USING HERBAL GRIPE WATER

Ingredients:
- 1 teaspoon dried peppermint leaves, crushed
- 1 teaspoon fennel seeds, crushed
- 1 teaspoon sugar made from cane
- 1 teaspoon fresh ginger root, diced
- 1 cup of hot water

Directions:
1. Combine the herbs and water in a mug.
2. Bring the water to a boil in a small saucepan and pour it into the mug.
3. Cover the mug with a lid and let the herbs soak.
4. Place the substance in a sterilized jar and utilize it.
5. You can give it to your child with a dropper and have him or her consume it orally.
6. Your youngster will quickly feel relieved.
7. To achieve optimum outcomes, take the medication twice a day.

8.GARGLE

Combine 1/4 cup warm water, 2 tablespoons of raw honey, and the juice of half a lemon. This is excellent for relieving sore throats and reducing swelling.

9.CONGESTION RELIEF

Make a paste with 2 teaspoons of powdered ginger, marshmallow root, and enough hot water. Stir well until it has the consistency of toothpaste, then apply with your fingertips directly to the chest. This can assist in loosening mucus and increasing the cough reflex.

10.SLEEPY TIME TEA

Combine 2 teaspoons of chamomile, lavender, and lemon balm in a tea ball with boiling water. This is excellent for assisting your child in falling asleep quickly.

11.TUMMY RELIEF

Make a paste with 1 teaspoon of fennel seeds, ginger powder, and enough boiling water. Stir until it has the consistency of toothpaste, then apply with your fingertips directly to the tummy. This can help reduce stomach cramps and gas discomfort.

12.BANANA MANGO SMOOTHIE RECIPE

1 banana, 1/2 cup diced mango, 2 tablespoons honey, 1 teaspoon chia seeds, and 1/2 cup ice cubes are required to make this banana mango smoothie. Put all of the ingredients in a blender to make a wonderful drink for your youngster to enjoy.

13.SOUR APPLE JUICE RECIPE

Pour a cup of apple cider vinegar into a measuring cup and add enough water to make 1 cup of sour apple juice. Then add a handful of fresh mint, a couple celery stalks, and up to 2 tablespoons of honey and powdered ginger. You can give this to your baby immediately after feeding them or as a supplement to their usual milk feedings.

14.BANANA MILK RECIPE

Mash two bananas with 1/4 teaspoon cinnamon powder and 2 teaspoons honey to make banana milk. After blending this combination for about 10 minutes, you should have around 1 pint of banana mil.

15.COLD AND COUGH SYRUP FOR YOUR 12 MONTH - 5-YEAR-OLD CHILD

Eucalyptus - 2 tbsp. to help freshen your child's breath. In a saucepan, combine all ingredients and cook for 15 minutes, allowing the ingredients to steep while you prepare your child for bed. When the mixture has finished simmering, ensure the children drink it immediately.

Dandelion Root - 3 tbsp. + 1/8 teaspoon salt (for flavor) to help with soothes nasal passage irritation. In a saucepan, combine all of the ingredients and cook for 10 minutes. Add 1 tablespoon of honey once the mixture has simmered to enhance the flavor. Remove from the stove and set aside to cool before serving to your toddler. Keep the leftover mixture in a container for later use.

Peppermint - 4 tsp. + 2 tbsp Honey (for flavor) to relieve nasal congestion and discomfort. Combine all ingredients in a pot and cook for 15 minutes on low heat. Remove from the stove and set aside to cool before serving to your toddler.

16.SORE THROAT TEA WITH SAGE, PEPPERMINT, AND COMFREY

Ingredients:
- 1 teaspoon dried comfrey
- 1 teaspoon dried peppermint
- 1 tsp. sage (dried form)
- 1 cup of water

Directions:
1. Half-fill a cup with boiling water.
2. Fill the cup halfway with sage, peppermint, and comfrey herbs and cover with a lid for a few minutes.
3. Drink the tea After the herbs have pleasantly blended in the water.
4. Drink this tea three to four times daily to treat your child's sore throat.

For Children aged 5 to 12 years

Nowadays, children are continuously exposed to hazardous toxins. Many beverages, snacks, and even home contaminants can affect children's health. Parents must be informed of the potential side effects to assist their child in avoiding them without having to purchase a tonic pouch at the shop.

Herbal medicines are a natural way to counteract the detrimental impacts of contemporary living; try creating one of the herbal treatments listed below for your child the next time they are unwell or looks to be under the weather.

17. BODY BATH MADE FROM LICORICE AND COMFREY FOR CHICKENPOX

Ingredients:
- Licorice root tincture (half teaspoon)
- 4 cups apple cider vinegar, unfiltered and organic
- Comfrey herbs, half tsp. tincture

Directions:
1. Combine the vinegar and tinctures in a clean, dry container.
2. Keep it in a dark/dry area until it's ready to use.
3. Combine one cup of the prepared mixture with one cup of water for spectacular results.

18. MULLEIN AND GARLIC INFUSED OIL FOR EAR PAIN

Ingredients:
- 2 tbsps. olive oil (mild)
- 1 ounce of dried mullein
- 2 tsp. garlic (dry form)

Directions:
1. Combine all ingredients in a pan and place it over a double boiler filled with water, continually stirring. Allow at least three to five hours to cook. The water will properly interact with the herbs, allowing the herbal extracts to enter the oil and deliver therapeutic effects.
2. Before pouring the mixture into the jar, drain it through cheesecloth into it. Twist and push it firmly enough to get every last drop of extract into the dish.
3. Remove and discard any residual debris from the cheesecloth.
4. Put two to three drops of this oil in your child's ear to ease the pain.
5. Keep it in a cold, dry location.

19. SOOTHE STOMACHACHES

As seen in this recipe, Native Americans used ajwain for medicinal purposes. Ajwain is a multipurpose plant with numerous applications. Plant parts of ajwain are used to manufacture a range of medications and syrups. Because of its strong aroma, ajwain is known as Ugargandha in Sanskrit, which means "powerfully fragrant."

Humans consume the plant's leaves as well as the seedlike fruit (also known as seeds). "Bishop's weed" is a common name for various plants. The "seed" (the fruit) is occasionally confused with the "seed" of lovage. The active enzymes in ajwain promote the flow of stomach acids, which can help with bloating, indigestion, and gas. This plant can be used to treat peptic ulcers and lesions in the esophagus, intestines, and stomach.

Ingredients:
- Ajwain 2 tsp

Directions:
1. Roast two tablespoons of ajwain on a flat pan (Tawa).
2. Once the aroma has been released, place it on a clean muslin cloth or a handkerchief.
3. Wrap the bundle securely around the navel and secure it in place.
4. However, be certain that it is not too hot.

20. SORE THROAT

There are around 12,000 different varieties of bees worldwide, but only a few, known as Apis mellifica, preserve honey. Until the early 1600s, North America had a plethora of native bees but only a few honeybees. They were termed "a white man's fly" by indigenous peoples. By 1800, honeybees had migrated into the wild, built their hives, and reached the Mississippi River.
American Indians ate unique honey before the arrival of Spanish conquistadors. The Mayans and Aztecs drank honey from Melipona beecheii, a bee that lived in hollow logs.

The Mayans and Aztecs devoured these settlements. Today's honeybees primarily consume clover and alfalfa nectar. Modern beekeepers experiment with orange blossom, raspberry, buckwheat, linden, sage blossom, and other innovative varieties. Honey has applications that extend beyond gastronomy and medicine. According to legend, Cupid is thought to have dipped his little arrows in honey before striking unsuspecting lovebirds. Wounds and burns are being treated, acid reflux and infection are being controlled, and cold and cough symptoms are being eased.

Ingredients:
- Honey 1 tbsp
- Lemon 1 tbsp

Directions:
1. Combine one tablespoon of each item, microwave for 20 seconds or until warm (not hot), and have your child swallow one teaspoon at a time.
2. Honey is not recommended for babies under one year old.

21. DIARRHEA

According to a 2015 research, ginger can treat diarrhea and other stomach disorders. Ginger is supposed to aid in treating diarrhea caused by contaminated foods. It also helps to prevent vomiting, nausea, and abdominal cramps. It also relieves flatulence and promotes appropriate digestion. Native Americans used the plant as a medicinal herb to cure dysentery, swollen breasts, digestive troubles, typhus, coughs and colds, nerves, scarlet fever, cramps, sore throats, heaves, headaches, earaches, asthma, urinary disorders, convulsions, tuberculosis, and venereal disease.

Ingredients:
- Grated nutmeg 2 tbsp
- Water 2 tbsp
- Jaggery 2 pinches
- Ginger powder ½ tsp
- Ghee ½ tsp

Directions:
1. Fill two spoons halfway with stone-ground/ shredded nutmeg and water.
2. Combine this in a small steel bowl with 2 pinches of jaggery (cane sugar), 1/2 teaspoon ginger powder, and half a teaspoon of handcrafted (genuine) ghee.
3. Bring to a boil, then remove from heat and set aside to cool.
4. Consume it gradually.

22. DIAPER RASH SPRAY

Since Roman times, lavender has been used in teas, balms, gastronomy, and medical remedies. If you suffer from anxiety, you've probably been prescribed lavender essential oil, and for good reason. It was used to treat anxiety disorders by Native Americans. Lavender has been demonstrated to be soothing in dental patients, and it was also appreciated for its soothing properties, which helped people sleep better.

Ingredients:
- Melaleuca 10 drops
- Lavender 10 drops
- Coconut oil (for rest filling)

Directions:
1. In a 15 ml container, combine the first two ingredients. Fill the rest of the bottle with coconut oil.
2. While changing the diaper, spray it on the baby's bum.

23. FOR A COMMON COLD

1/4 cup hot water with 1 lemon squeezed in. Stir in 2 teaspoons honey and 1 teaspoon ginger until thoroughly combined. Because honey is still a sugar, have this cure on hand for when your child has a cold or is fighting one. Add 1 teaspoon of mint leaf to the mixture if you have sinus issues.

24. MILKWEED FOR EYEWASH

Several Native Americans have used the latex fluid extracted from milkweed roots, stems, and plant tops for medicinal purposes. The Miwoks utilized latex to get rid of warts. To treat snow blindness, the Cheyenne made a decoction from dried plant tops and used it as eyewash. Although the plant is potentially harmful, it has been used for therapeutic purposes. Milkweed sap was used to treat warts, and the roots were taken by many indigenous Americans to alleviate diarrhea. Salves and infusions were also used to treat inflammation, rashes, fevers, cough, and asthma.

Ingredients:
- 1 tsp milkweed dried
- ½ cup water

Directions:
1. In a pan, combine the ingredients.
2. Cook for 3–5 minutes.

25. WILLOW FOR TEETH

Native Americans used a toothbrush constructed from a small willow twig. The tannins' astringency would keep their gums healthy while cleaning their teeth. For millennia, willow bark has been used to treat fevers and colds. Taken 2-3 times daily, white willow tea can help with minor fevers, colds, and flu.
Willow bark has a pain-relieving action that can help with menstrual discomfort. The bark of white willow trees contains salicin, a chemical similar to aspirin. When paired with the herb's potent anti-inflammatory plant compounds, salicin is thought to be responsible for the herb's pain-relieving and anti-inflammatory capabilities.

Ingredients:
- 3-inch willow stick

Directions:
1. To make the stick bushy, bite it and chew it for a while.
2. Use the bushy edge like a brush to clean your teeth.

26. EASE ECZEMA

An amulet constructed from turmeric rhizome is used to ward off evil spirits. Turmeric has been used to dye cloth and thread for centuries due to its vivid yellow natural hue (it is used to color Buddhist clothes that are saffron in color).

Curcumin can help the brain in several ways. Other neurological diseases, such as dementia, multiple sclerosis, Huntington's disease, and Parkinson's disease, may benefit from polyphenols' antioxidant and anti-inflammatory properties.

Ingredients:
- Turmeric 1 tbsp
- Jaggery 1 tbsp

Directions:
1. Apply a paste of jaggery and turmeric to the affected area.

2. Make a bandage from one thick wheat-flour flatbread and bind it with cloth.
3. The jaggery warms the illness, forcing it to ooze out, while the turmeric disinfects and the roti keeps the heat going.

27.BUG BITES

Native Americans used baking soda in conjunction with sour milk to leaven bread. The leavening mixture was carried back to Ireland by Irish immigrant.

Ingredients:
- Baking soda 1 tsp
- Water 4-5 drops

Directions:
1. Make a thick paste with one teaspoon of baking soda and just enough water to cover the bits, then dry.

28.HEALING SALVE

Rose geranium oil is extracted from the leaves and stems of the rose geranium plant. Certain people may benefit from rose geranium oil to treat depression, nerve discomfort (neuropathy), and diarrhea. It can also be applied topically to the skin to reduce the nerve pain caused by shingles.

Ingredients:
- Calendula-infused Almond Sweet oil 1/3 cup (75 g)
- Comfrey-infused Almond Sweet oil 1/3 cup (75 g)
- Plantain-infused Almond Sweet oil 1/3 cup (75 g)
- Beeswax 1 oz (28 g)
- Rose Geranium essential oil 1/2 tsp (optional)

Directions:
1. Create your infused oil.
2. Combine plantain leaves, dried calendula blossoms, and comfrey leaves to fill a pint jar two-thirds full.
3. Drizzle sweet almond oil over the herbs and within one-quarter inch of the jars' tops. Seal the jars, shake them well, and store them somewhere warm and out of direct sunlight. If you want to set them on a window sill, wrap them in a paper bag to protect the oil from the sun's rays.
4. Give the jars a vigorous shake daily, then strain the plant material oil through cheesecloth after three to six weeks. Take the plant material out of the jars and pour the oils into new, sterilized jars. The infused oil has a shelf life of one year or until the oil's best-by date, whichever comes first. Keep it at room temperature in a dark place.
   Make a Herbal Healing Salve.
5. Bring the water in the larger pan to a boil.
6. Place the beeswax in the smaller pan on top of the hot water. This method evenly distributes the heat because beeswax should never be melted over direct heat.
7. Pour the melted beeswax over the herb-infused oils. Using a spatula, stir in the oils until they are just melted. Remove the pan from the heat and place it on a towel or potholder.
8. Allow the tins/containers to cool after adding the essential oil (optional). The temperature would approach room temperature in about four hours. Cover the containers at this time to avoid moisture on

the inside of the lid. Cover them with lids once the balm has cooled.

9. The salve is now ready to use. Shelf life could be up to a year or until the best-by date of the components, whichever comes first. Check the back of all of your bottles for them; remember that fresh oil is always best when cooking or making cosmetic products.

29. GINGER TEA FOR THE CAR SICKNESS

Wild ginger has been used for various purposes by many Native American tribes. When steeped in tea, wild ginger was used as a contraceptive. The herb was a well-known carminative that was used to calm upset stomachs. It was also used to treat digestive issues, stomach aches, cramps, and indigestion and to cure colic, garnering the moniker "Colic Root" among many others.

The pioneers utilized wild ginger to treat open wounds. When the roots are chopped up and placed on a plantain leaf, they contain antibiotic chemicals that could be used as a poultice to treat skin inflammations. Meriweather Lewis is supposed to have received this therapy while on tour in Louisiana in 1806. Pioneers used the plant to treat chest aches and heart palpitations, generate perspiration to reduce fever, as a tonic, and to stimulate appetite.

Ingredients:
- Ginger 1 tsp
- Water 4 ounces

Directions:
1. For children aged 2 years and up, place one teaspoon of grated fresh ginger in four ounces of boiling water and steep for four to five minutes.
2. A little honey could be used to enhance the flavor.
3. Allow your child to eat it for a half-hour after it has cooled before putting it in the car.

30. JUNIPER BERRY OIL FOR SKIN

To tone the skin, massage Juniper oil into it after exercise or dry brushing.
Mix it with your favorite body cream or a facial moisturizer to nourish the appearance of your skin. Use it topically to reduce the appearance of blemishes.
Juniper can be diffused to promote relaxation and spiritual awareness. Juniper berry essential oil is extracted from the plant's berries, while Juniper leaf essential oil is extracted from the plant's branches and leaves. Although they have similar therapeutic properties, their compositions differ.

Ingredients:
- Juniper berries 3 cups
- Oil 4 cups

Directions:
1. Juniper berries should be placed in a clean, sterilized jar. Fill the container three-quarters of the way.
2. Fill the container with the oil of your choice. Select a healthy oil, such as olive or coconut oil.
3. Close the jar tightly and store it in a cool, dark place.

31. SLIPPERY ELM FOR SORE THROAT

Slippery elm is one of the best herbs for sore throats. It comes from the inner barks of trees and the Native Americans have employed it for ages as a treatment. Mucilage, the active ingredient, is a sticky substance that, when coupled with water makes a slick gel. The gel covers and soothes inflamed mucous membranes while suppressing cough receptors in the throat and larynx, producing a protective barrier all the way down the digestive system and throat. For older children, slippery elm throat lozenges are available.

Ingredients:
- 2 tablespoon powdered bark
- 2 cups boiling water

Directions:
1. Fill a jar halfway with boiling water.
2. Mix in the powdered bark.
3. Allow it to steep for 3 to 5 minutes.
4. You may mask the flavor of the powdered bark by mixing it with orange juice.

32. GOOSEBERRY TEA FOR GARGLES

Currants and gooseberries have long been used medicinally by indigenous peoples in North America.

The continent of North America. The Comanche used berry tea gargles to treat sore throats. The Prairie Potawatomi made a decoction from the root that was useful in eliminating foreign particles and relaxing tired or inflamed eyes. The Muscogee people drank a potent tea made from the root bark to get rid of intestinal worms.
Gooseberry juice had been used also as a wash to soothe inflamed and swollen skin tissue.

Ingredients:
- 2 cups water
- 1 teaspoon ginger
- 1 teaspoon dried gooseberry powder
- 2 leaves of tulsi

Directions:
1. To make the tea, fill a pitcher halfway with water.
2. Add the ginger, dried gooseberry powder, and tulsi leaves when the water boils.
3. Bring to a boil this mixture. After straining it, gargle with it

33.CAYENNE PEPPER FOR THE NOSEBLEEDS

Native Americans have used cayenne (Capsicum annuum) as both medicine and food for around 9,000 years. Cayenne pepper gets its fiery and spicy flavor from capsaicin, which aids in pain relief. Capsaicin has anti-inflammatory properties when applied to the skin.

Powerful pain-relieving properties. It reduces the amount of substance P in your body, which is a chemical that sends pain signals to your brain. Pain signals do not access the brain when substance P levels are low, and you feel soothed. Capsaicin is commonly recommended for the following conditions:

Joint or muscle pain caused by fibromyalgia or other conditions, osteoarthritis, and rheumatoid arthritis. Postherpetic neuralgia is a type of nerve pain caused by shingles and other serious skin illnesses that lasts after the skin blisters have healed.

Capsaicin cream alleviates lower back pain. Psoriasis is a chronic skin disease characterized by raised, red skin patches covered by a flaky white coating. Capsaicin cream may help relieve itching and discomfort.

Ingredients:
- Ground cayenne pepper one pinch cotton swab

Directions:
2. Hold your child's head erect and his nostrils together for several minutes.
3. Then, with a damp cotton swab, dab a pinch of ground cayenne pepper into the bleeding location in the nose.
4. It appears to sting, but it does not.

34.JUNIPER BERRY TEA FOR COUGH AND FEVER

Juniper berries were also used as female contraception by Native Americans. Some Plateau tribes prepared an infusion of juniper berry inner bark and leaves to treat coughs and colds.

Children's fevers. The berries were cooked into a drink that was used to treat colds and as a laxative. Juniper is a diuretic that aids in the removal of excess fluids while also stimulating the kidneys by boosting urine flow. This allows the body to cleanse itself of uric acid and excess crystals that can cause gout, kidney stones, and arthritis.

Ingredients:
- Juniper berries
- Water
- Honey

Directions:
1. Arrange some dried juniper berries in a tea ball or directly in the mug in a large cup.
2. Half-fill the cup with boiling water. Allow for 15 minutes of steeping time. Take out the tea ball or strain the berries.
3. If preferred, top with a teaspoon of raw honey.

35.FOR BURNS

Because they are both safe and natural, eco-friendly burn cures are ideal for every type of burn injury. Apply aloe vera gel to the wound for minor burns. If you don't have any, select an aloe vera leaf and scrape off the clear gel within. Before applying aloe vera to a burn, prevent your child's hands and face from becoming burned.

If you don't have any gel or your child is allergic to it, use a cool, moist towel or sponge wrapped in gauze to treat more serious burns. This will assist in minimizing inflammation and swelling while also preventing additional skin damage.

36.FOR A TOOTHACHE

To warm water, combine 1 tablespoon of lemon juice, 1 teaspoon of honey, and 1 teaspoon of baking soda to make tea.

37.FOR A STOMACHACHE

Warm salt water should be used to rinse your child's mouth. If this doesn't work or you don't have any on hand, make a gentle, calming herbal treatment for their stomach pain. Boil two eggs in a saucepan.

Pour one cup of chilly water through two cups of water. Allow 2 teaspoons of ginger, 1 teaspoon of peppermint leaves, and 1 teaspoon of cinnamon bark to steep for 10 minutes before draining into a cup. This can be consumed hot or cold as your child needs until the pain lessens.

38.FOR A SORE THROAT

1 teaspoon lemon juice, 1 teaspoon salt and 1 cup warm water. For optimal results, gargle with this mixture. The salt will soothe your child's throat while also aiding in removing any bacteria that may be causing their sore throat. Your child can also gargle with warm salt water as needed, but no more than once every 30 minutes to avoid salt irritation.

39.FOR MINOR CUTS AND SCRAPES

Add 1 teaspoon crushed cloves, 1 teaspoon ground thyme, 2 tablespoons coconut oil, 1/2 cup mashed avocado, 3 teaspoons lemon juice, and 1 whisked egg white to make the ointment.

40.FOR INSECT BITES

Use 1 tablespoon of rubbed mint leaves with equal parts honey and raw potato flake and combine all of the ingredients. For relief, apply it to the skin.

41.EASE EAR PAIN

Marigold is a multipurpose plant with numerous therapeutic benefits. All of this is made possible by the essential oils and resins found in the bright yellow flowers.The pleasant blossom's eagerness to bloom is palpable. The Romans named it calendula after the first day of its month because its petals sparkled in dazzling yellow and gold each month from June to October.Marigold's most prevalent medical use are for skin problems of various types, such as bruises, contusions, and varicose veins. Minor skin abrasions and irritation could also be adequately addressed. Marigold ointment promotes faster healing of eczema and sunburn lesions. Fresh flowers should be kept in olive oil and stored in a cool, dark place.

The filtered oil could be combined with wax to make the ointment after three weeks. The ointment can now be decanted and stored in the jar for several months.The inclusion of the blooms, which bring color and a moderate flavor to beverages, soups, and pesto, benefits many recipes. Marigold is utilized as a natural hue in the food industry to make cheese and butter look more appealing. Dried blooms are frequently used to enhance Some teas.

Fried marigold is a culinary delight that is sure to impress. After dipping the blooms in the honey-sweetened batter, deep-fry them until golden brown. In the summer, the crispy tidbits are utilized as finger food and in salads.Marigold tea has numerous applications. When taken three times a day, it relieves cramps and improves digestion. It also relieves nausea, stomach ulcers, and menstrual cramps. Marigold tincture alleviates headaches and promotes sound sleep. As an anti-inflammatory and relaxing, the tea can also be used in cold compresses and baths.Despite substantial research in alternative medicine, the origin of marigold remains unknown. However, it appears that it is now a truly European plant.

What isn't to love about a low-maintenance beauty? It comes as no surprise that it has spread across the continent. The marigold blooms only once a year. However, because it is adaptable, it cultivates itself for the next year if it remains in the garden until seed maturation.

Ingredients:
- Genda (marigold) leaves 10

Directions:
1. Crush the agenda (marigold) leaves, extract the juice, and place a few drops in each ear.
2. The juice aids in the release of the wax.
3. This treatment should not be used to treat other types of ear pain.

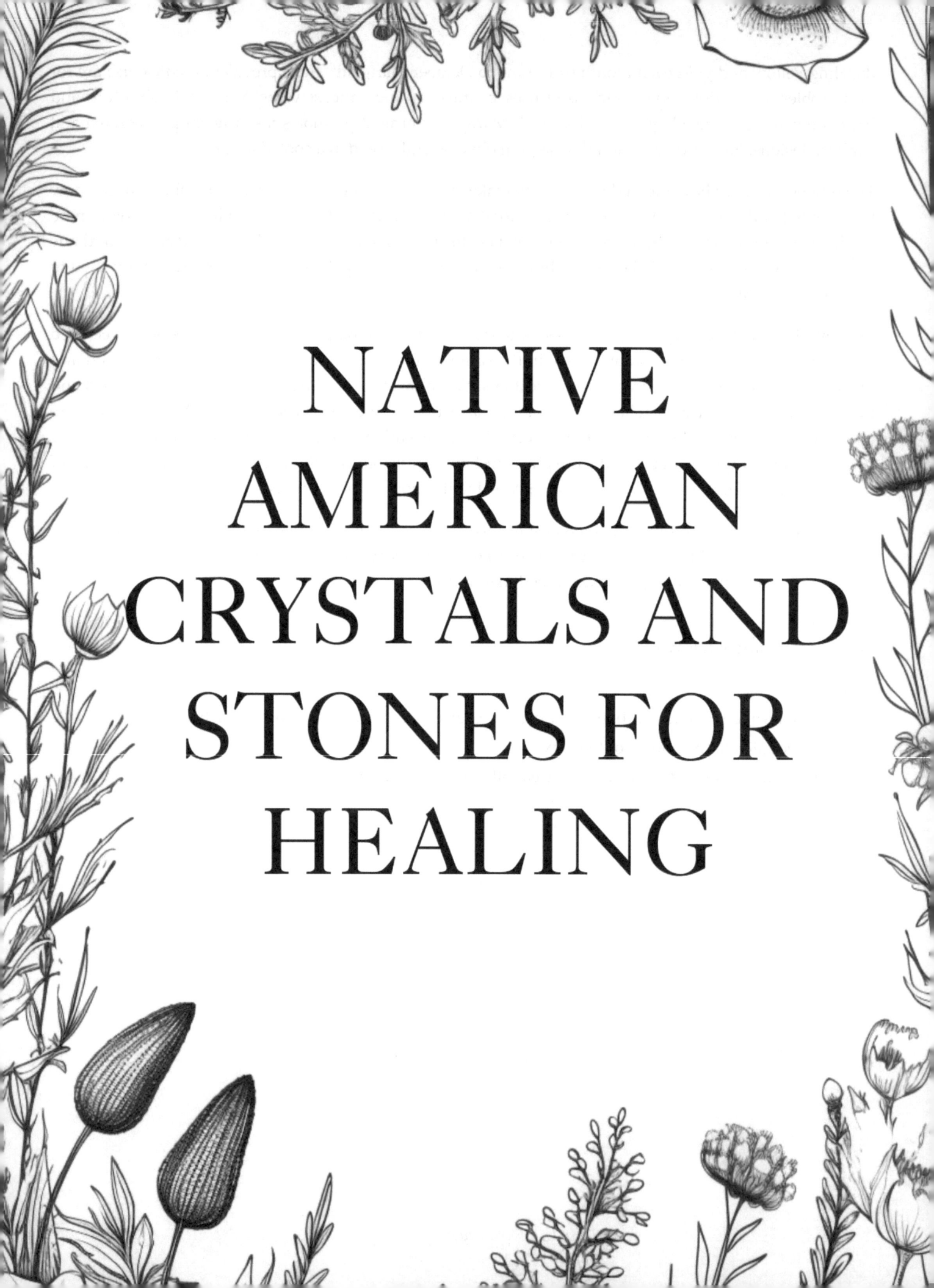

NATIVE AMERICAN CRYSTALS AND STONES FOR HEALING

INTRODUCTION

Welcome to the captivating world of Native American crystals and stones, where ancient wisdom meets the profound power of Earth's treasures. In this book, we embark on a journey through the sacred landscapes of Native American cultures, exploring the profound connection they shared with crystals and stones for healing, spirituality, and transformation. Here, we delve into the rich tapestry of indigenous traditions, unlocking the secrets of these sacred tools and their ability to bring balance, harmony, and well-being into our lives.

For countless generations, Native American cultures have revered crystals and stones as potent allies in their spiritual practices and healing rituals. They recognized the inherent wisdom and energetic vibrations held within these natural formations, understanding that they were gifts from the Earth, carrying the essence of the divine. Crystals and stones were seen as mediators between the physical and spiritual realms, serving as conduits for healing energies and spiritual guidance.

In this book, we honor and celebrate the profound knowledge passed down by Native American tribes, who understood the unique properties and vibrations of each crystal and stone. We explore the fundamental principles of their teachings, the sacred ceremonies and practices they employed, and the deep spiritual connection they cultivated with the natural world.

Our journey begins with an exploration of the origins and significance of crystals and stones in Native American cultures. We discover the ancient wisdom embedded in their creation stories and folklore, gaining insight into the symbolic meanings and spiritual attributes associated with specific crystals and stones. From the luminous quartz to the iridescent labradorite, each gem holds a story waiting to be told.

Next, we delve into the healing properties and practices that have been cherished by Native American traditions for centuries. We examine how crystals and stones were used to restore energetic balance, address physical ailments, and support emotional well-being. From crystal layouts and grids to medicine pouches and talismans, we uncover the tools and techniques employed by Native Americans to harness the power of these sacred treasures.

Throughout the book, we explore the profound cultural significance of crystals and stones within specific Native American tribes. We discover the distinct rituals and ceremonies that were conducted to honor and engage with these sacred allies, and how they were integrated into everyday life. We also pay homage to the wisdom keepers and healers who carried the sacred knowledge of crystals and stones, passing it down through generations.

As we journey through these pages, it is important to approach the knowledge and practices of Native American cultures with deep respect and reverence. We honor their traditions and teachings, recognizing the immense value they hold in helping us reconnect with the Earth, our own inner wisdom, and the healing energies that surround us.

May this book serve as a bridge, connecting us to the ancient wisdom of Native American cultures and the transformative power of crystals and stones. Let us embark on this journey together, embracing the spiritual essence and healing potential that lie within these timeless gifts from the Earth. May we find inspiration, guidance, and healing as we embrace the teachings of Native American crystals and stones for our own well-being and the greater harmony of the world around us.

OVERVIEW

Welcome to "Native American Crystals and Stones for Healing," a comprehensive guide that explores the profound connection between Native American culture and the powerful energy of crystals and stones. By delving into the rich traditions and wisdom of Native American cultures, we will gain a deeper appreciation for the unique healing properties these natural treasures possess.

Native American Spirituality and Connection to the Earth

Native American spirituality is deeply rooted in a profound reverence for the natural world and the interconnectedness of all living beings. This holistic perspective recognizes that everything in the universe carries its own unique energy and spiritual essence. Crystals and stones, with their vibrant energy and distinct characteristics, have played a significant role in Native American cultures as sacred tools for healing, protection, and spiritual guidance. We will explore how this reverence for the Earth and its gifts shaped the Native American approach to crystal and stone healing.

The Significance of Crystals and Stones in Native American Culture

Throughout history, Native American tribes have utilized crystals and stones in various rituals, ceremonies, and healing practices. These revered gems were believed to embody the wisdom and power of the Earth, acting as conduits for spiritual energy and healing vibrations. Each crystal and stone holds its own unique properties, resonating with specific intentions and healing qualities. We will delve into the symbolism, cultural significance, and traditional uses of a selection of crystals and stones cherished by Native American tribes.

Traditional Native American Crystal and Stone Healing Techniques

Native American crystal and stone healing techniques are rooted in ancient wisdom and passed down through generations. These practices encompass a holistic approach, recognizing the physical, emotional, mental, and spiritual aspects of well-being. From crystal layouts and grids to spiritual cleansings and offerings, we will explore a range of traditional Native American healing techniques that can be used to harness the energy of crystals and stones for personal transformation and spiritual growth.

Ethical Considerations and Respect for Native American Culture

As we explore the profound connection between Native American culture and crystal healing, it is crucial to approach this subject with respect, sensitivity, and ethical awareness. Native American traditions and spiritual practices are sacred and should be honored with utmost reverence. We will discuss the importance of cultural sensitivity, responsible sourcing of crystals and stones, and the need to appreciate and support Native American communities in preserving their cultural heritage.

We have discovered the deep-rooted spirituality of Native American culture, its reverence for the Earth, and the integral role of crystals and stones in their healing practices. As we continue our journey, we will dive deeper into the specific crystals and stones revered by Native American tribes, their properties, and the profound healing potential they hold. By blending ancient wisdom with contemporary understanding, we can harness the transformative power of these precious gifts from the Earth and embark on our own personal healing journeys.

SCAN THE QR CODE TO UNVEIL VIBRANT, FULL-COLOR IMAGES OF ALL THE HEALING STONES AND DISCOVER THEIR BEAUTY IN ALL ITS MAGNIFICENCE!

HEALING STONES

1. AMAZONITE

Healing Properties: Amazonite is a soothing and calming stone. It is associated with harmony, balance, and communication.

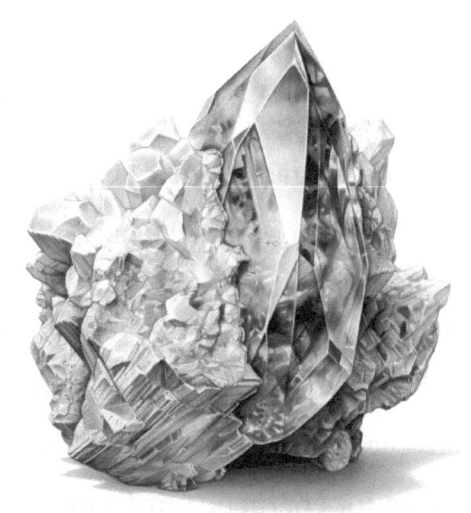

Benefits: Amazonite is believed to enhance clarity of thought, promote emotional healing, and facilitate effective communication.

Practical Applications: Amazonite can be used in meditation for relaxation and stress relief, worn as jewelry for emotional support, or placed in a living space to promote harmonious relationships.

2. AMETHYST

Healing Properties: Amethyst is known for its calming and protective qualities. It is often used to enhance spiritual awareness, promote relaxation, and alleviate stress and anxiety.

Benefits: Amethyst is believed to aid in sleep and dream work, support emotional balance, and enhance intuition.

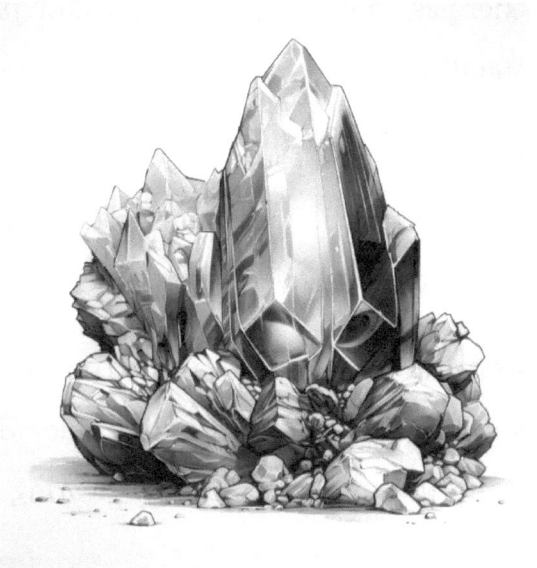

Practical Applications: Amethyst can be placed under a pillow for restful sleep, used in meditation, or worn as jewelry.

3. BLACK OBSIDIAN

Healing Properties: Black Obsidian is a stone of protection and purification. It is associated with grounding, shielding against negativity, and releasing emotional blockages.

Benefits: Black Obsidian is believed to absorb and transmute negative energies, promote self-awareness, and support emotional healing.

Practical Applications: Black Obsidian can be used in meditation for grounding and protection, placed near electronic devices for EMF shielding, or carried as a talisman for energetic purification.

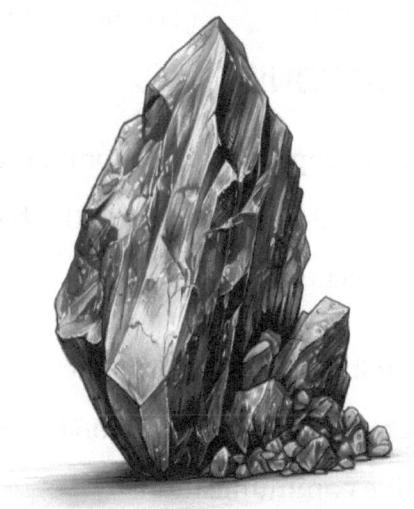

4. BLACK TOURMALINE

Healing Properties: Black Tourmaline is a powerful protective stone. It is often used to absorb negative energies, provide grounding, and promote emotional stability.

Benefits: Black Tourmaline is believed to protect against electromagnetic radiation, promote a sense of security, and cleanse the energy field.

Practical Applications: Black Tourmaline can be worn as jewelry, placed near electronic devices for EMF protection, or used in energy-clearing rituals.

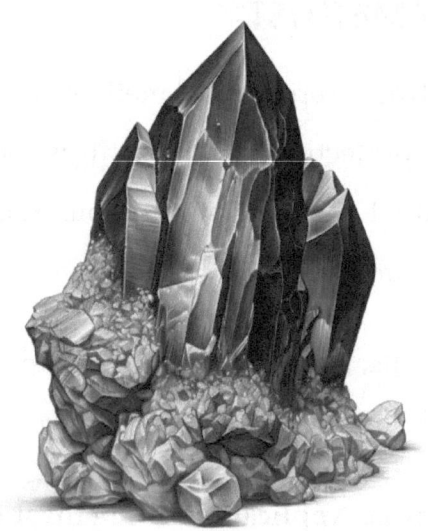

5. CARNELIAN

Healing Properties: Carnelian is a stone of vitality and motivation. It is associated with courage, creativity, and passion.

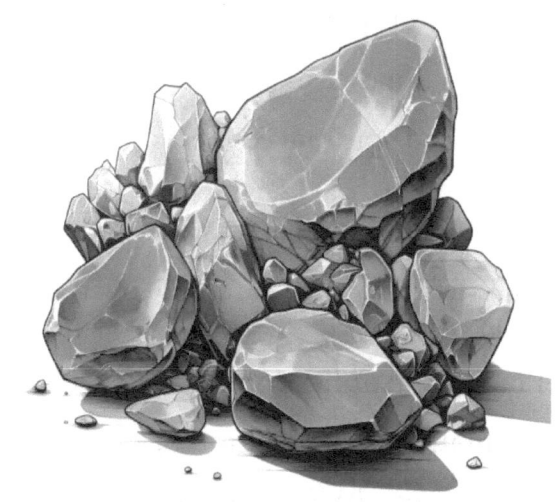

Benefits: Carnelian is believed to enhance confidence, stimulate creativity, and boost energy levels.

Practical Applications: Carnelian can be worn as jewelry for motivation, used during creative pursuits, or placed on the sacral chakra for emotional healing.

6. CHAROITE

Healing Properties: Charoite is a stone of transformation and spiritual insight. It is associated with personal growth, inner vision, and healing.

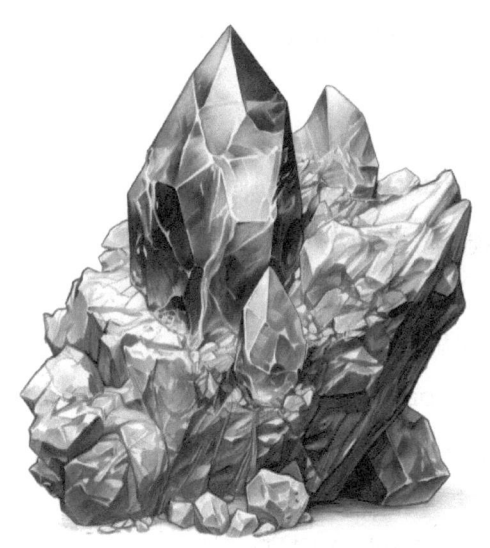

Benefits: Charoite is believed to facilitate spiritual transformation, enhance intuition, and support inner healing and purification.

Practical Applications: Charoite can be used in meditation for accessing higher realms of consciousness, worn as jewelry for personal growth, or placed on the third eye chakra for enhancing intuition.

7. CLEAR QUARTZ

Healing Properties: Clear Quartz is a powerful energy amplifier and cleanser. It is often used to enhance clarity, focus, and spiritual connection.

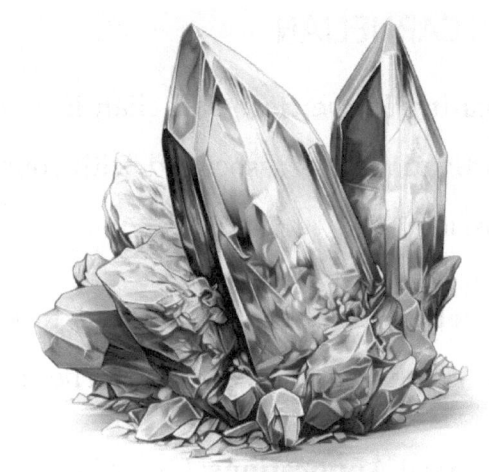

Benefits: Clear Quartz is believed to strengthen the aura, balance energy, and promote overall well-being.

Practical Applications: Clear Quartz can be used in meditation, placed in a room for energy purification, or worn as jewelry for daily energetic support.

8. CITRINE

Healing Properties: Citrine is a stone of abundance and joy. It is associated with vitality, prosperity, and positive energy.

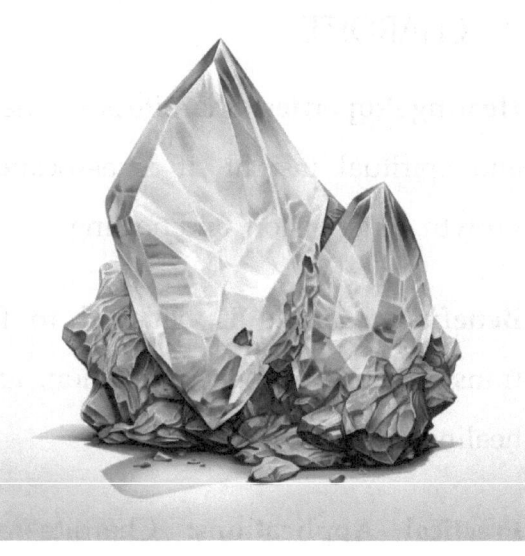

Benefits: Citrine is believed to promote confidence, attract success, and dispel negativity.

Practical Applications: Citrine can be placed in a workspace or business area for prosperity, used during manifestation rituals, or carried as a talisman for motivation.

9. GREEN AVENTURINE

Healing Properties: Green Aventurine is a stone of luck and abundance. It is associated with prosperity, growth, and optimism.

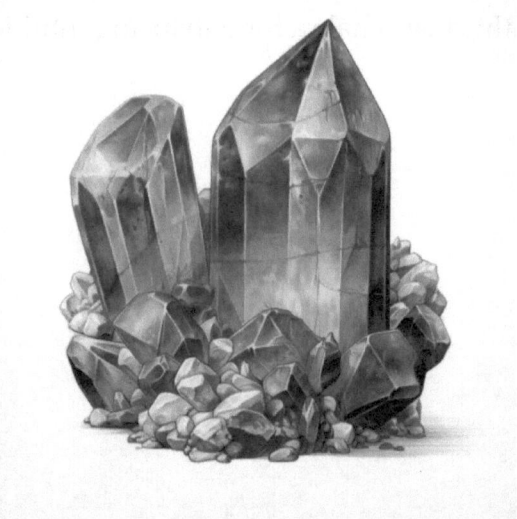

Benefits: Green Aventurine is believed to attract good fortune, promote emotional healing, and enhance vitality and overall well-being.

Practical Applications: Green Aventurine can be carried

as a talisman for luck and success, used in manifestation rituals, or placed in a workspace for increased productivity and abundance.

10. HEMATITE

Healing Properties: Hematite is a grounding and protective stone. It is known for its ability to absorb negative energy and promote balance and stability.

Benefits: Hematite is believed to enhance courage, strengthen the physical body, and promote mental clarity and focus.

Practical Applications: Hematite can be used in meditation for grounding, worn as jewelry for energetic protection, or placed on the body to alleviate pain and inflammation.

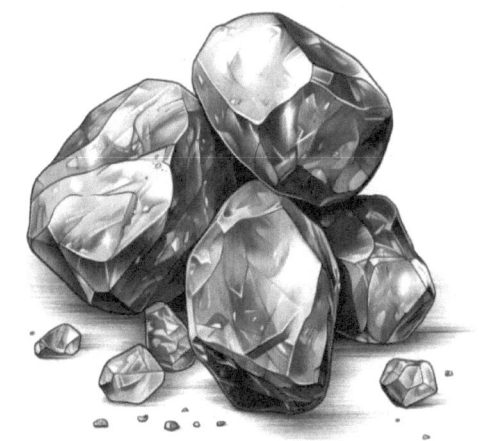

11. LABRADORITE

Healing Properties: Labradorite is a stone of transformation and protection. It is associated with intuition, spiritual awakening, and psychic abilities.

Benefits: Labradorite is believed to enhance intuition, promote spiritual growth, and protect against negative energies.

Practical Applications: Labradorite can be used in meditation to explore higher realms of consciousness, worn as jewelry for energetic protection, or placed on a desk for enhanced creativity.

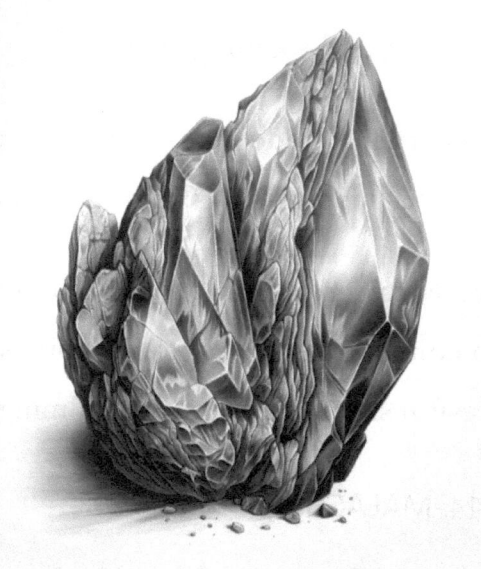

12. LAPIS LAZULI

Healing Properties: Lapis Lazuli is a stone of wisdom and truth. It is associated with inner peace, intuition, and spiritual enlightenment.

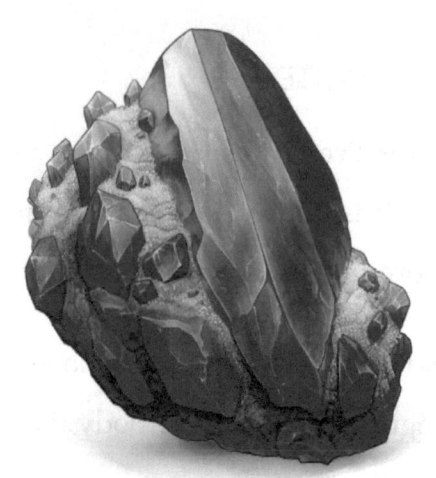

Benefits: Lapis Lazuli is believed to enhance clarity of thought, promote self-expression, and stimulate psychic abilities.

Practical Applications: Lapis Lazuli can be used in meditation for deepening spiritual connections, worn as jewelry for self-expression, or placed in a living space to promote a calm and harmonious environment.

13. LEPIDOLITE

Healing Properties: Lepidolite is a stone of calmness and balance. It is associated with stress relief, emotional healing, and soothing anxiety.

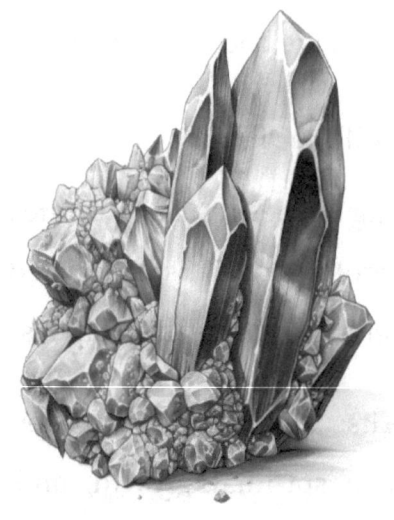

Benefits: Lepidolite is believed to promote relaxation, balance mood swings, and support emotional stability.

Practical Applications: Lepidolite can be used in meditation for stress relief, placed under a pillow for restful sleep, or carried as a calming talisman.

14. MALACHITE

Healing Properties: Malachite is a stone of transformation and emotional healing. It is known for its vibrant green color and unique banding patterns.

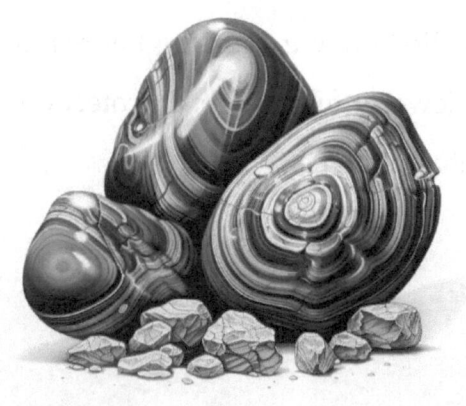

Benefits: Malachite is believed to promote emotional balance, release negative patterns, and stimulate personal growth and spiritual evolution.

Practical Applications: Malachite can be used in meditation to facilitate emotional healing, worn as jewelry for protection, or placed in a living or workspace to absorb negative energies.

15. MOLDAVITE

Healing Properties: Moldavite is a rare and powerful stone of transformation and spiritual awakening. It is associated with accelerated growth and higher consciousness.

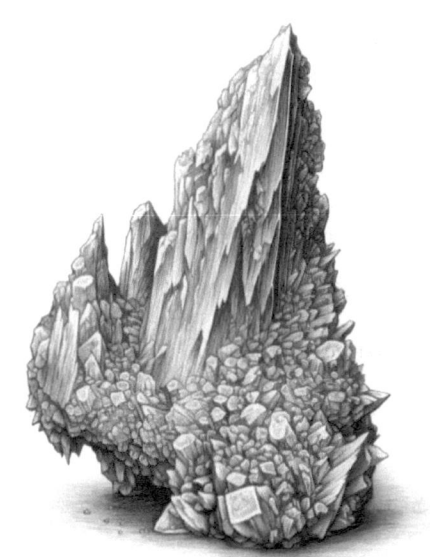

Benefits: Moldavite is believed to facilitate spiritual evolution, enhance psychic abilities, and promote deep spiritual experiences.

Practical Applications: Moldavite can be used in meditation for spiritual exploration, worn as jewelry for personal transformation, or placed on the third eye chakra for enhanced intuition.

16. RHODONITE

Healing Properties: Rhodonite is a stone of compassion and emotional healing. It is known for its pink color with black or brown veins.

Benefits: Rhodonite is believed to promote forgiveness, emotional healing, and unconditional love for oneself and others.

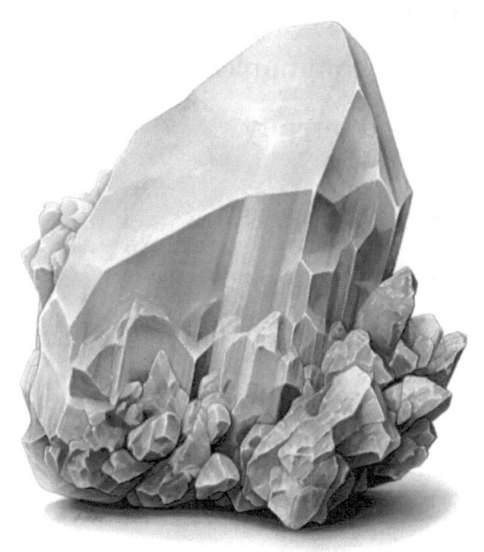

Practical Applications: Rhodonite can be used in meditation for emotional healing, worn as jewelry for self-love and acceptance, or placed in a living space to create a harmonious environment.

17. ROSE QUARTZ

Healing Properties: Rose Quartz is the stone of love and compassion. It is associated with emotional healing, self-love, and nurturing.

Benefits: Rose Quartz is believed to enhance relationships, promote forgiveness, and attract love and harmony.

Practical Applications: Rose Quartz can be placed in the bedroom for a soothing ambiance, used in self-care rituals, or carried as a heartwarming talisman.

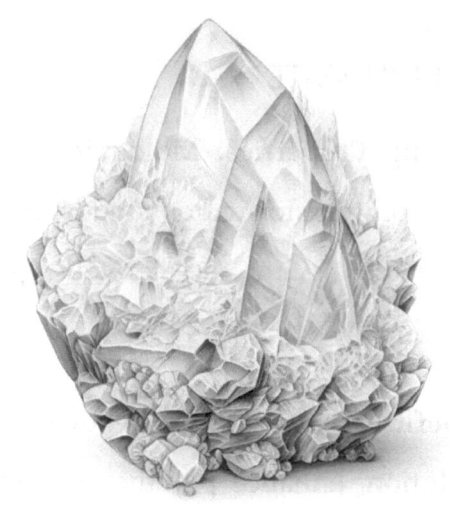

18. SELENITE

Healing Properties: Selenite is known for its cleansing and purifying properties. It is often used to clear energy blockages, promote mental clarity, and access higher consciousness.

Benefits: Selenite is believed to enhance spiritual growth, facilitate communication with spirit guides, and bring peace and serenity.

Practical Applications: Selenite can be used to cleanse other crystals, placed in a sacred space for energetic purification, or used in meditation for mental clarity.

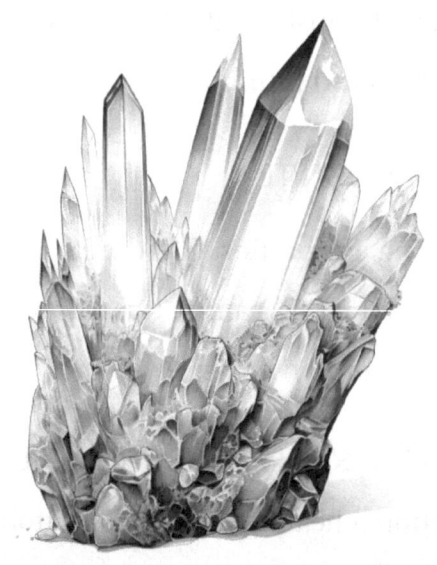

19. SHUNGITE

Healing Properties: Shungite is a powerful stone of protection and purification. It is associated with electromagnetic field (EMF) shielding and detoxification.

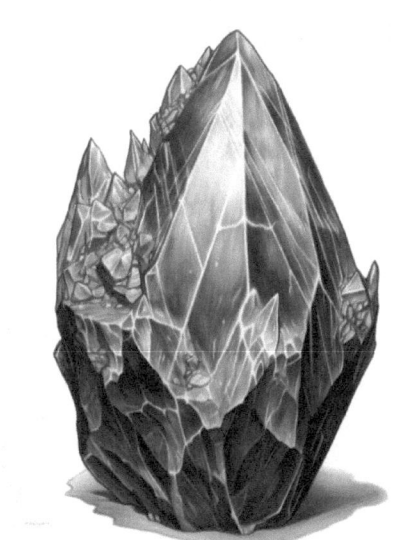

Benefits: Shungite is believed to absorb and neutralize harmful energies, support physical healing, and enhance vitality.

Practical Applications: Shungite can be placed near electronic devices to absorb EMF radiation, used in water filtration systems for purifying drinking water, or worn as jewelry for personal protection.

20. SNOWFLAKE OBSIDIAN

Healing Properties: Snowflake Obsidian is a stone of purity and balance. It is associated with grounding, protection, and emotional healing.

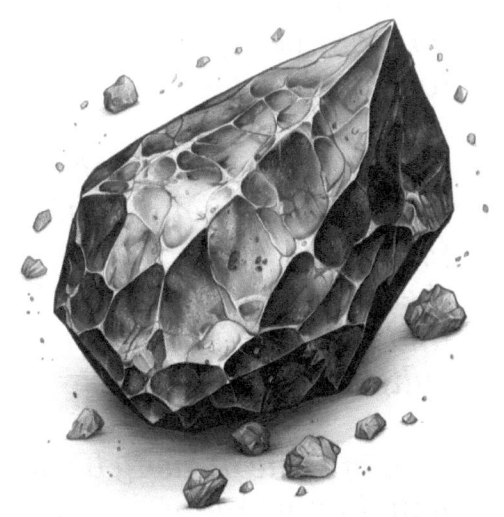

Benefits: Snowflake Obsidian is believed to promote inner harmony, balance yin and yang energies, and release negative patterns.

Practical Applications: Snowflake Obsidian can be used in meditation for grounding and stability, worn as jewelry for protection, or placed in a living space to absorb negative energies.

Journey's End and a Path Forward from Aiyana Tessay

As we turn the final page of
"Native American Herbalists Bible: 13 Books in 1," *my hope is that it has sown seeds of wisdom and curiosity within you about the rich traditions of Native American herbalism.*

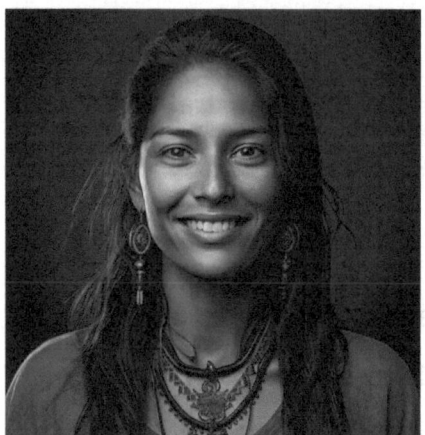

Allow me to share a reflection that truly resonates with the spirit of our exploration:

> *" This biblical book is quite extensive and interesting, where you can go from being a beginner to an expert, as it covers a wide range of topics related to Native American culture and medicine.*
>
> *The book focuses on the deep connection between Native Americans and nature, highlighting how their spirituality, religion and daily practices are related to the natural environment. In its extensive theory and information, the book explores the importance of animism and wild plant gathering in their culture and how we can adopt those cultures.*
>
> *Also in some of his 13 books he delves into the figure of the shaman and how important he is to understanding native medicine and how they used the myriad of herbs in traditional medicine. Also, of course, I learned a lot as he offers information on specific medicinal plants such as cardamom, bramble and white willow among a myriad of other herbs that have healing properties that you can't even imagine.*
>
> *I highly recommend this book if you are a lover of indigenous culture related to herbs and natural medicine. You will learn a lot with the amount of natural recipes that you will find, very beneficial and easy to prepare."*

Nicholas

Should you feel a similar sense of inspiration and enlightenment, I warmly encourage you to extend the circle of knowledge by sharing your thoughts on Amazon. Your reflections can enhance the value of this book, serving as a guiding light for others on their path to discovering the depth of Native American herbalism.

Leaving your feedback is a simple gesture of support that can have a lasting impact. Navigate to the ORDERS section of your Amazon account and click on the "Write a product review" button, or scan this QR Code:

Your journey with us may have reached a pause, but the path of learning and growth continues. It has been an honor to guide you through these teachings, and I look forward to hearing about your adventures in herbalism.

Should you wish to share your journey or seek further guidance, feel free to reach out at info [at] herbfulharmony [dot] com.

With deepest gratitude and encouragement for your continued exploration,
Aiyana Tessay.

Made in United States
Troutdale, OR
04/08/2024

19038165R10179